T0229014

Randomized Clinical Trials in Surgical Oncology

Guest Editors

ADAM C. YOPP, MD
RONALD P. DeMATTEO, MD

SURGICAL ONCOLOGY CLINICS OF NORTH AMERICA

www.surgonc.theclinics.com

Consulting Editor
NICHOLAS J. PETRELLI, MD

January 2010 • Volume 19 • Number 1

SAUNDERS an imprint of ELSEVIER, Inc.

W.B. SAUNDERS COMPANY

A Division of Elsevier Inc.

1600 John F. Kennedy Boulevard ● Suite 1800 ● Philadelphia, PA 19103-2899

http://www.theclinics.com

SURGICAL ONCOLOGY CLINICS OF NORTH AMERICA Volume 19, Number 1
January 2010 ISSN 1055-3207, ISBN-13: 978-1-4377-1878-2

Editor: Catherine Bewick
Developmental Editor: Theresa Collier

Surgical Oncology Clinics of North America (ISSN 1055-3207) is published quarterly by Elsevier Inc., 360 Park Avenue South, New York, NY 10010-1710. Months of issue are January, April, July and October. Business and Editorial Offices: 1600 John F. Kennedy Blvd., Ste. 1800, Philadelphia, PA 19103-2899. Customer Service Office: 3251 Riverport Lane, Maryland Heights, MO 63043. Periodicals postage paid at New York, NY and additional mailing offices. Subscription prices are $225.00 per year (US individuals), $340.00 (US institutions) $113.00 (US student/resident), $259.00 (Canadian individuals), $423.00 (Canadian institutions), $163.00 (Canadian student/resident), $323.00 (foreign individuals), $423.00 (foreign institutions), and $163.00 (foreign student/resident). Foreign air speed delivery is included in all *Clinics* subscription prices. All prices are subject to change without notice. **POSTMASTER:** Send address changes to *Surgical Oncology Clinics of North America*, Elsevier Health Sciences Division, Subscription Customer Service, 3251 Riverport Lane, Maryland Heights, MO 63043. **Customer Service: 1-800-654-2452 (U.S. and Canada); 314-447-8871 (outside U.S. and Canada). Fax: 314-447-8029. E-mail: journalscustomerservice-usa@elsevier.com** (for print support); **journalsonline support-usa@elsevier.com** (for online support).

Reprints. For copies of 100 or more, of articles in this publication, please contact the Commercial Reprints Department, Elsevier Inc., 360 Park Avenue South, New York, New York 10010-1710. Tel. 212-633-3813; Fax: 212-462-1935; E-mail: reprints@elsevier.com.

Surgical Oncology Clinics of North America is covered in *MEDLINE/PubMed (Index Medicus)* and *EMBASE/ Excerpta Medica, Current Contents/Clinical Medicine,* and *ISI/BIOMED.*

Printed and bound by CPI Group (UK) Ltd, Croydon, CR0 4YY

Transferred to Digital Print 2011

Contributors

CONSULTING EDITOR

NICHOLAS J. PETRELLI, MD
Bank of America Endowed Medical Director, Helen F. Graham Cancer Center at Christiana Care Health System, Newark, Delaware; Professor of Surgery, Department of Surgery, Jefferson Medical College, Philadelphia, Pennsylvania

GUEST EDITORS

ADAM C. YOPP, MD
Assistant Professor of Surgery, Department of Surgery, Division of Surgical Oncology, University of Texas Southwestern Medical Center, Dallas, Texas

RONALD P. DeMATTEO, MD
Vice Chair, Department of Surgery, Head, Division of General Surgical Oncology and Attending Surgeon, Hepatopancreatobiliary Service, Memorial Sloan-Kettering Cancer Center, New York, New York

AUTHORS

PETER J. ALLEN, MD
Attending Surgeon, Department of Surgery, Memorial Sloan-Kettering Cancer Center, New York, New York

CHARLOTTE ARIYAN, MD, PhD
Assistant Attending, Department of Surgery, Memorial Sloan-Kettering Cancer Center, New York, New York

MICHELLE AZU, MD
Fellow, Department of Surgery, Division of Breast Surgery, Memorial Sloan-Kettering Cancer Center, New York, New York

STEPHEN A. BARNETT, MD
Thoracic Surgery Fellow, Department of Surgery, Memorial Sloan-Kettering Cancer Center, New York, New York

MURRAY F. BRENNAN, MD
Attending Surgeon and Benno C. Schmidt Chair of Clinical Oncology, Department of Surgery, Memorial Sloan-Kettering Cancer Center, New York, New York

DANIEL G. COIT, MD
Attending Physician, Department of Surgery, Memorial Sloan-Kettering Cancer Center, New York, New York

AIMEE M. CRAGO, MD, PhD
Fellow, Department of Surgery, Division of Surgical Oncology, Memorial Sloan-Kettering Cancer Center, New York, New York

MICHAEL I. D'ANGELICA, MD
Associate Attending, Department of Surgery, Hepatopancreatobiliary Service, Memorial Sloan-Kettering Cancer Center; Associate Professor, Department of Surgery, Cornell University, Weill Medical College, New York, New York

RONALD P. DeMATTEO, MD
Vice Chair, Department of Surgery, Head, Division of General Surgical Oncology and Attending Surgeon, Hepatopancreatobiliary Service, Memorial Sloan-Kettering Cancer Center, New York, New York

WILLIAM R. JARNAGIN, MD
Professor of Surgery, Department of Surgery, Division of Hepatobiliary Surgery, Memorial Sloan-Kettering Cancer Center, New York, New York

GIORGOS KARAKOUSIS, MD
Surgical Oncology Fellow, Department of Surgery, Memorial Sloan-Kettering Cancer Center, New York, New York

STEVEN C. KATZ, MD
Department of Surgery, Roger Williams Medical Center, Providence, Rhode Island

T. PETER KINGHAM, MD
Surgical Oncology Fellow, Department of Surgery, Memorial Sloan-Kettering Cancer Center, New York, New York

PETER A. LEARN, MD
Department of Surgery, Memorial Sloan-Kettering Cancer Center, New York, New York

SHISHIR K. MAITHEL, MD
Surgical Fellow, Department of Surgery, Hepatopancreatobiliary Service, Memorial Sloan-Kettering Cancer Center, New York, New York

AJAY V. MAKER, MD
Department of Surgery, Memorial Sloan-Kettering Cancer Center, New York, New York

JAMES J. MEZHIR, MD
Surgical Oncology Fellow, Department of Surgery, Memorial Sloan-Kettering Cancer Center, New York, New York

MONICA MORROW, MD
Chief of Breast Service and Anne Burnett Windfohr Chair of Clinical Oncology, Department of Surgery, Division of Breast Surgery, Memorial Sloan-Kettering Cancer Center, New York, New York

HEATHER B. NEUMAN, MD, MS
Assistant Professor, Department of Surgery, Section of Surgical Oncology, University of Wisconsin, Madison, Wisconsin

JASON PARK, MD, MEd
Assistant Professor, Department of Surgery, University of Manitoba, Winnipeg, Manitoba, Canada

VENU G. PILLARISETTY, MD
Surgical Oncology Fellow, Department of Surgery, Memorial Sloan-Kettering Cancer Center, New York, New York

NABIL P. RIZK, MD, MS
Attending Surgeon, Thoracic Service, Department of Surgery, Memorial Sloan-Kettering Cancer Center, New York, New York

UDO RUDLOFF, MD, PhD
Department of Surgery, Memorial Sloan-Kettering Cancer Center, New York, New York

MANISH A. SHAH, MD
Attending Physician, Department of Medicine, Memorial Sloan-Kettering Cancer Center, New York, New York

JASON K. SICKLICK, MD
Department of Surgery, Memorial Sloan-Kettering Cancer Center, New York, New York

SHANNON TIERNEY, MD
Fellow, Department of Surgery, Division of Breast Surgery, Memorial Sloan-Kettering Cancer Center, New York, New York

MARTIN R. WEISER, MD
Associate Attending, Department of Surgery, Colorectal Service, Memorial Sloan-Kettering Cancer Center, New York, New York

W. DOUGLAS WONG, MD
Chief, Department of Surgery, Colorectal Service, Memorial Sloan-Kettering Cancer Center; Professor of Surgery, Cornell University-Weill Medical College, New York, New York

ADAM C. YOPP, MD
Assistant Professor of Surgery, Department of Surgery, Division of Surgical Oncology, University of Texas Southwestern Medical Center, Dallas, Texas

Contents

> Soft tissue sarcomas (STS) are rare, but potentially lethal, extraskeletal mesenchymal neoplasms. It is estimated that approximately 12,000 cases of STS are reported annually in the United States, with 3,500 STS deaths. Few randomized controlled trials (RCTs) have been conducted since the previous issue of this publication. The current understanding of STS biology and, hence, ability to provide safe, effective therapy is predicated upon seminal trials performed in the 1980s and 1990s. The authors briefly summarize the trials presented in the previous issue and then critically assess the more recent publications that have addressed the management of STS.

> The incidence of melanoma is increasing and it is estimated that, in the United States, the lifetime risk of developing melanoma is 1 in 55. There have been many randomized trials that have refined the treatment and minimized the morbidity of the intervention of this prevalent disease. From 1975 to 2000, there were 154 prospective randomized trials on the treatment of local, regional, and metastatic melanoma. Between 2001 and the end of 2008, there were 52 randomized controlled trials relating to the treatment of patients with malignant melanoma. This article reviews the results of the major studies included in the prior article, and provides a detailed description of selected randomized controlled trials performed from 2001 to 2008.

> Breast cancer remains the most common cancer diagnosed in women and the second leading cause of cancer-related deaths in this group.

Significant advances in the treatment of breast cancer and in the ability to screen for the disease mean that it is also one of the most curable forms of cancer. Long-term updates of the trials reviewed in the previous edition of this article have demonstrated that breast-conserving therapy remains a viable option for most patients, and that local control is related to over-all survival. New chemotherapeutic options and endocrine therapies are available to select subsets of patients, and the use of endocrine therapy in breast cancer prevention has been shown to be of clear benefit. The sheer number of breast cancer-related randomized, controlled trials makes it impossible to review all level Ia evidence in this article but, where possible, extensive referencing and tabular review of related trials are used to provide the reader with a clear outline of the central data dictating current standard of care.

The treatment of esophageal cancer with curative intent remains highly controversial, with advocates of surgery alone, chemoradiotherapy alone, surgery with adjuvant therapy (including neoadjuvant and postoperative), and trimodality therapy each contributing prospective randomized con-trolled trials (PRCTs) to the body of scientific publications between 2000 and 2008. Any improvements in survival have been small in absolute per-centage terms, and as such PRCTs published over the last decade have met the same primary obstacle encountered by the studies from the two prior decades, namely lack of power to detect small differences in out-come. Variations in staging methods, surgical technique, radiotherapy technique, and chemotherapy regime have in turn been the subject of PRCTs over the last nine years. In many cases primary end points have not been survival but rather rates of complication or response. As well as giving an overview of PRCTs, this article collates the level Ia evidence published to date.

Minimally invasive resection has emerged as a surgical technique for gas-tric cancer, and there has been continued investigation to determine the appropriate extent of lymphadenectomy in gastric cancer patients. There has also been significant progress in evaluating the role of chemothera-peutic regimens used in the neoadjuvant and adjuvant settings for patients with resectable disease. We also summarize a selection of RCT trials fo-cused on the perioperative care of the gastric cancer patient.

Gastrointestinal (GI) stromal tumor (GIST) is the most common mesenchy-mal tumor of the GI tract, constituting 80% of all GI mesenchymal tumors and approximately 20% of all small bowel malignancies, excluding lym-phomas. This article provides a summary of recent randomized clinical tri-als of these tumors.

improving the surgical staging of patients with colon cancer, and improving adjuvant treatment regimens. We review those randomized controlled trials that have most impacted the clinical management of patients with colon cancer in 2009.

This article reviews randomized clinical trials (RCTs) published between April 2001 and November 2008 on the management of patients with rectal cancer. In total, the authors reviewed 78 RCTs on therapy for rectal cancer. Of these, five met the authors' criteria for level 1a evidence. The article discusses the major RCTs and relevant findings that have impacted clinical management most and includes most but not all RCTs on therapy for rectal cancer published during this period.

RELATED INTEREST

Perioperative Nursing Clinics, September 2009 (Vol. 4, Issue 3, Pages 201–316)
Research
Robin Froman, RN, PhD, FAAN, *Guest Editor*

THE CLINICS ARE NOW AVAILABLE ONLINE!

Access your subscription at:
www.theclinics.com

Foreword

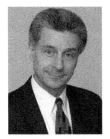

Nicholas J. Petrelli, MD
Consulting Editor

This issue of the *Surgical Oncology Clinics of North America* is devoted to randomized control trials. The guest editors are Ronald DeMatteo, MD, Professor of Surgery, Head, Division of Surgical Oncology, Leslie H. Blumgard Chair in Surgery, Memorial Sloan-Kettering Cancer Center; and Adam C. Yopp, MD, Assistant Professor of Surgery, Division of Surgical Oncology, University of Texas Southwestern Medical Center, Dallas, Texas. As we are reminded in the commentary by Murray Brennan, MD, Benno C. Schmidt Chair in Clinical Oncology in the Department of Surgery at Memorial Sloan-Kettering Cancer Center, the fellows and staff at Memorial 5 years ago completed an issue on the same subject.

Since 5 years have passed, I felt it was time for an update of the recent randomized clinical trials in surgical oncology. This subject required an extreme amount of time and effort to put together, and I congratulate both Drs. Yopp and DeMatteo for their efforts in this successful endeavor. As mentioned in their preface, Drs. Yopp and DeMatteo emphasize that the "randomized clinical trial is the gold standard for proving the relative value of a medical intervention." Without question, progress in the last 20 years in cancer care of the patient is due to the randomized clinical trial, especially those completed by the National Cancer Institute (NCI) Cooperative Groups. Unfortunately, only 3% to 4% of oncology patients are placed on NCI clinical trials. Many barriers to improving this accrual rate have been reported in the literature. Lack of resources, strict eligibility criteria, and obstacles to insurance coverage are just some of the issues that have resulted in this low national accrual rate.

Individuals who read this issue of the *Surgical Oncology Clinics of North America* will certainly learn about the results of recent randomized clinical trials in surgical oncology. However, I also hope this issue will stimulate our readers to become more involved in accruing patients to clinical trials. It is hoped that trainees in the three major disciplines of surgery, radiation, and medical oncology will seek out additional information on how to become involved in national cooperative group clinical trials. This information can be found on the NCI web site at http://www.cancer.gov/CLINICALTRIALS. I can't emphasize enough how important it is to become involved in the thought

Surg Oncol Clin N Am 19 (2010) xiii–xiv
doi:10.1016/j.soc.2009.09.015   **surgonc.theclinics.com**
1055-3207/09/$ – see front matter © 2010 Elsevier Inc. All rights reserved.

process of developing clinical trials in the NCI Cooperative Group setting. My introduction to the randomized clinical trial was during my surgical oncology fellowship under the mentorship of such individuals as Harold Douglass, MD, and Arnold Mittleman, MD, in Buffalo, New York, and Edward Mansour, MD, in Cleveland, Ohio, during annual meetings of the Eastern Cooperative Oncology Group (ECOG). Every clinician, starting in residency and continuing throughout his or her career, should learn the importance of clinical trials, understand the process of formulating a trial, and develop skills in interpreting trial results. I would like to thank Dr. Yopp and Dr. DeMatteo, for putting together this issue of the *Surgical Oncology Clinics of North America*, and also Dr. Murray Brennan, for his excellent commentary. I know the readers will find this issue educational and stimulating.

Nicholas J. Petrelli, MD
Helen F. Graham Cancer Center
4701 Ogletown-Stanton Road, Suite 1213
Newark, DE 19713, USA
Department of Surgery
Jefferson Medical College
Philadelphia, PA 19107, USA

E-mail address:
npetrelli@christianacare.org

Preface

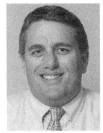 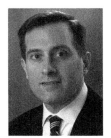

Adam C. Yopp, MD   Ronald P. DeMatteo, MD
Guest Editors

The randomized clinical trial (RCT) is the gold standard for proving the relative value of a medical intervention. Patients are assigned randomly by chance to different therapies so that the investigator cannot select patients for one particular treatment arm. Randomization also tends to distribute known, prognostic factors (as well as those that are unrecognized) equally between or among the study arms. Currently, there are over 350 active phase 3 trials in cancer therapy in the United States (http://www.cancer.gov).

The design of an RCT is paramount. In general, simpler is better. Witness the confusion over the results of the ESPAC-1 (European Study Group for Pancreatic Cancer) trial that used a two-by-two design to test adjuvant chemotherapy and radiation in pancreatic cancer (see article by Rudloff, Maker, Brennan, and Allen). While most trials have multiple end points, a trial is typically only powered to assess the primary end point. All other analyses are relegated to be "ad hoc" or "retrospective." In metastatic cancer, progression-free survival is often accepted as a primary end point and used as a surrogate for overall survival. In adjuvant therapy, it is controversial as to whether recurrence-free survival is an acceptable primary end point in lieu of the traditional gold standard of overall survival. We agree with Elfenbein[1] (New Engl J Med 2003;349:80–2) that "The absence of a relapse is the best indicator of the efficacy of an antitumor strategy because it is directly related to the treatment." Furthermore, "… it is inappropriate to conclude that a primary strategy yields no benefit if overall survival is not prolonged," since salvage therapies confound analysis of overall survival. Most RCTs are currently analyzed on an intention-to-treat basis to minimize the effects of patient dropout and crossover between the study arms.

Over the last 2 decades, the reporting of trials has become standardized because of the widespread acceptance of the CONSORT (Consolidated Standards of Reporting Trials) guidelines (http://www.consort-statement.org). A flow diagram is used to show patient enrollment, intervention allocation, follow up, and analysis. A 22-item checklist is used to facilitate a uniform style of manuscript presentation. Whether the results of a particular trial are actually implemented depends on a multitude of factors. Notably, the magnitude of the difference in outcome between the arms does not

Surg Oncol Clin N Am 19 (2010) xv–xvii
doi:10.1016/j.soc.2009.09.014
1055-3207/09/$ – see front matter

necessarily correlate with the clinical impact of a trial. For instance, sorafenib achieved limited improvement in overall survival (10.7 months vs. 7.9 months) and did not alter time to symptomatic progression compared with placebo in advanced hepatocellular carcinoma. Nevertheless, the Food and Drug Administration approved sorafenib, which, because of a lack of effective agents, is now the standard of care (see article by Yopp and Jarnagin). Results from similar trials often conflict when the treatment effect is small or statistical power is low because of limited sample size. For example, the data are inconsistent as to whether neoadjuvant therapy should be performed prior to the resection of esophageal cancer (see article by Barnett and Rizk). In cases where a question remains unresolved despite numerous trials, a meta-analysis may provide clarification. Accordingly, a large meta-analysis was required to show a slight survival advantage with adjuvant doxorubicin in sarcoma (see article by Katz and Brennan).

Surgeons are appropriately focused on technical factors that may provide the basis for an RCT. For instance, the COST (Comparison of Laparoscopically Assisted and Open Colectomy for Colon Cancer) study showed that recurrence was similar after laparoscopically-assisted colectomy compared with open colectomy (see article by Neuman, Park, and Weiser). The extent of lymphadenectomy in gastric cancer has not consistently been found to improve survival (see article by Mezhir, Pillarisetty, Shah, and Coit). Meanwhile pylorus-preserving pancreaticoduodenectomy achieves survival similar to that of classic pancreaticoduodenectomy (see article by Rudloff, Maker, Brennan, and Allen). In many circumstances, though, patient demand (and corporate encouragement) now drive new techniques and technology, despite the lack of evidence of superiority. For instance, laparoscopic prostatectomy is now widely practiced but has not been formally established in terms of oncologic efficacy or safety. However, most of the critical questions in surgical oncology pertain to the selection and timing of multimodality therapy. For many solid tumors, improvements in patient outcome depend on the development of more effective nonsurgical therapies. Although these therapies may not necessarily be curative, they may be used to enable more cancer patients to undergo surgical resection or prevent (or at least delay) tumor recurrence after removal of the primary tumor.

While the surgical literature is replete with retrospective analyses, it is imperative that surgical oncologists avoid a defeatist attitude regarding their ability to participate in, or even lead, an RCT. Despite the complexities of institutional review boards and regulatory oversight, an RCT provides the opportunity to redefine the standard of care around the world. Recently, adjuvant imatinib mesylate increased 1-year recurrence-free survival (98% vs. 83%) compared with placebo following the resection of primary gastrointestinal stromal tumor, culminating in approval by the American and European health authorities (see article by Learn, Sicklick, and DeMatteo). Surgeons have played critical leadership roles in many other cancers, including breast cancer and melanoma (see articles by Crago, Azu, Tierney, and Morrow; and by Kingham, Karakousis, and Ariyan). So how do surgeons become more involved? It has to start with education in clinical trials, which is clearly lacking during surgical training. While medical oncology fellows routinely become facile in trial design and methodology, it is uncommon for surgeons to be familiar with protocol writing by the time they reach the level of assistant professor (which is not the optimal time to start learning). It seems that there is now a shift away from basic research during surgical residency as more trainees opt for advanced degrees in epidemiology and public health. It is imperative that surgical oncology fellowships provide training and encourage interested fellows to pursue prospective clinical research. Attendance at cooperative group meetings, such as those of the American College of Surgeons Oncology Group, is essential to understand the development process for multicenter protocols. In this issue of the *Surgical Oncology Clinics of North America*, surgical fellows and staff members of the Memorial Sloan-Kettering Cancer Center provide a comprehensive review of recent RCTs in surgical oncology. Earlier RCTs were reviewed in a 2002 issue, which was edited by David Jaques, who originated the initial endeavor. We hope that the reader of this text will gain an understanding of the basis for many current practices in surgical oncology and, more importantly, be inspired to rise to the challenge of posing new questions.

Adam C. Yopp, MD
Assistant Professor of Surgery
Department of Surgery
Division of Surgical Oncology
University of Texas Southwestern Medical Center
5323 Harry Hines Boulevard
Dallas, TX 75390, USA

Ronald P. DeMatteo, MD
Vice Chair, Department of Surgery
Head, Division of Surgical Oncology
Attending, Hepatopancreatobiliary Service
Memorial Sloan-Kettering Cancer Center
1275 York Avenue, New York, NY 10065, USA

E-mail addresses:
adam.yopp@utsouthwestern.edu (A.C. Yopp)
dematter@mskcc.org (R.P. DeMatteo)

REFERENCE

1. Elfenbein GJ. Stem-cell transplantation for high-risk breast cancer. New Engl J Med 2003; 349:80–2.

Commentary: Randomized Controlled Trials

In 2002, the fellows and staff at Memorial Sloan-Kettering put together an issue of *Surgical Oncology Clinics of North America* on randomized clinical trials in oncology. At that time, I emphasized the importance of that endeavor and expressed the hope that the results of such trials would translate into meaningful changes in practice. The present symposium reviews trials performed since that time. What progress has been made in randomized controlled trials since 2002? A broad table of disease-specific sites is examined and one is challenged as to whether the glass is half full or half empty. On one hand, we have, as a community, embraced the concept of randomized control trials as less than perfect, but the best alternative to evaluate clinical practice. We have come to realize that trials are both a gift and a curse. Those well done, well stratified, with adequate numbers and appropriate end points, generally add to what we know about the efficacy, or lack thereof, of what we do. Others, while idling behind the euphemism of "randomized," are little more than efforts in sciolism.

We imagined 8 years ago that this was a start. Has there been any progress? When one looks at the relative dearth of meaningful trials, the glass appears too empty, but important surgical questions have been addressed, as in the case, for example, of melanoma. The more troublesome question, however, is: Why do trials, when even if well done, fail to change behavior? At this stage in my career, I would settle for them provoking the willingness to think, the willingness to question, and the willingness to change. I have great faith in the present generation, as represented by the authors of this text, but then again I have had great faith in their colleagues at all stages of their earlier careers. Why do we find it so difficult to change? Why is it that we cannot accept that nasogastric tubes are unnecessary for routine upper gastrointestinal malignancy? Why is it that we have such difficulty accepting that 100 mL of water will not change significantly the 800 mL of saliva that disappears down into the partially or completely resected stomach? Why do we continue to punish all patients with mechanical bowel preparation? Why do we justify adjuvant treatment for pancreas cancer based on underpowered trials performed 30 years ago as a substitute for investigational approaches to this lethal disease?

The authors provide an excellent summary of randomized trials in multiple areas, but unless we take the next step and find out why we are not willing to challenge our self-conceived notions even when randomized trials suggest that we should, then once again we will lose the opportunity to make the kind of progress we all desperately want.

This seminar series provides information that should allow realistic judgments to be made. These summaries, by a cadre of young, enthusiastic, and thoughtful

Surg Oncol Clin N Am 19 (2010) xix–xx
doi:10.1016/j.soc.2009.09.016
1055-3207/09/$ – see front matter © 2010 Elsevier Inc. All rights reserved.

surgonc.theclinics.com

surgical oncologists, should challenge us all to continue our lifelong education. Fellowship is not a finishing school, just a methodology to gain the tools to continue to grow.

Murray F. Brennan, MD
Attending Surgeon and Benno C. Schmidt Chair of Clinical Oncology
Department of Surgery
Memorial Sloan-Kettering Cancer Center
1275 York Avenue
New York, NY 10021, USA

E-mail address:
brennanm@mskcc.org

Randomized Clinical Trials in Soft Tissue Sarcoma

Steven C. Katz, MD[a], Murray F. Brennan, MD[b],*

KEYWORDS

- Soft-tissue sarcoma • Surgery • Chemotherapy
- Radiation therapy

Soft tissue sarcomas (STS) are a heterogeneous group of rare but potentially lethal, extraskeletal mesenchymal neoplasms. Although the absolute incidence is unknown, it is estimated that approximately 12,000 cases of STS are reported annually in the United States, with 3,500 STS deaths.[1] The rarity of these diseases explains, in large part, why few randomized controlled trials (RCTs) have been conducted since the previous issue of this publication. The current understanding of STS biology and, hence, ability to provide safe, effective therapy is predicated upon seminal trials performed in the 1980s and 1990s. The authors briefly summarize the trials presented in the previous issue and then critically assess the more recent publications that have addressed the management of STS. This review does not include pediatric sarcomas or gastrointestinal stromal tumors, the latter of which are covered in a separate article.

SURGERY

The original RCT addressing the surgical management of STS had a profound impact, despite being small. Rosenberg and colleagues[2] reported that when compared with amputation, wide excision with external beam radiation therapy was associated with equivalent 5-year disease-free and overall survival. Demonstration of equivalence for limb preservation clearly has had important functional and quality of life implications for patients with extremity STS. This trial illustrated that while local recurrence may be associated with distant metastases and death from disease, the relationship is not necessarily causative. Recent retrospective studies have provided additional guidance for our surgical treatment of STS.[3]

Disclosure: See last page of article.
[a] Department of Surgery, Roger Williams Medical Center, 825 Chalkstone Avenue, Providence, RI 02908, USA
[b] Department of Surgery, Memorial Sloan-Kettering Cancer Center, 1275 York Avenue, New York, NY 10065, USA
* Corresponding author.
E-mail address: brennanm@mskcc.org (M.F. Brennan).

Surg Oncol Clin N Am 19 (2010) 1–11
doi:10.1016/j.soc.2009.09.006
1055-3207/09/$ – see front matter © 2010 Elsevier Inc. All rights reserved.

surgonc.theclinics.com

RADIATION THERAPY

The impact of postoperative radiation therapy on STS was largely defined by two RCTs. Pisters and colleagues[4] reported that adjuvant brachytherapy decreased local recurrence following resection of extremity STS, with the greatest benefit being conferred to patients with high-grade tumors. Yang and colleagues[5] demonstrated the effectiveness of external beam radiation in limiting local recurrence for both high and low-grade extremity STS. A more recent report addressed preoperative external beam radiation therapy. O'Sullivan and colleagues[6] reported a multicenter randomized trial that demonstrated that neoadjuvant external beam radiation therapy is associated with a higher rate of complications than postoperative adjuvant therapy.[6] A subsequent article from the same authors demonstrated that, despite the higher rate of wound complications, neoadjuvant radiation therapy leads to better functional outcomes.[7] A small survival advantage was associated with preoperative radiation therapy, yet there was no difference in either local or distant recurrence.

CHEMOTHERAPY

The level 1 chemotherapy trials summarized in the previous issue indicated some improvements in recurrence-free intervals or response rates, but not survival.[8–11] A recent meta-analysis which included 1953 patients from 18 trials indicated significant recurrence-free and survival advantages associated with adjuvant doxorubicin-based regimens (**Table 1**).[12] The small absolute recurrence and survival benefits (3%–10%) presented in the meta-analysis must be tempered against the known toxicities of doxorubicin-based systemic regimens. Furthermore, the vast majority of the individual trials included in the meta-analysis failed to demonstrate a significant survival benefit.

In a small RCT that closed after 12 years because of poor accrual, Petrioli and colleagues[13] found a statistically significant recurrence-free advantage for epirubicin-based postoperative chemotherapy, but no significant difference with respect to overall survival. A single trial with a small number of patients found no benefit to the addition of intraperitoneal chemotherapy following cytoreduction for peritoneal sarcomatosis.[14] Mace and colleagues[15] showed that, in a small group of patients receiving ifosfamide for STS, a regimen incorporating oral mesna as opposed to exclusively intravenous (IV) mesna was as effective in providing uroprotection. In a large phase III trial, Lorigan and colleagues[16] found that single agent ifosfamide should not replace doxorubicin as the first-line agent for advanced STS. A randomized phase II trial of neoadjuvant doxorubicin with ifosfamide for high-risk STS demonstrated that preoperative therapy afforded no survival or recurrence benefit compared with surgery alone.[17]

Table 1 Meta-analysis of RCTs of adjuvant chemotherapy for localized resectable soft-tissue sarcoma[12]				
Outcome	OR (95% CI)	p	ARR (95% CI)	NNT
Local recurrence	0.73 (0.56–0.94)	0.02	3% (0%–7%)	25
Distant recurrence	0.67 (0.56–0.86)	<0.01	9% (5%–14%)	12
Overall recurrence	0.67 (0.56–0.82)	<0.01	10% (5%–15%)	10
Overall survival	0.77 (0.64–0.93)	0.01	6% (2%–11%)	17

Abbreviations: ARR, absolute risk reduction; OR, odds ratio; NNT, number needed to treat.

SUMMARY

The lessons learned from the trials discussed above have influenced our management of STS in meaningful ways. Limb-sparing surgery offers an equivalent chance of cure and a clear functional advantage when compared with amputation for extremity STS. Adjuvant radiation therapy for extremity STS significantly decreases the chance of local recurrence. Preoperative radiation therapy increases the risk of wound complications but is associated with better functional outcomes than postoperative radiation treatment. The decrease in local recurrence afforded by radiation therapy does not affect survival time because most patients who succumb to extremity STS die from disseminated disease. Local recurrence is an important cause of death in cases of retroperitoneal sarcoma,[18] yet the evidence supporting a role for radiation therapy in these cases is lacking. Trials addressing the impact of modern, more targeted delivery of external beam radiation for retroperitoneal sarcoma are warranted. With regard to systemic therapy, the body of evidence does not indicate a compelling long-term survival benefit for any systemic regimen. More sophisticated predictors of response are needed, in addition to the identification of novel targets and agents. Slight modifications of approaches already proven to have marginal or no survival benefit will not lead to meaningful progress.

FUTURE DIRECTIONS

The rarity of soft tissue sarcomas makes conducting RCTs for these diseases extraordinarily challenging. Multi-institutional trials are needed to define the role of neoadjuvant chemotherapy and radiation therapy for high-risk soft tissue sarcomas, including those arising in the retroperitoneum. More importantly, our increasingly sophisticated understanding of the biologic differences among soft tissue sarcoma subtypes, along with tumor heterogeneity within subtypes, should be incorporated into treatment strategies. The success of future trials for soft tissue sarcoma chemotherapy may depend, in large part, on our ability to define inclusion criteria to focus on more biologically homogeneous groups of patients.

LEVEL I EVIDENCE: RANDOMIZED CLINICAL TRIALS

1. Preoperative versus postoperative radiotherapy in soft-tissue sarcoma of the limbs: a randomised trial. O'Sullivan B, Davis AM, Turcotte R, et al. Lancet 2002;359:2235–41.[6]

Hypothesis: The use of preoperative radiation therapy would be associated with a higher rate of wound complications.

# Patients Randomized	Study Groups	Stratification	Significance Demonstrated	Change Identified in Trial
190	Preoperative (N=94) Postoperative (N=96)	Tumor size (10cm)	Yes	18% absolute increase in wound complication rate with neoadjuvant therapy

Published abstract: BACKGROUND: External-beam radiotherapy (delivered either preoperatively or postoperatively) is frequently used in local management of sarcomas in the soft tissue of limbs, but the two approaches differ substantially in their potential toxic effects. We aimed to determine whether the timing of external-beam radiotherapy affected the number of wound healing complications in soft-tissue sarcoma in the limbs of adults. METHODS: After stratification by tumor size (≤ 10 cm or >10 cm), we randomly allocated 94 patients to preoperative radiotherapy (50 Gy in 25 fractions) and 96 to postoperative radiotherapy (66 Gy in 33 fractions). The primary endpoint was rate of wound complications within 120 days of surgery. Analyses were per protocol for primary outcomes and by intention to treat for secondary outcomes. FINDINGS: Median follow-up was $3\cdot3$ years (range $0\cdot27$–$5\cdot6$). Four patients, all in the preoperative group, did not undergo protocol surgery and were not evaluable for the primary outcome. Of those patients who were eligible and evaluable, wound complications were recorded in 31 (35%) of 88 in the preoperative group and 16 (17%) of 94 in the postoperative group (difference 18% [95% CI 5–30], $P = 0\cdot01$). Tumor size and anatomic site were also significant risk factors in multivariate analysis. Overall survival was slightly better in patients who had preoperative radiotherapy than in those who had postoperative treatment ($P = 0\cdot0481$). INTERPRETATION: Because preoperative radiotherapy is associated with a greater risk of wound complications than postoperative radiotherapy, the choice of regimen for patients with soft-tissue sarcoma should take into account the timing of surgery and radiotherapy, and the size and anatomic site of the tumor. (Copyright Elsevier 2002.)

Editor's summary and comments: The principal question posed by the authors was adequately addressed. Patients who received radiation therapy before surgery had a clinically and statistically significant increase in the rate of wound complications. Forty-five percent of the patients in the neoadjuvant group who developed a wound complication required reoperation for management. Lower extremity sites and tumors larger than 10cm were associated with a greater risk of wound complications. The two groups did not differ with respect to recurrence- or progression-free survival. A small 3-year overall survival advantage ($P = .05$) was noted in the preoperative group (85%) compared with the postoperative group (72%). The short duration of follow-up and the use of overall survival as an endpoint warrant caution because 19% of the deaths in the postoperative group were not due to disease, compared with only 7% in the preoperative group. The authors also note that the study was not adequately powered to detect this difference in a secondary endpoint such as overall survival. In a follow-up article, patients who received postoperative radiation therapy were found to have significantly worse functional outcomes with respect to fibrosis, joint stiffness, edema, and functional scores.[7]

2. Adjuvant epirubicin with or without ifosfamide for adult soft-tissue sarcoma.
Petrioli R, Coratti A, Correale P, et al. Am J Clin Oncol 2002;25:468–73.[13]

Hypothesis: The use of epirubicin with or without ifosfamide after local therapy for STS would improve the disease-free interval and overall survival duration.

# Patients Randomized	Study Groups	Stratification	Significance Demonstrated	Change Identified in Trial
88	Epiriubicin ± Ifosfamide (N=45) Observation (N=43)	None	Yes	Absolute DFS benefit at 5 years of 25% ($P = .01$) with a trend toward improved OS ($P = .06$)

Abbreviations: DFS, disease-free survival: OS, overall survival.

Published abstract: BACKGROUND: This randomized study compared the efficacy of epirubicin-based adjuvant chemotherapy on the disease-free interval (DFI) and overall survival of patients with high-risk soft-tissue sarcomas. METHODS: After cura-tive surgery, 43 of the 88 enrolled patients were assigned to surgery with or without radiotherapy and 45 to surgery plus chemotherapy (26 epirubicin, 19 epirubicin and ifosfamide) with or without radiotherapy. The trial closed prematurely because of poor patient accrual. FINDINGS: There was a statistically significant difference in the 5-year disease-free survival of the patients receiving adjuvant chemotherapy with or without radiotherapy (69%) and that of those treated with surgery with or without radiotherapy (44%) (P = .01). The 5-year survival of the patients treated with adjuvant chemotherapy with or without radiotherapy was 72% as against 47% of those treated with surgery with or without radiotherapy (P = .06). The power of the study was 0.65 for both the DFI and overall survival. INTERPRETATION: The results of the study suggest a possible advantage of epirubicin-based adjuvant chemotherapy in patients with soft-tissue sarcoma at high risk of relapse. (Copyright 2002 Lippincott Williams & Wilkins. Reprinted with permission.)

Editor's summary and comments: Although the results of this study indicate a disease-free benefit to epirubicin-based systemic therapy after resection of STS with or without radiation therapy, several important limitations warrant discussion. The authors appropriately exercise caution in interpreting their data by stating that their findings only suggest a benefit to the systemic regimen. Over the course of 12 years, the trial accrued only 88 patients. The small sample size and potential variability in diagnostic and treatment modalities over such a prolonged period are problematic. While 72% of the group that received adjuvant systemic therapy survived for 5 years compared with 47% of the control arm, the result was not significant (P = .06). A signif-icant (P = .01) overall survival advantage was found when comparing only those patients who received epirubicin plus ifosfamide (84%) to controls (57%). The groups were imbalanced with respect to histologic subtypes and potentially sensitivity to cytotoxic agents. The difference (25%) for disease-free survival was significant (P = .01), but the authors found no difference when analyzing local or distant recurrence separately. The findings with respect to a benefit for combination chemotherapy are encouraging, but do not sit well in the context of results from previous, larger RCTs.

3. Randomized trial of cytoreduction followed by intraperitoneal chemo-therapy versus cytoreduction alone in patients with peritoneal sarcomatosis. Bonvalot S, Cavalcanti A, Le Péchoux C, et al. Eur J Surg Onc 2005;31:917–23.[14]

Hypothesis: The use of intraperitoneal chemotherapy would be associated with a decrease in locoregional recurrence and increase in survival after optimal cytoreduc-tion for peritoneal carcinomatosis.

# Patients Randomized	Study Groups	Stratification	Significance Demonstrated	Change Identified in Trial
38	IP chemotherapy (n=19) No chemotherapy (n=19)	None	No	No differences in recurrence-free or overall survival

Published abstract: BACKGROUND: To decrease loco-regional relapse after complete resection of peritoneal sarcomatosis (PS), the role of intraperitoneal chemotherapy (IPEC) was prospectively evaluated. METHODS: Patients (pts) with completely resected PS were randomized between adjunction of IPEC or not. IPEC consisted of doxorubicin, 0.1 mg/kg and cisplatin, 15 mg/m2 per day for 5 consecutive days. FINDINGS: Thirty-eight consecutive pts have been randomized, 19 in each group. Ratio of retroperitoneal (RPS) and visceral (VS) sarcomatosis were 9/10 and 6/13 in IPEC- and IPEC+ groups, respectively. Histoprognostic grade, Sugarbaker's score and mean number of resected organs were similar in both groups. There were no toxic deaths and morbidity was similar in both groups (four pts in each group). The median follow-up is 60 months. The median local relapse-free, metastatic relapse-free survival and overall survival were identical in both groups (12.5, 18 and 29 months, respectively), with no difference between RPS and VERSUS sarcomatosis. INTERPRETATION: Administration of IPEC after a macroscopically complete surgery did not allow increasing greatly the outcome of pts. Complete surgery remains the cornerstone of the treatment of patients with sarcomatosis with best results for low-grade sarcomatosis. (Copyright Elsevier 2005.)

Editor's summary and comments: Based upon the variable success of intraperitoneal chemotherapy (IPEC) with or without hyperthermia for carcinomatosis, the authors attempted to define the role of IPEC following optimal cytoreduction of sarcomatosis. The identical median overall survival time of 29 months in both groups leaves little room for rationalizing the use of IPEC after surgical treatment of sarcomatosis. However, this trial included a very small number of patients and the breakdown of histologic subtypes is not provided. Larger trials with the inclusion of hyperthermia warrant consideration given the high likelihood of locoregional relapse in patients with sarcomatosis.

4. Crossover randomized comparison of intravenous versus intravenous/oral mesna in soft tissue sarcoma treated with high-dose ifosfamide. Mace JR, Keohan ML, Bernardy H, et al. Clin Can Res 2003;9:5829–34.[15]

Hypothesis: The use of oral plus IV mesna in patients receiving ifosfamide for STS would be equivalent to IV mesna.

# Patients Randomized	Study Groups	Stratification	Significance Demonstrated	Change Identified in Trial
17	Crossover comparison	None	No	No difference in the rate of hemorrhagic cystitis with either mesna formulation

Published abstract: BACKGROUND: We conducted our study to determine the pharmacokinetics (PK) and clinical efficacy of oral mesna in patients receiving ifosfamide for soft tissue sarcoma. METHODS: Seventeen patients were enrolled in a randomized prospective Phase I/II study. Seventeen patients were exposed to study medication. Ifosfamide was given at a dose of 2 g/m^2/day for 5 days on a 21-day cycle. Before the first cycle, all patients were randomized onto a crossover design and received either the approved i.v. or i.v./oral mesna regimen, with crossover for the second cycle of chemotherapy. The i.v. mesna regimen consisted of dosings (20% ifosfamide dose) at 0, 4, and 8 h. The i.v./oral arm consisted of an i.v. mesna dosing (20% ifosfamide dose) at 0 h, followed by oral tablet dosing (40% ifosfamide dose) at 2 and 6 h. In-patient clinical monitoring and phlebotomy and urine sampling for mesna, dimesna, and ifosfamide PK were performed on all chemotherapy days. FINDINGS: Thirteen patients were evaluable for PK and 17 for efficacy and toxicity. No significant differences were detected in the plasma PK of the concomitantly infused ifosfamide. Rates of hemorrhagic cystitis were similar across mesna schedules. Four of 10 evaluable patients demonstrated objective response.

INTERPRETATION: On the basis of our study, an i.v./oral mesna regimen is at least as uroprotective as the approved i.v. regimen. The i.v./oral regimen will improve patient tolerance and convenience, allow for a reduction in elective hospitalizations for ifosfamide chemotherapy, reduce the potential morbidity associated with inpatient administration of chemotherapy, and likely result in decreased costs of care. (Copyright 2003 by the American Association for Cancer Research. Reprinted with permission.)

Editor's summary and comments: This small study suggested that substituting a portion of the IV mesna regimen for tablets in STS patients receiving ifosfamide yields an equivalent approach. In turn, patients may require less inpatient care for systemic therapy administration.

5. Phase III trial of two investigational schedules of ifosfamide compared with standard-dose doxorubicin in advanced or metastatic soft tissue sarcoma: a European Organisation for Research and Treatment of Cancer Soft Tissue and Bone Sarcoma group study. Lorigan P, Verweij J, Papai Z, et al. J Clin Onc 2007;25:3144–50.[16]

Hypothesis: Single-agent ifosfamide would be associated with equivalent progression-free survival compared with doxorubicin for the treatment of advanced STS.

# Patients Randomized	Study Groups	Stratification	Significance Demonstrated	Change Identified in Trial
326	Doxorubicin (N=110) Ifosfamide 3g/m^2 (N=109) Ifosfamide 9g/m^2 (N=107)	None	No	None

Published abstract: BACKGROUND: Single-agent doxorubicin remains the standard treatment for advanced soft tissue sarcomas. Combining doxorubicin with standard-dose ifosfamide has not been shown to improve survival and is associated with a significantly increased toxicity; it is not known whether higher dose single-agent ifosfamide is superior to doxorubicin. METHODS: This randomized prospective multicenter phase III trial was designed to compare progression-free survival of patients with advanced soft tissue sarcoma receiving either regimen of standard doxorubicin 75 mg/m2 every 21 days, ifosfamide 9 g/m2 over 3 days continuous infusion, or ifosfamide 3 g/m2 per day in 3 hours over 3 days. The primary end point was progression-free survival. Secondary end points included overall survival, response rate, and toxicity. FINDINGS: The study included 326 patients. Grade 4 leukopenia, neutropenia, febrile neutropenia, and encephalopathy were more frequent in the ifosfamide arms. Progression-free survival, overall survival, and response rates were not significantly different between the three arms. An independent data monitoring committee reviewed the interim data and recommended early closure of the trial for futility (ie, no significant difference would be shown). INTERPRETATION: Single-agent doxorubicin remains the treatment of choice for patients with advanced soft tissue sarcoma. (Copyright 2007 American Society of Clinical Oncology. Reprinted with permission.)

Editor's summary and comments: This RCT conducted by the European Organization for the Research and Treatment of Cancer (EORTC) and Soft-tissue and Bone Sarcoma Group (STBSG) established that ifosfamide alone should not be considered as a first-line therapy for patients with advanced STS. An important message from this well-conducted trial is that novel therapeutic approaches are sorely needed.

6. A randomized phase ii study on neo-adjuvant chemotherapy for 'high-risk' adult soft-tissue sarcoma. Gortzak E, Azzarelli A, Buesa J, et al. Eur J Cancer 2001;37:1096–103.[17]

Hypothesis: Neoadjuvant chemotherapy for high-risk STS is safe and feasible.

# Patients Randomized	Study Groups	Stratification	Significance Demonstrated	Change Identified in Trial
150	Local treatment only (N = 75) Preoperative chemotherapy (N=75)	<8cm, high grade >8cm, low grade >8cm, high grade Incomplete resection Local recurrence	No	Similar 5-year survival rates in both arms

Published abstract: BACKGROUND: The aim of this study was to examine the strategy, feasibility and outcome of neo-adjuvant chemotherapy, with doxorubicin and ifosfamide, in adult patients with 'high-risk' soft-tissue sarcomas. METHODS: Patients with 'high-risk' soft-tissue sarcomas, defined as tumors ≥ 8 cm of any grade, or grade II/III tumors <8 cm, or grade II/III locally recurrent tumors, or grade II/III tumors with inadequate surgery performed in the previous 6 weeks and therefore requiring further surgery, were randomized between either surgery alone or three cycles of 3-weekly doxorubicin 50 mg/m2 intravenous (i.v.) bolus and ifosfamide 5 g/m2 (24 h infusion) before surgery. The type of surgery had to be planned at randomization. Tumors were to be amenable to surgery by amputation, compartmental resection, wide or marginal excision. If chemotherapy was given, surgery had to be performed within 21 days after the last chemotherapy. Patients received postoperative radiotherapy in cases of marginal surgery, microscopically incomplete resection and no further possibility for surgery, and in cases of surgery because of local recurrence. FINDINGS: 150 patients were entered into the study and 134 were eligible, 67 in each arm. The most frequent side-effects of chemotherapy were alopecia, nausea and vomiting (95%), and leukocytopenia (32%). One patient died of neutropenic fever after the first cycle of chemotherapy. Chemotherapy did not interfere with planned surgery and did not affect postoperative wound healing. Limb-salvage was achieved in 88%, amputation was necessary in 12% (all according to the plan at randomization). The trial was closed after completion of phase II, since accrual was too slow to justify expanding the study into the scheduled phase III study. At a median follow-up of 7.3 years, the 5 year disease free survival is estimated at 52% for the no chemotherapy and 56% for the chemotherapy arm (standard error: 7%) ($P = .3548$). The 5 year overall survival for both arms is 64 and 65%, respectively (standard error 7%) ($P = .2204$). INTERPRETATION: Neo-adjuvant-chemotherapy with doxorubicin and ifosfamide at these doses and with this schedule was feasible and did not compromise subsequent treatment, surgery with or without radiotherapy. Although not powered to draw definitive conclusions on benefit, but with an at least 7 year median follow-up, the results render it less likely that major survival benefits will be achieved with this type of chemotherapy. (Copyright Elsevier 2001.)

Editor's summary and comments: Although not designed or powered to determine definitively whether neoadjuvant chemotherapy confers a survival benefit, the 5-year survival rates of both arms were nearly identical. The neoadjuvant regimen was reasonably well tolerated in that not a single patient failed to receive definitive local therapy. However, 18% of patients did progress while receiving neoadjuvant treatment. Whether this is a group of patients who would have been better served by immediate resection or who had extremely aggressive disease biology is a matter for conjecture. The response rate of only 28% to combined doxorubicin and ifosfamide therapy once again points to the need for more targeted and effective systemic agents.

7. Randomized phase ii study of gemcitabine and docetaxel compared with gemcitabine alone in patients with metastatic soft tissue sarcomas: results of Sarcoma Alliance for Research Through Collaboration Study 002. Maki RG, Wathen JK, Patel SR, et al. J Clin Onc 2007;19:2755–63.[19]

Hypothesis: Gemcitabine in combination with docetaxel is superior to gemcitabine alone for recurrent or progressive STS.

# Patients Randomized	Study Groups	Stratification	Significance Demonstrated	Change Identified in Trial
122	Gemcitabine (N=75) Gemcitabine + docetaxel (N=75)	Bayesian adaptive randomization	Yes (0.999 posterior probability)	Median overall survival of 17.9 months in the dual-drug regimen compared with 11.5 months

Published abstract: BACKGROUND: Gemcitabine as a single agent and the combination of gemcitabine and docetaxel have activity in patients with metastatic soft tissue sarcoma. To determine if the addition of docetaxel to gemcitabine improved clinical outcome of patients with metastatic soft tissue sarcomas, we compared a fixed dose rate infusion of gemcitabine versus a lower dose of gemcitabine with docetaxel. METHODS: In this open-label phase II clinical trial, the primary end point was tumor response, defined as complete or partial response or stable disease lasting at least 24 weeks. A Bayesian adaptive randomization procedure was used to produce an imbalance in the randomization in favor of the superior treatment, accounting for treatment-subgroup interactions. FINDINGS: One hundred nineteen of 122 randomly assigned patients had assessable outcomes. The adaptive randomization assigned 73 patients (60%) to gemcitabine-docetaxel and 49 patients (40%) to gemcitabine alone, indicating gemcitabine-docetaxel was superior. The objective Response Evaluation Criteria in Solid Tumors response rates were 16% (gemcitabine-docetaxel) and 8% (gemcitabine). Given the data, the posterior probabilities that gemcitabine-docetaxel was superior for progression-free and overall survival were 0.98 and 0.97, respectively. Median progression-free survival was 6.2 months for gemcitabine-docetaxel and 3.0 months for gemcitabine alone; median overall survival was 17.9 months for gemcitabine-docetaxel and 11.5 months for gemcitabine. The posterior probability that patients receiving gemcitabine-docetaxel had a shorter time to discontinuation for toxicity compared with gemcitabine alone was .999. INTERPRETATION: Gemcitabine-docetaxel yielded superior progression-free and overall survival to gemcitabine alone, but with increased toxicity. Adaptive randomization is an effective method to reduce the number of patients receiving inferior therapy. (Copyright 2007 American Society of Clinical Oncology. Reprinted with permission.)

Editor's summary and comments: The response rates were 8% and 17% to the gemcitabine and gemcitabine-docetaxel regimens, respectively. Although the dual-drug arm had a significantly longer survival time, the group did contain a higher proportion of patients with leiomyosarcoma, which were more sensitive to the regimen.

DISCLOSURE

Authors have nothing to disclose.

REFERENCES

1. Cancer facts and figures. In: American Cancer Society. Available at: http://www.cancer.org. 2006. Accessed April 26, 2009.
2. Rosenberg SA, Tepper J, Glatstein E, et al. The treatment of soft-tissue sarcomas of the extremities: prospective randomized evaluations of (1) limb-sparing surgery plus radiation therapy compared with amputation and (2) the role of adjuvant chemotherapy. Ann Surg 1982;196:305.
3. Singer S, Antonescu CR, Riedel E, et al. Histologic subtype and margin of resection predict pattern of recurrence and survival for retroperitoneal liposarcoma. Ann Surg 2003;238:358.
4. Pisters PW, Harrison LB, Leung DH, et al. Long-term results of a prospective randomized trial of adjuvant brachytherapy in soft tissue sarcoma. J Clin Oncol 1996;14:859.
5. Yang JC, Chang AE, Baker AR, et al. Randomized prospective study of the benefit of adjuvant radiation therapy in the treatment of soft tissue sarcomas of the extremity. J Clin Oncol 1998;16:197.
6. O'Sullivan B, Davis AM, Turcotte R, et al. Preoperative versus postoperative radiotherapy in soft-tissue sarcoma of the limbs: a randomised trial. Lancet 2002;359:2235.
7. Davis AM, O'Sullivan B, Turcotte R, et al. Late radiation morbidity following randomization to preoperative versus postoperative radiotherapy in extremity soft tissue sarcoma. Radiother Oncol 2005;75:48.
8. Antman K, Crowley J, Balcerzak SP, et al. An intergroup phase III randomized study of doxorubicin and dacarbazine with or without ifosfamide and mesna in advanced soft tissue and bone sarcomas. J Clin Oncol 1993;11:1276.
9. Bramwell V, Rouesse J, Steward W, et al. Adjuvant CYVADIC chemotherapy for adult soft tissue sarcoma–reduced local recurrence but no improvement in survival: a study of the European Organization for Research and Treatment of Cancer Soft Tissue and Bone Sarcoma Group. J Clin Oncol 1994;12:1137.
10. Frustaci S, Gherlinzoni F, De Paoli A, et al. Adjuvant chemotherapy for adult soft tissue sarcomas of the extremities and girdles: results of the Italian randomized cooperative trial. J Clin Oncol 2001;19:1238.
11. Santoro A, Tursz T, Mouridsen H, et al. Doxorubicin versus CYVADIC versus doxorubicin plus ifosfamide in first-line treatment of advanced soft tissue sarcomas: a randomized study of the European Organization for Research and Treatment of Cancer Soft Tissue and Bone Sarcoma Group. J Clin Oncol 1995;13:1537.
12. Pervaiz N, Colterjohn N, Farrokhyar F, et al. A systematic meta-analysis of randomized controlled trials of adjuvant chemotherapy for localized resectable soft-tissue sarcoma. Cancer 2008;113:573.

13. Petrioli R, Coratti A, Correale P, et al. Adjuvant epirubicin with or without Ifosfamide for adult soft-tissue sarcoma. Am J Clin Oncol 2002;25:468.
14. Bonvalot S, Cavalcanti A, Le Pechoux C, et al. Randomized trial of cytoreduction followed by intraperitoneal chemotherapy versus cytoreduction alone in patients with peritoneal sarcomatosis. Eur J Surg Oncol 2005;31:917.
15. Mace JR, Keohan ML, Bernardy H, et al. Crossover randomized comparison of intravenous versus intravenous/oral mesna in soft tissue sarcoma treated with high-dose ifosfamide. Clin Cancer Res 2003;9:5829.
16. Lorigan P, Verweij J, Papai Z, et al. Phase III trial of two investigational schedules of ifosfamide compared with standard-dose doxorubicin in advanced or metastatic soft tissue sarcoma: a European Organisation for Research and Treatment of Cancer Soft Tissue and Bone Sarcoma Group Study. J Clin Oncol 2007;25: 3144.
17. Gortzak E, Azzarelli A, Buesa J, et al. A randomized phase II study on neo-adjuvant chemotherapy for 'high-risk' adult soft-tissue sarcoma. Eur J Cancer 2001;37:1096–103.
18. Canter RJ, Qin LX, Ferrone CR, et al. Why do patients with low-grade soft tissue sarcoma die? Ann Surg Oncol 2008;15:3550.
19. Maki RG, Wathen KJ, Patel SR, et al. Randomized phase II study of gemcitabine and docetaxel compared with gemcitabine alone in patients with metastatic soft tissue sarcomas: results of sarcoma alliance for research through collaboration study 002. J Clin Onc 2007;19:2755–63.

Randomized Clinical Trials in Melanoma

T. Peter Kingham, MD*, Giorgos Karakousis, MD,
Charlotte Ariyan, MD, PhD

KEYWORDS

• Melanoma • Management • Randomized controlled trials

The incidence of melanoma is increasing and it is estimated that, in the United States, the lifetime risk of developing melanoma is 1 in 55.[1] There have been many randomized trials that have refined the treatment and minimized the morbidity of the intervention of this prevalent disease. From 1975 to 2000, there were 154 prospective randomized trials on the treatment of local, regional, and metastatic melanoma. Between 2001 and the end of 2008, there were 52 randomized controlled trials (RCTs) relating to the treatment of patients with malignant melanoma. This article reviews the results of the major studies included in the prior article, and provides a detailed description of selected RCTs performed from 2001 to 2008.

PRIMARY MELANOMA

Current surgical margins are based on several randomized trials that were described in the 2002 review article and are listed in **Table 1**. These studies demonstrated increased local recurrence rates as the melanoma increases in thickness and the excision margin decreases. No trial has clearly demonstrated a difference in survival with more aggressive surgical margins, and yet local recurrence is associated with poor overall survival,[7] therefore investigation into the appropriate margin has continued. Since 2001, there have been two additional randomized trials addressing the effect of excision margins of the primary lesion on outcome in patients with melanoma. A large European multicentric phase 3 study from nine European centers investigated the difference between 2-cm and 5-cm excision margins for melanomas less than 2.1 mm thick.[5] No significant difference was found in the number of recurrences, recurrence-free survival, or overall survival between the two excision margin groups. Another trial from the UK studied patients with melanomas 2 mm or greater in thickness, randomized to 1-cm or 3-cm margins.[6] This trial demonstrated no significant difference in overall survival or melanoma-specific survival, but did demonstrate an increase in LR in the 1-cm margin group compared with the 3-cm margin group

Disclosure: See last page of article.
Department of Surgery, Memorial Sloan-Kettering Cancer Center, NY, NY, USA
* Corresponding author.
E-mail address: kinghamt@mskcc.org (T.P. Kingham).

Surg Oncol Clin N Am 19 (2010) 13–31
doi:10.1016/j.soc.2009.09.008
1055-3207/09/$ – see front matter © 2010 Elsevier Inc. All rights reserved.

Table 1 Surgical margin randomized trials before 2002			
Trial	Thickness of Melanoma	Margin	Comments
WHO[2]	<2 mm	1 cm vs 3 cm	1-cm margin safe for melanoma <1 mm, increased local recurrence with 1-cm excision in melanoma >1 mm
Intergroup[3]	1–4 mm	2 cm versus 4 cm	2-cm margin safe for intermediate-thickness melanoma
Swedish[4]	0.8–2 mm	2 cm vs 5 cm	2 cm margin safe
European phase III[5]	<2.1 mm	2 cm vs 5 cm	2 cm safe
UK[6]	>2 mm	1 cm vs 3 cm	Increased LR rate with 1-cm excision, no SLN biopsy performed

(hazard ratio [HR] 1.26; $P = .05$). The results of all the randomized trials on excision margins suggest that reasonable practice is still a 1-cm margin for lesions less than 1 mm in thickness, and 2-cm margins for thicker lesions. Whether 1-cm margins may yield equivalent outcomes to those of 2-cm margins for 1- to 2-mm lesions remains to be addressed specifically by a randomized trial.

REGIONAL METASTATIC DISEASE

As shown in **Table 2**, elective lymph node dissection (ELND) has not been shown to improve survival in patients with melanoma. Only the long-term follow-up of the Intergroup trial suggested a survival benefit in younger patients with nonulcerated, intermediate-thickness melanomas.[3] The sentinel lymph node (SLN) biopsy technique has supplanted the need for further investigations into the merits of ELND. SLN biopsy is the standard approach to evaluate clinically negative lymphatic basins. The Melanoma Selective Lymphadenectomy Trial (MSLT)-1 trial randomized patients with intermediate-thickness melanomas to either wide local excision (WLE) with nodal observation, or WLE in combination with SLN biopsy. Those patients with metastatic disease detected in the sentinel node underwent immediate completion lymph node dissection, whereas the patients in the observation arm underwent a therapeutic lymphadenectomy for clinically evident nodal disease. The study confirmed the high prognostic value of the sentinel-node status for patients with intermediate-thickness melanomas. MSLT-I did not demonstrate any difference in melanoma-specific survival between the two groups, which was the primary end point of the trial. In a subset analysis of all patients with nodal metastases, however, there was a statistically significant improved 5-year survival rate in those patients who underwent SLN biopsy and immediate lymphadenectomy versus those who underwent delayed lymphadenectomy on clinically evident disease (72.3% vs 52.4%).

The benefits of prophylactic regional hyperthermic isolated limb perfusion (ILP) for patients with high-risk melanomas were examined in a cooperative-group trial that randomized 832 patients to ILP with melphalan.[13] No significant difference in survival was reported at the conclusion of the trial. Since 2001, the results of one additional randomized trial have been performed using ILP in the treatment of locally advanced

Table 2
Results of randomized ELND trials before 2002

Study	N	Site	Thickness (mm)	F/U (y)	OS: WLE	OS: WLE + ELND	P value
Sim[8]	173	Excluded midline trunk, head, and neck	Any	NR	85	85	NS
Veronesi[9]	553	Extremity	Any	8.2	72	74	NS
Balch[10] (intergroup)	740	All	1–4	7.4	82	86	.25
Intergroup f/u[3]				10	73	77	.12
Cascinelli[11,12]	240	Trunk	>1.5	11	51	62	.09

melanoma (ACOSOG trial Z0020).[14,15] This trial randomized patients with locally advanced melanoma to standard hyperthermic limb perfusion with either melphalan alone or melphalan in combination with tumor necrosis factor (TNF). The trial was stopped early because of an increase in grade 4 toxicities, including amputations, in the combined treatment arm. The survival data, with short follow-up, was not different between the two groups.

ADJUVANT TREATMENT OF HIGH-RISK MELANOMA

Chemotherapies are toxic and ineffective in melanoma, and therefore adjuvant strategies have focused on immunotherapy. The rationale for immunotherapy in the treatment of melanoma stems from observations of rare, but spontaneous, regression of melanoma in patients. In addition, patients with tumor infiltrating lymphocytes, vitiligo, or other evidence of immune activation, may have improved survival. Therefore, adjuvant immunotherapies aim to activate the host immune system through vaccines, interferons (IFNs), and compounds such as bacillus Calmette-Guérin (BCG).

IFN is a protein that is produced by the immune system in response to viral infection and foreign proteins. Exogenous administration of this compound is intended to stimulate the immune system to recognize melanoma antigens. The results of adjuvant IFN treatment usually fail to demonstrate a survival benefit, but do demonstrate a modest improvement in recurrence-free survival. Investigations have therefore continued to attempt to identify whether there is a subset of patients and a dosing regimen that will improve outcomes. IFN α-2b was approved by the US Food and Drug Administration (FDA) as adjuvant treatment of high-risk patients with deep primary melanomas or regional lymph node metastatic disease after ECOG trial E1684.[16] This trial compared high-dose IFN α-2b with observation, and found a significant improvement in disease-free and overall survival. The follow-up study compared observation, low-dose IFN α-2b, and high-dose IFN α-2b, and found improved relapse-free survival but no overall survival difference.[17]

The continued inconsistency in results of IFN trials is demonstrated by two recent studies with no significant results: the AIM HIGH Study and EORTC 18952. The AIM HIGH Study randomized patients to long-term low-dose IFN or observation after resection of stage IIB or III melanoma.[18,19] In this trial there was an initial benefit in recurrence-free survival that disappeared after 3 years of follow-up and was not significant. Fifteen percent of patients in the IFN group withdrew from the study, and toxicities were modest. These results are similar to those of the EORTC 18952 trial which randomized patients after resection with stage IIb or III melanoma to 13 months or 25 months of intermediate dose IFN or observation.[20] Recent results from EORTC 18991,[21] which randomized patients with stage III melanoma after resection to pegylated IFN or observation, also demonstrated additional promise for this immunotherapy. The trial demonstrated a small (6% at 4 years) improvement in recurrence-free survival with the pegylated IFN, which is potentially best noted in the subgroup of patients with N1 disease. It is possible that long-term follow-up of pegylated IFN will continue to show an improvement in patients with early stage III disease, and, therefore, it may have a more definitive role in the adjuvant setting than standard IFN, because it is also better tolerated.

IFN has also been combined with other immunologic and chemotherapeutic agents. Garbe and colleagues[22–24] randomized patients with stage III disease following surgery to adjuvant low-dose IFN, with or without dacarbazine, or to observation. Overall survival was significantly higher by multivariate analysis in patients with adjuvant low-dose IFN compared with surgery alone, but the addition of dacarbazine removed this survival benefit. In another trial, high-dose IFN was compared with a ganglioside vaccine, GM2-KLH/QS-21, in patients with resected stage IIB and III melanomas.[25,26] The trial was halted on an interim analysis because of a significant recurrence-free survival, and overall survival, benefit in the high-dose IFN arm. In 2007, Mitchell reported on 604 patients who were randomized to 2 years of treatment with an allogeneic melanoma lysate and low-dose IFN or high-dose IFN.[27] Overall and recurrence-free survival were the same between the two arms, providing another trial without any clear benefit to vaccine use in the adjuvant setting. Other immunotherapy trials have examined BCG in the adjuvant setting. Early trials reported improvements in disease-free survival (DFS) with BCG use. To test this hypothesis, Agarwala randomized 734 patients with stage I to III melanoma into four groups that were assembled into two cohorts: (1) BCG versus BCG plus dacarbazine; and (2) BCG versus. observation.[28] There was no benefit to BCG or BCG plus dacarbazine with any patients in the stage I to III categories of melanoma patients.

The Canvaxin vaccine consisted of allogeneic melanoma cells with high antigen expression. Phase 2 studies showed an improvement in survival when used as an adjuvant in stage III patients, which generated considerable interest.[29,30] However, a multicenter randomized phase 3 trial failed to confirm these results, and this therapy is no longer used.[31]

TREATMENT OF METASTATIC MELANOMA

In the prior review, the Dartmouth regimen (cisplatin, carmustine, dimethyltriazenyl imidazole carboxamide [DTIC], and tamoxifen) and its components were the most commonly studied regimen in several large prospective RCTs. The only positive trial was Cocconi's[16] study, which showed improved response rates and median survival with DTIC plus tamoxifen compared with DTIC alone. Chapman then performed a study that showed no difference between the Dartmouth regimen and DTIC regarding tumor response, toxicity, or survival.[32] At that time, DTIC alone was felt to be the optimal treatment. Temozolamide has also been used to treat patients with metastatic melanoma, and DTIC was compared with temozolomide in a study by the Royal Marsden Hospital.[33] Patients treated with temozolomide demonstrated equivalent progression-free survival, response rates, toxicity, and survival. Temozolomide was also studied in combination with cisplatin, with no benefit found in the combined regimen.[34] Recently, imatinib mesylate was also used in a phase 2 trial with 21 patients who had melanoma cells that expressed c-kit.[35] At 400 mg twice a day, imatinib had little clinical efficacy, although it did have individual responders, suggesting a possible role for imatinib in patients with specific kit mutations.

Additional agents that have been investigated outside the published randomized trials include sorafenib and bevacizumab. Sorafenib was evaluated by Eisen[36] and found to be well tolerated but with little to no antitumor activity in patients with advanced melanoma. Bevacizumab was studied in a trial that randomized to bevacizumab with or without low-dose IFN α-2b.[37] There was no benefit to combining IFN with bevacizumab, but bevacizumab alone caused prolonged disease stabilization in approximately 25% of patients in the bevacizumab-alone group. Currently, the benefits of using this drug are limited. Trials using anti-CTLA-4 for the treatment of patients with metastatic disease, and as an adjuvant in stage III disease, are in progress. Although not FDA approved, durable clinical responses have been noted with CTLA-4 blockade, and there is hope that this field will continue to evolve.[38]

Investigators have combined treatments with biologic agents and chemotherapies in an effort to maximize activity against melanoma. Unfortunately, most of these studies have not improved survival. As reviewed in the previous article, studies comparing IL-2/IFN α and chemotherapy to IL-2/IFN α alone, or IL-2 to IL-2/IFN α, showed no difference in overall survival.[39–41] This review includes a biochemotherapy trial that is similar to other trials, such as EORTC 18951, in structure and outcomes, in that it compared cisplatin, vinblastine, dacarbazine with cisplatin, vinblastine, dacarbazine, IL-2, and IFN α and found no significant alteration in overall survival or durable responses.[42] There were higher response rates and a longer median progression-free survival rate with the biochemotherapy, but there were significant toxicities associated with these regimens. The conclusion from these trials is that biochemotherapy with IL-2 and IFN α are not recommended for treating metastatic melanoma.

LEVEL IA EVIDENCE IN MELANOMA
Surgical Trials

1. Surgical margins in cutaneous melanoma (2-cm versus 5-cm for lesions measuring less than 2.1-mm thick). Khayat D, Rixe O, Martin G, et al. Cancer 2003 Apr 15;97(8):1941–6.[5]

Hypothesis: A smaller excision margin (2-cm) of the primary tumor for patients with melanomas less than 2.1 mm in thickness may yield similar outcomes regarding disease recurrence and survival to a wider (5-cm) excision margin.

Number of Patients Randomized	Study Groups	Stratification	Significance Demonstrated	% Change Identified in Trial
337	2-cm margins N = 161	Histology	None Equivalent	None
	5-cm margins N = 165			

Published abstract: BACKGROUND: This study addressed the question of whether limited surgery for primary malignant melanoma with a 2-cm margin is as good as a 5-cm margin. An update of a 16-year follow-up is provided. METHODS: Nine European Centers, over a period of 5 years, prospectively randomized 337 patients with melanoma measuring less than 2.1 mm in thickness to undergo a local excision with either a 2-cm or a 5-cm margin. Three hundred twenty-six patients were eligible for statistical analysis. Excluded from the trial were patients older than 70 years; those with melanomas from the toe, nail, or finger; and those with acral-lentiginous melanoma. A separate randomization was performed to independently test an adjuvant treatment with a nonspecific immunostimulant, isoprinosine, compared with observation. The median follow-up time was 192 months (16 years) for the estimation of survival and disease recurrences. RESULTS: There were 22 tumor recurrences in the 2-cm arm and 33 in the 5-cm arm. The median time to disease recurrence was 43 months and 37.6 months, respectively. The 10-year disease-free survival rates were 85% for the group with a 2-cm margin and 83% for the group with a 5-cm margin. There was no difference in the 10-year overall survival rates (87% vs. 86%). Isoprinosine did not demonstrate any activity in this setting. CONCLUSIONS: The authors concluded that for melanoma less than 2.1-mm thick, a margin of excision of 2 cm is sufficient. A larger margin of 5 cm does not appear to have any impact on either the rate or the time to disease recurrence or on survival. (Copyright 2003 American Cancer Society. Reprinted with permission.)

Editor's summary and comments: This multicenter European trial investigated the role of surgical margins for melanoma lesions less than 2.1 mm in thickness by randomizing patients to either 2-cm or 5-cm excisional margins in patients (those >70 years and with acral-lentiginous lesions were excluded). There was no difference in local tumor recurrence rates, DFS or overall survival between the two excision margin groups, with a median follow-up of 16 years. This study reinforces the results of the Swedish Melanoma Study group (2-cm versus 5-cm margin groups for 0.8-mm to 2-mm thickness lesions), and the WHO trial discussed earlier. As a secondary randomization, patients in each excisional margin arm were assigned to receive isoprinosine, shown to have immunostimulation properties toward natural killer cells against melanoma in vitro, or to observation. No difference was seen in median overall survival or DFS between the groups receiving adjuvant immunotherapy and those followed with observation alone, using any subgroup analysis of tumor characteristics or surgery extent, although the numbers in each final randomized group were fairly small (76–89 patients).

2. Excision margins in high-risk malignant melanoma. Thomas JM, Newton-Bishop J, A'Hern R, et al. N Engl J Med 2004 Feb 19;350(8):757–66.[6]

Hypothesis: Narrow (1-cm) excision margins for high-risk melanoma lesions (>2 mm) may be insufficient compared with wider (3-cm) margins.

Number of Patients Randomized	Study Groups	Stratification	Significance Demonstrated	% Change Identified in Trial
453	1-cm margin (N = 453)	Histology	Increase in locoregional recurrence (LR) with 1-cm margin	HR 1.26 for LR in 1-cm vs 3-cm margin group (P = .05)
	3-cm margin (N = 447)			

Published abstract: BACKGROUND: Controversy exists concerning the necessary margin of excision for cutaneous melanoma 2 mm or greater in thickness. METHODS: We conducted a randomized clinical trial comparing 1-cm and 3-cm margins. RESULTS: Of the 900 patients who were enrolled, 453 were randomly assigned to undergo surgery with a 1-cm margin of excision and 447 with a 3-cm margin of excision; the median follow-up was 60 months. A 1-cm margin of excision was associated with a significantly increased risk of locoregional recurrence. There were 168 locoregional recurrences (as first events) in the group with 1-cm margins of excision, as compared with 142 in the group with 3-cm margins (hazard ratio, 1.26; 95 percent confidence interval, 1.00 to 1.59; P = .05). There were 128 deaths attributable to melanoma in the group with 1-cm margins, as compared with 105 in the group with 3-cm margins (hazard ratio, 1.24; 95 percent confidence interval, 0.96 to 1.61; P = .1); overall survival was similar in the two groups (hazard ratio for death, 1.07; 95 percent confidence interval, 0.85 to 1.36; P = .6). CONCLUSIONS: A 1-cm margin of excision for melanoma with a poor prognosis (as defined by a tumor thickness of at least 2 mm) is associated with a significantly greater risk of regional recurrence than is a 3-cm margin, but with a similar overall survival rate. (Copyright [2004] Massachusetts Medical Society. All rights reserved.)

Editor's summary and comments: This well-designed randomized trial addresses the important question of whether 1-cm margins are adequate for higher risk melanoma lesions greater than 2 mm in thickness. The comparison arm to the 1-cm margin is a 3-cm margin, and not 2-cm, which is the standard margin size routinely performed for intermediate-thickness lesions (adapted largely from the results of the Intergroup trial). The study design directly complements the design of the WHO trial, which compared 1-cm to 3-cm margins for lesions less than 2 mm. The investigators found a decrease in the incidence of locoregional recurrence (which included local, in transit or regional nodal recurrences) favoring the 3-cm margin group. However, this finding did not translate into a statistically different DFS, or overall survival, between the two randomized arms, although there was a trend toward an increased disease-specific mortality associated with the narrow margin (HR 1.24, P = .1). Patients in the study were not permitted to undergo SLN biopsy, and it remains unclear how the use of this technique, which is routinely performed in this patient population, would have affected the results.

3. Sentinel-node biopsy or nodal observation in melanoma. Morton DL, Thompson JF, Cochran AJ, et al. N Engl J Med 2006 Sep 28;355(13):1307–17.[43]

Hypothesis: Patients with intermediate-thickness melanomas undergoing SLN biopsy for staging with immediate lymphadenectomy for SLN metastases would have an improved survival compared with patients with simple excision of their primary lesion and therapeutic lymphadenectomy on detection of clinically evident regional nodal disease.

Number of Patients Randomized	Study Groups	Stratification	Significance Demonstrated	% Change Identified in Trial
1347	Nodal observation with therapeutic lymphadenec-tomy for clinically evident disease (N = 500)	Histology	None	None (see editor's comments)
	SLN biopsy and immediate lymphadenec-tomy for SLN metastases (N =769)			

Published abstract: BACKGROUND: We evaluated the contribution of sentinel-node biopsy to outcomes in patients with newly diagnosed melanoma. METHODS: Patients with a primary cutaneous melanoma were randomly assigned to wide excision and postoperative observation of regional lymph nodes with lymphadenectomy if nodal relapse occurred, or to wide excision and sentinel-node biopsy with immediate lymphadenectomy if nodal micrometastases were detected on biopsy. RESULTS: Among 1269 patients with an intermediate-thickness primary melanoma, the mean (±SE) estimated 5-year disease-free survival rate for the population was 78.3 ± 1.6% in the biopsy group and 73.1 ± 2.1% in the observation group (hazard ratio for recurrence [corrected], 0.74; 95% confidence interval [CI], 0.59 to 0.93; $P =$ .009). Five-year melanoma-specific survival rates were similar in the two groups (87.1 ± 1.3% and 86.6 ± 1.6%, respectively). In the biopsy group, the presence of metastases in the sentinel node was the most important prognostic factor; the 5-year survival rate was 72.3 ± 4.6% among patients with tumor-positive sentinel nodes and 90.2 ± 1.3% among those with tumor-negative sentinel nodes (hazard ratio for death, 2.48; 95% CI, 1.54 to 3.98; $P<.001$). The incidence of sentinel-node micrometastases was 16.0% (122 of 764 patients), and the rate of nodal relapse in the observation group was 15.6% (78 of 500 patients). The corresponding mean number of tumor-involved nodes was 1.4 in the biopsy group and 3.3 in the observation group ($P<.001$), indicating disease progression during observation. Among patients with nodal metastases, the 5-year survival rate was higher among those who underwent immediate lymphadenectomy than among those in whom lymphadenectomy was delayed (72.3 ± 4.6% vs. 52.4 ± 5.9%; hazard ratio for death, 0.51; 95% CI, 0.32 to 0.81; $P = .004$). CONCLUSIONS: The staging of intermediate-thickness (1.2 to 3.5 mm) primary melanomas according to the results of sentinel-node biopsy provides important prognostic information and identifies patients with nodal metastases whose survival can be prolonged by immediate lymphadenectomy. (Copyright [2006] Massachusetts Medical Society. All rights reserved.)

Editor's summary and comments: This trial randomizes patients with intermediate-thickness melanomas to SLN biopsy and immediate lymphadenectomy for those patients with metastatic disease in the SLNs, versus observation and therapeutic lymphadenectomy for patients who develop clinically evident nodal disease. Several important conclusions can be drawn from this well-designed study, which required considerable international efforts for its implementation. First, the study confirms the prognostic role of SLN status in patients with intermediate-thickness melanomas. On Cox multivariate analysis, SLN status conferred an HR (positive vs negative) of 3.04 ($P<.001$) for disease recurrence, and 2.48 for melanoma-specific mortality ($P<.001$). Secondly, the incidence of SLN positivity and clinically evident disease in the observation group were almost identical (16% vs 15.6% respectively), suggesting that the patients randomized in the two groups shared similar characteristics and that the natural progression of SLN positivity would be the development of clinically evident nodal disease. Finally, although the study showed no difference in melanoma-specific survival between the two randomized arms (primary end point), in a subset analysis focusing on patients with nodal metastases, those patients with positive SLN biopsy who underwent immediate lymphadenectomy demonstrated an improved melanoma-specific survival compared with patients in the observation group with clinically evident nodal disease who underwent a therapeutic lymphadenectomy. The results of the subset analysis have been the subject of ongoing controversy among various experts in the field. Moreover, the therapeutic role of SLN biopsy in melanoma remains undefined. The role of completion lymph node dissection following SLN biopsy has therefore served as the foundation for the MSLT-II trial, which is currently accruing patients.

4. Prospective Randomized Trial of Interferon Alfa-2b and Interleukin-2 as Adjuvant Treatment for Resected Intermediate- and High-Risk Primary Melanoma Without Clinically Detectable Node Metastasis. Hauschild A, Weichenthal B, diger Balda BR, et al. J Clin Oncol 2003;21:2883–8.[44]

Hypothesis: The addition of low-dose IL-2 to adjuvant low-dose IFN α-2b will improve survival.

Number of Patients Randomized	Study Groups	Stratification	Significance Demonstrated	% Change Identified in Trial
225	Surgery, low-dose IFN α, low-dose IL-2		None	None
	Surgery, observation			

Published abstract: BACKGROUND: Low-dose interferon alfa (IFN A) has been shown to have limited effects in the adjuvant treatment of patients with intermediate- and high-risk primary melanoma. We hypothesized that a combination regimen with low-dose interleukin-2 (IL-2) may improve survival prospects in these patients. PATIENTS AND METHODS: After wide excision of primary melanoma without clinically detectable lymph node metastasis (pT3 to 4, cN0, M0), 225 patients from 10 participating centers were randomly assigned to receive either subcutaneous low-dose IFN alpha-2b (3 million international units [MU]/m²/d, days 1 to 7, week 1; three times weekly, weeks 3 to 6, repeated all 6 weeks) plus IL-2 (9 MU/m²/d, days 1 to 4, week 2 of each cycle) for 48 weeks, or observation alone. The primary end point was prolongation of a relapse-free interval. RESULTS: Of the 225 enrolled patients, 223 were found to be eligible. Median follow-up time was 79 months. All evaluated prognostic factors were well balanced between the two arms of the study. Relapses were noticed in 36 of 113 patients treated with IFN alpha-2b plus IL-2 and in 34 of 110 patients with observation alone. Five-year disease-free survival of those who had routine surgery supplemented by IFN alpha-2b and IL-2 treatment was 70.1% (95% confidence interval [CI], 61.3% to 78.9%), compared with 69.9% in those receiving surgery and observation alone (95% CI, 60.7% to 79.1%) in the intention-to-treat analysis. Evaluation of the overall survival did not show any difference between treated and untreated melanoma patients ($P = .93$). CONCLUSION: Adjuvant treatment of intermediate- and high-risk melanoma patients with low-dose IFN alpha-2b and IL-2 is safe and well tolerated by most patients, but it does not improve disease-free or overall survival. (Copyright 2003 American Society of Clinical Oncology. Reprinted with permission.)

Editor's summary and comments: Prior studies showed that low-dose IFN α improved relapse-free survival, but not overall survival, in patients with resectable melanoma. This trial randomized patients to receive adjuvant low-dose IFN and IL-2 or observation. At a median follow-up of 79 months, 5-year DFS was 70% in the treatment arm and 69.9% in the observation arm. Although the therapy was tolerated well, with 104 patients receiving more than 90% of the intended therapy, there was no benefit in the adjuvant setting.

5. Adjuvant Immunotherapy of Resected, Intermediate-Thickness, Node-Negative Melanoma With an Allogeneic Tumor Vaccine: Overall Results of a Randomized Trial of the Southwest Oncology Group. Sondak V, Liu PY, Tuthill RJ, et al. J Clin Oncol 2002;20:2058–66.[45]

Hypothesis: Adjuvant allogeneic melanoma vaccine will improve recurrence-free survival in patients with node-negative intermediate-thickness melanoma.

Number of Patients Randomized	Study groups	Stratification	Significance Demonstrated	% Change Identified in Trial
689	Surgery plus allogeneic melanoma vaccine for 2 y	Sex Thickness Nodal stage	None	None
	Surgery alone			

Published abstract: BACKGROUND: Patients with clinically negative nodes constitute over 85% of new melanoma cases. There is no adjuvant therapy for intermediate-thickness, node-negative melanoma patients. PATIENTS AND METHODS: The Southwest Oncology Group conducted a randomized phase III trial of an allogeneic melanoma vaccine for 2 years versus observation in patients with intermediate-thickness (1.5 to 4.0 mm or Clark's level IV if thickness unknown), clinically or pathologically node-negative melanoma (T3N0M0). RESULTS: Six hundred eighty-nine patients were accrued over 4.5 years; 89 patients (13%) were ineligible. Surgical node staging was performed in 24%, the remainder were clinical N0. Thirteen eligible patients refused assigned treatment: seven on the observation arm and six on the vaccine arm. Most vaccine patients experienced mild to moderate local toxicity, but 26 (9%) experienced grade 3 toxicity. After a median follow-up of 5.6 years, there were 107 events (tumor recurrences or deaths) among the 300 eligible patients randomized to vaccine compared with 114 among the 300 eligible patients randomized to observation (hazard ratio, 0.92; Cox-adjusted $P_2 = 0.51$). There was no difference in vaccine efficacy among patients with tumors <3 mm or >3 mm. CONCLUSION: This represents one of the largest randomized, controlled trials of adjuvant vaccine therapy in human cancer reported to date. Compliance with randomization was excellent, with only 2% refusing assigned therapy. There is no evidence of improved disease-free survival among patients randomized to receive vaccine, although the power to detect a small but clinically significant difference was low. Future investigations of adjuvant vaccine approaches for patients with intermediate-thickness melanoma should involve larger numbers of patients and ideally should include sentinel node biopsy staging. (Copyright 2002 American Society of Clinical Oncology. Reprinted with permission.)

Editor's summary and comments: A prior phase 3 study showed that an allogeneic melanoma cell lysate had a slightly improved response rate and survival (although not significantly so) compared with a group treated with the Dartmouth Regimen. There was, however, no control arm of surgery alone, so this trial was developed to answer the question of the benefit of an allogeneic melanoma cell lysate used in the adjuvant setting compared with the control arm of surgery alone. The vaccine consisted of 15 melanoma-associated antigens. The primary outcome of the trial, DFS, showed no difference between the two groups. Secondary analyses of groups with different thicknesses also showed no difference.

Adjuvant Treatment (Nodal Disease/High-risk Primaries)

6. Adjuvant low-dose interferon {alpha}2a with or without dacarbazine compared with surgery alone: a prospective-randomized phase III DeCOG trial in melanoma patients with regional lymph node metastasis. Garbe C, Radny P, Linse R, et al. Annals of Oncology 2008;19:1195–201.[22]

Hypothesis: IFN α 2a with or without dacarbazine improves DFS and overall survival in patients after nodal dissection with positive lymph nodes.

Number of Patients Randomized	Study Groups	Stratification	Significance Demonstrated	% Change Identified in Trial
444	Adjuvant IFN α 2a (n = 146)	none	DFS	59% (IFN) vs 45% (combination) vs 42% (observation) (P = .0045. IFN vs observation, P = .76 for combination vs observation)
	Adjuvant IFN α 2a plus DTIC (n = 148)		Overall survival	IFN alone HR .609 (P = .005)
	Observation (n = 147)			

Published abstract: BACKGROUND: More than half of patients with melanoma that has spread to regional lymph nodes develop recurrent disease within the first 3 years after surgery. The aim of the study was to improve disease-free survival (DFS) and overall survival (OS) with interferon (IFN) alpha2a with or without dacarbazine (DTIC) compared with observation alone. PATIENTS AND METHODS: A total of 444 patients from 42 centers of the German Dermatologic Cooperative Oncology Group who had received a complete lymph node dissection for pathologically proven regional node involvement were randomized to receive either 3 MU s.c. of IFN alpha 2a three times a week for 2 years (Arm A) or combined treatment with same doses of IFN alpha 2a plus DTIC 850 mg/m(2) every 4–8 weeks for 2 years (Arm B) or to observation alone (Arm C). Treatment was discontinued at first sign of relapse. RESULTS: A total of 441 patients were eligible for intention-to-treat analysis. Kaplan-Meier 4-year OS rate of those who had received IFN alpha 2a was 59%. For those with surgery alone, survival was 42% (A versus C, P = .0045). No improvement of survival was found for the combined treatment Arm B with 45% survival rate (B versus C, P = .76). Similarly, DFS rates showed significant benefit for Arm A, and not for Arm B. Multivariate Cox model confirmed that Arm A has an impact on OS (P = .005) but not Arm B (P = .34). CONCLUSIONS: 3 MU interferon alpha 2a given s.c. three times a week for 2 years significantly improved OS and DFS in patients with melanoma that had spread to the regional lymph nodes. Interestingly, the addition of DTIC reversed the beneficial effect of adjuvant interferon alpha 2a therapy. (Copyright 2008 by Oxford University Press. Reprinted with permission.)

Editor's summary and comments: Given the high mortality rates of patients with metastatic melanoma, the goal of this trial was to attempt to improve on DFS and overall survival in patients with positive lymph nodes by using a combination of low-dose IFN α 2a, dacarbazine, and observation. The study was well powered, with 441 total patients, and designed to detect a significant difference of 15% in the 4-year survival rate. The overall survival of patients in the IFNα 2a group was significantly higher than the surgery alone group (59% vs 42%, P = .0045). There was a lower overall survival in the combination group, with an overall survival rate of 45%. These trends were similar with multivariate analysis, with an HR of .609 for the IFN-alone group (P = .005) and .854 for the combination group (P = .343). These findings are relevant for two reasons: (1) low-dose IFN α in this study showed an increase in disease-specific and overall survival after 2 years of treatment; and (2) the addition of dacarbazine to low-dose IFN negated the benefit of low-dose IFN. The 5-year overall survival in Hancock's[18] low-dose IFN group was 44% for all patients, which is lower than the 59% overall survival at 4 years in this year, raising questions about the patient populations in both studies.

7. Adjuvant Interferon in High-Risk Melanoma: The AIM HIGH Study—United Kingdom Coordinating Committee on Cancer Research Randomized Study of Adjuvant Low-Dose Extended-Duration Interferon Alfa- 2a in High-Risk Resected Malignant Melanoma. Hancock BW, Wheatley K, Harris S, et al. J Clin Oncol 2004;22:53–61.[18]

Hypothesis: Low-dose extended adjuvant IFN α-2a improves recurrence-free survival and overall survival in patients with resected high-risk melanomas.

Number of Patients Randomized	Study Groups	Stratification	Significance Demonstrated	% Change Identified in Trial
674	IFN α (n = 338)	None	None	None
	Observation (n = 336)			

Published abstract: PURPOSE: To evaluate low-dose extended-duration interferon alfa-2a as adjuvant therapy in patients with thick (>4 mm) primary cutaneous melanoma and/or locoregional metastases. PATIENTS AND METHODS: In this randomized controlled trial involving 674 patients, the effect of interferon alfa-2a (3 megaunits three times per week for 2 years or until recurrence) on overall survival (OS) and recurrence-free survival (RFS) was compared with that of no further treatment in radically resected stage IIB and stage III cutaneous malignant melanoma. RESULTS: The OS and RFS rates at 5 years were 44% (SE, 2.6) and 32% (SE, 2.1), respectively. There was no significant difference in OS or RFS between the interferon-treated and control arms (odds ratio [OR], 0.94; 95% CI, 0.75 to 1.18; $P = .6$; and OR, 0.91; 95% CI, 0.75 to 1.10; $P = .3$; respectively). Male sex ($P = .003$) and regional lymph node involvement ($P = .0009$), but not age ($P = .7$), were statistically significant adverse features for OS. Subgroup analysis by disease stage, age, and sex did not show any clear differences between interferon-treated and control groups in either OS or RFS. Interferon-related toxicities were modest: grade 3 (and in only one case, grade 4) fatigue or mood disturbance was seen in 7% and 4% respectively, of patients. However, there were 50 withdrawals (15%) from interferon treatment due to toxicity. CONCLUSION: The results from this study, taken in isolation, do not indicate that extended-duration low-dose interferon is significantly better than observation alone in the initial treatment of completely resected high-risk malignant melanoma. (Copyright 2004 American Society of Clinical Oncology. Reprinted with permission.)

Editor's summary and comments: This study was initiated in response to several phase 1 and phase 2 trials that showed some improvement in recurrence-free survival in patients with metastatic melanoma who were treated with IFN α. The original target accrual was 1000 patients to achieve a 90% chance of detecting a 10% absolute difference in recurrence-free survival and overall survival, but accrual was halted after 674 patients due to the belief that additional patients would not change the preliminary analysis. Patients were randomized to low-dose IFN α for 2 years, or until disease recurrence, after resection of high-risk melanomas (≥4 mm or locoregional metastases). Similar to prior RCTs that examined adjuvant IFN, there was an initial benefit in recurrence-free survival that disappeared after 3 years of follow-up and was not significant. In addition, 15% of patients in the IFN group withdrew from the study, and toxicities were modest. Given that no effect on overall survival was demonstrated with low-dose IFN, there is no clear benefit to using it as treatment of high-risk melanoma patients in the adjuvant setting.

8. Adjuvant therapy with pegylated interferon alfa-2b versus observation alone in resected stage III melanoma: final results of EORTC 18991, a randomized phase III trial. Eggermont AMM, Suciu S, Santinami M, et al. Lancet; 2008;372:117–26.[21]

Hypothesis: Pegylated IFN α-2b is well tolerated and will improve recurrence-free survival in patients after resection of stage III melanoma.

Number of Patients Randomized	Study Groups	Stratification	Significance Demonstrated	% Change Identified in Trial
1256	Observation (n = 629)	Microscopic vs macroscopic nodal involvement	Recurrence-free survival	45.6% vs 38.9% at 4 y (HR .82, P = .01)
	Pegylated IFN α-2b (n = 627)	Number of positive nodes		
		Ulceration		
		Tumor thickness		

Published abstract: BACKGROUND: Any benefit of adjuvant interferon alfa-2b for melanoma could depend on dose and duration of treatment. Our aim was to determine whether pegylated interferon alfa-2b can facilitate prolonged exposure while maintaining tolerability. METHODS: 1256 patients with resected stage III melanoma were randomly assigned to observation (n = 629) or pegylated interferon alfa-2b (n = 627) 6 μg/kg per week for 8 weeks (induction) then 3 μg/kg per week (maintenance) for an intended duration of 5 years. Randomization was stratified for microscopic (N1) versus macroscopic (N2) nodal involvement, number of positive nodes, ulceration and tumor thickness, sex, and center. Randomization was done with a minimization technique. The primary endpoint was recurrence-free survival. Analyses were done by intention to treat. This study is registered with ClinicalTrials.gov, number NCT00006249. RESULTS: All randomized patients were included in the primary efficacy analysis. Six hundred and eight patients in the interferon group and 613 patients in the observation group were included in safety analyses. The median length of treatment with pegylated interferon alfa-2b was 12 (IQR 3.8–33.4) months. At 3.8 (3.2–4.2) years median follow-up, 328 recurrence events had occurred in the interferon group compared with 368 in the observation group (hazard ratio 0.82, 95% CI 0.71–0.96; P = .01); the 4-year rate of recurrence-free survival was 45.6% (SE 2.2) in the interferon group and 38.9% (2.2) in the observation group. There was no difference in overall survival between the groups. Grade 3 adverse events occurred in 246 (40%) patients in the interferon group and 60 (10%) in the observation group; grade 4 adverse events occurred in 32 (5%) patients in the interferon group and 14 (2%) in the observation group. In the interferon group, the most common grade 3 or 4 adverse events were fatigue (97 patients, 16%), hepatotoxicity (66, 11%), and depression (39, 6%). Treatment with pegylated interferon alfa-2b was discontinued because of toxicity in 191 (31%) patients. CONCLUSIONS: Adjuvant pegylated interferon alfa-2b for stage III melanoma has a significant, sustained effect on recurrence-free survival. (Copyright Elsevier 2008).

Editor's summary and comments: In this trial patients were randomized to observation or adjuvant pegylated IFN α-2b after resection of stage III melanoma. This is the first randomized trial to examine the usefulness of pegylation in the adjuvant setting. The theoretical advantage to using pegylated IFN is that it is better tolerated, allows for a longer treatment period, and maintains maximum exposure of IFN. The study reported a significant difference in recurrence-free survival at 4 years, with 45.6% of the IFN group, compared with 38.9% of the observation group, free of recurrence. There was no difference in overall survival between the two groups. When the groups were broken down into subgroups, the greatest effect of IFN treatment was in the group with earlier stage III disease, specifically microscopic nodal disease or only one positive node. However, there was no statistically significant difference in overall survival in these groups. The only subgroup with a difference in overall survival was in the 96 patients treated with pegylated IFN who had an ulcerated lesion, among whom the overall survival was 65% compared with 45.4% (HR .61, $P = .03$). There was a large difference between the toxicities found in the two groups, as in the IFN group 40% of patients had grade 3 toxicities, compared with 10% of patients in the observation arm. Although the greatest benefit was in patients with limited N1 disease, this was at 4 years follow-up, which is too short a time period for patients with positive nodal disease. This regimen may be an alternative for patients who are offered high-dose adjuvant IFN, but its usefulness is not fully proven, and, again, there was no difference in overall survival outside of small subgroup analyses.

9. Randomized Trial of an Allogeneic Melanoma Lysate Vaccine With Low-Dose Interferon Alfa-2b Compared With High-Dose Interferon Alfa-2b for Resected Stage III Cutaneous Melanoma. Mitchell MS, Abrams J, Thompson JA, et al. J Clin Oncol 2007;25:2078–85.[27]

Hypothesis: Adjuvant allogeneic melanoma lysate vaccine and low-dose IFN α-2b will improve overall survival compared with high-dose IFN α-2b.

Number of Patients Randomized	Study Groups	Stratification	Significance Demonstrated	% Change Identified in Trial
604	Allogeneic lysates and low-dose IFN a-2b (n = 300)	Sex Number of nodes	None	None
	High-dose IFN a-2b (n = 300)			

Published abstract: BACKGROUND: To compare the overall survival (OS) of patients with resected stage III melanoma administered active specific immunotherapy and low-dose interferon alfa-2b (IFN a-2b) with the OS achieved using high-dose IFN a-2b. PATIENTS AND METHODS: An Ad Hoc Melanoma Working Group of 25 investigators treated 604 patients from April 1997 to January 2003. Patients were stratified by sex and number of nodes and were randomly assigned to receive either 2 years of treatment with active specific immunotherapy with allogeneic melanoma lysates and low-dose IFN a-2b (arm 1) or high-dose IFN a-2b alone for 1 year (arm 2). Active specific immunotherapy was injected subcutaneously (SC) weekly for 4 weeks, at week 8, and bimonthly thereafter. IFN a-2b SC was begun on week 4 and continued thrice weekly at 5 MU/m^2 for 2 years. IFN a-2b in arm 2 was administered according to the Eastern Cooperative Oncology Group 1684 study regimen. RESULTS: Median follow-up time was 32 months for all patients and 42 months for surviving patients. Median OS time exceeds 84 months in arm 1 and is 83 months in arm 2 ($P = .56$). Five-year OS rate is 61% in arm 1 and 57% in arm 2. Estimated 5-year relapse-free survival (RFS) rate is 50% in arm 1 and 48% in arm 2, with median RFS times of 58 and 50 months, respectively. The incidence of serious adverse events as a result of treatment was the same in both arms, but more severe neuropsychiatric toxicity was seen in arm 2. CONCLUSION: OS and RFS achieved by active specific immunotherapy and low-dose IFN a-2b were indistinguishable from those achieved by high-dose IFN a-2b. Long RFS and OS times were observed in both treatment arms. (Copyright 2007 American Society of Clinical Oncology. Reprinted with permission.)

Editor's summary and comments: This trial examined the difference in recurrence-free survival and overall survival in patients with stage III melanoma. The study was powered to detect a 1-year difference in recurrence-free survival with 90% statistical power. At a median follow-up of 32 months, overall survival and relapse-free survival were similar between the two groups. There were also similar toxicities between the two treatment regimens. The survival times in both arms of this trial were longer than historical controls (eg, ECOG 1684), as approximately 70% of patients in this study were alive at 36 to 42 months. This study, however, is probably more representative of modern survival rates, as many patients had microscopically positive nodal disease due to the sentinel-node procedure. One difficulty in analyzing the results of this trial is that there was no control arm without IFN. In addition, the study was not powered to show equivalence between the two groups, so it is not clear that the results of this study can be used to argue for low-dose IFN and allogeneic melanoma lysate.

Systemic Treatments (Metastatic Disease)

10. Phase III Trial Comparing Concurrent Biochemotherapy With Cisplatin, Vinblastine, Dacarbazine, Interleukin-2, and Interferon Alfa-2b With Cisplatin, Vinblastine, and Dacarbazine Alone in Patients With Metastatic Malignant Melanoma (E3695): A Trial Coordinated by the Eastern Cooperative Oncology Group. Atkins MB, Hsu J, Lee S, et al. J Clin Oncol 2008;26:5748–54.[42]

Hypothesis: Biochemotherapy with IL-2 and IFN α-2b added to a regimen of cisplatin, vinblastine, and dacarbazine will improve survival.

Number of Patients Randomized	Study Groups	Stratification	Significance Demonstrated	% Change Identified in Trial
415	Cisplatin, vinblastine, and dacarbazine (n = 195)	None	Median progression-free survival	4.8 mo vs 2.9 mo ($P = .015$)
	Cisplatin, vinblastine, dacarbazine, IL-2, IFN α-2b (n = 200)		Rate of grade 3 or worse toxicities	95% vs 73% ($P = .001$)

Published abstract: BACKGROUND: Phase II trials with biochemotherapy (BCT) have shown encouraging response rates in metastatic melanoma, and meta-analyses and one phase 3 trial have suggested a survival benefit. In an effort to determine the relative efficacy of BCT compared with chemotherapy alone, a phase III trial was performed within the United States Intergroup. PATIENTS AND METHODS: Patients were randomly assigned to receive cisplatin, vinblastine, and dacarbazine (CVD) either alone or concurrent with interleukin-2 and interferon alfa-2b (BCT). Treatment cycles were repeated at 21-day intervals for a maximum of four cycles. Tumor response was assessed after cycles 2 and 4, then every 3 months. RESULTS: Four hundred fifteen patients were enrolled, and 395 patients (CVD, n = 195; BCT, n = 200) were deemed eligible and assessable. The two study arms were well balanced for stratification factors and other prognostic factors. Response rate was 19.5% for BCT and 13.8% for CVD (P = .140). Median progression-free survival was significantly longer for BCT than for CVD (4.8 v 2.9 months); (P = .015), although this did not translate into an advantage in either median overall survival (9.0 v 8.7 months) or the percentage of patients alive at 1 year (41% v 36.9%). More patients experienced grade 3 or worse toxic events with BCT than CVD (95% v 73%; P = .001). CONCLUSION: Although BCT produced slightly higher response rates and longer median progression-free survival than CVD alone, this was not associated with either improved overall survival or durable responses. Considering the extra toxicity and complexity, this concurrent BCT regimen cannot be recommended for patients with metastatic melanoma. (Copyright 2008 American Society of Clinical Oncology. Reprinted with permission.)

Editor's summary and comments: This phase 3 trial was initiated in response to phase 2 trials that showed encouraging response rates with biochemotherapy in patients with metastatic melanoma. The only significant finding in this trial was a longer median time to progression (4.8 months compared with 2.9 months, P = .015). However, this finding did not translate into any difference in overall survival or percentage of patients alive at 1 year. Given that 95% of the patients in the biochemotherapy group experienced a toxicity that was grade 3 or higher, the conclusion of this trial is that biochemotherapy is not indicated for treatment of patients with metastatic melanoma. These treatments need further optimization to balance quality of life with treatment in patients with metastatic melanoma.

DISCLOSURE

Authors have nothing to disclose.

REFERENCES

1. Available at: http://www.cancer.gov. National Cancer Institute. Accessed April 10, 2009.
2. Veronesi U, Cascinelli N. Narrow excision (1-cm margin). A safe procedure for thin cutaneous melanoma. Arch Surg 1991;126:438.
3. Balch CM, Soong S, Ross MI, et al. Long-term results of a multi-institutional randomized trial comparing prognostic factors and surgical results for intermediate thickness melanomas (1.0 to 4.0 mm). Intergroup Melanoma Surgical Trial. Ann Surg Oncol 2000;7:87.
4. Ringborg U, Andersson R, Eldh J, et al. Resection margins of 2 versus 5 cm for cutaneous malignant melanoma with a tumor thickness of 0.8 to 2.0 mm: randomized study by the Swedish Melanoma Study Group. Cancer 1809;77:1996.
5. Khayat D, Rixe O, Martin G, et al. Surgical margins in cutaneous melanoma (2 cm versus 5 cm for lesions measuring less than 2.1-mm thick). Cancer 1941;97:2003.
6. Thomas JM, Newton-Bishop J, A'Hern R, et al. Excision margins in high-risk malignant melanoma. N Engl J Med 2004;350:757.
7. Dong XD, Tyler D, Johnson JL, et al. Analysis of prognosis and disease progression after local recurrence of melanoma. Cancer 2000;88:1063.
8. Sim FH, Taylor WF, Ivins JC, et al. A prospective randomized study of the efficacy of routine elective lymphadenectomy in management of malignant melanoma. Preliminary results. Cancer 1978;41:948.

 9. Veronesi U, Adamus J, Bandiera DC, et al. Delayed regional lymph node dissection in stage I melanoma of the skin of the lower extremities. Cancer 1982;49: 2420.
10. Balch CM, Soong SJ, Bartolucci AA, et al. Efficacy of an elective regional lymph node dissection of 1 to 4 mm thick melanomas for patients 60 years of age and younger. Ann Surg 1996;224:255.
11. Cascinelli N, Bufalino R, Morabito A, et al. Results of adjuvant interferon study in WHO melanoma programme. Lancet 1994;343:913.
12. Cascinelli N, Morabito A, Santinami M, et al. Immediate or delayed dissection of regional nodes in patients with melanoma of the trunk: a randomised trial. WHO Melanoma Programme. Lancet 1998;351:793.
13. Koops HS, Vaglini M, Suciu S, et al. Prophylactic isolated limb perfusion for localized, high-risk limb melanoma: results of a multicenter randomized phase III trial. European Organization for Research and Treatment of Cancer Malignant Melanoma Cooperative Group Protocol 18832, the World Health Organization Melanoma Program Trial 15, and the North American Perfusion Group Southwest Oncology Group-8593. J Clin Oncol 1998;16:2906.
14. Cornett WR, McCall LM, Petersen RP, et al. Randomized multicenter trial of hyperthermic isolated limb perfusion with melphalan alone compared with melphalan plus tumor necrosis factor: American College of Surgeons Oncology Group Trial Z0020. J Clin Oncol 2006;24:4196.
15. Creagan ET, Dalton RJ, Ahmann DL, et al. Randomized, surgical adjuvant clinical trial of recombinant interferon alfa-2a in selected patients with malignant melanoma. J Clin Oncol 1995;13:2776.
16. Cocconi G, Bella M, Calabresi F, et al. Treatment of metastatic malignant melanoma with dacarbazine plus tamoxifen. N Engl J Med 1992;327:516.
17. Kirkwood JM, Ibrahim JG, Sondak VK, et al. High- and low-dose interferon alfa-2b in high-risk melanoma: first analysis of intergroup trial E1690/S9111/C9190. J Clin Oncol 2000;18:2444.
18. Hancock BW, Wheatley K, Harris S, et al. Adjuvant interferon in high-risk melanoma: the AIM HIGH Study–United Kingdom Coordinating Committee on Cancer Research randomized study of adjuvant low-dose extended-duration interferon Alfa-2a in high-risk resected malignant melanoma. J Clin Oncol 2004;22:53.
19. Kaufmann R, Spieth K, Leiter U, et al. Temozolomide in combination with interferon-alfa versus temozolomide alone in patients with advanced metastatic melanoma: a randomized, phase III, multicenter study from the Dermatologic Cooperative Oncology Group. J Clin Oncol 2005;23:9001.
20. Eggermont AMM, Suciu S, MacKie R, et al. Post-surgery adjuvant therapy with intermediate doses of interferon alfa 2b versus observation in patients with stage IIb/III melanoma (EORTC 18952): randomised controlled trial. Lancet 2005;366: 1189.
21. Eggermont AMM, Suciu S, Santinami M, et al. Adjuvant therapy with pegylated interferon alfa-2b versus observation alone in resected stage III melanoma: final results of EORTC 18991, a randomised phase III trial. Lancet 2008;372: 117.
22. Garbe C, Radny P, Linse R, et al. Adjuvant low-dose interferon {alpha}2a with or without dacarbazine compared with surgery alone: a prospective-randomized phase III DeCOG trial in melanoma patients with regional lymph node metastasis. Ann Oncol 2008;19:1195.
23. Grob JJ, Dreno B, de la Salmoniere P, et al. Randomised trial of interferon alpha-2a as adjuvant therapy in resected primary melanoma thicker than 1.5 mm

without clinically detectable node metastases. French Cooperative Group on Melanoma. Lancet 1998;351:1905.

24. Grunhagen DJ, van Etten B, Brunstein F, et al. Efficacy of repeat isolated limb perfusions with tumor necrosis factor alpha and melphalan for multiple in-transit metastases in patients with prior isolated limb perfusion failure. Ann Surg Oncol 2005;12:609.

25. Kirkwood JM, Ibrahim JG, Sosman JA, et al. High-dose interferon alfa-2b significantly prolongs relapse-free and overall survival compared with the GM2-KLH/QS-21 vaccine in patients with resected stage IIB-III melanoma: results of intergroup trial E1694/S9512/C509801. J Clin Oncol 2001;19:2370.

26. Kirkwood JM, Strawderman MH, Ernstoff MS, et al. Interferon alfa-2b adjuvant therapy of high-risk resected cutaneous melanoma: the Eastern Cooperative Oncology Group Trial EST 1684. J Clin Oncol 1996;14:7.

27. Mitchell MS, Abrams J, Thompson JA, et al. Randomized trial of an allogeneic melanoma lysate vaccine with low-dose interferon Alfa-2b compared with high-dose interferon Alfa-2b for Resected stage III cutaneous melanoma. J Clin Oncol 2007;25:2078.

28. Agarwala SS, Neuberg D, Park Y, et al. Mature results of a phase III randomized trial of bacillus Calmette-Guerin (BCG) versus observation and BCG plus dacarbazine versus BCG in the adjuvant therapy of American Joint Committee on Cancer Stage I-III melanoma (E1673): a trial of the Eastern Oncology Group. Cancer 2004;100:1692.

29. Morton DL, Hsueh EC, Essner R, et al. Prolonged survival of patients receiving active immunotherapy with Canvaxin therapeutic polyvalent vaccine after complete resection of melanoma metastatic to regional lymph nodes. Ann Surg 2002;236:438.

30. Pehamberger H, Soyer HP, Steiner A, et al. Adjuvant interferon alfa-2a treatment in resected primary stage II cutaneous melanoma. Austrian Malignant Melanoma Cooperative Group. J Clin Oncol 1998;16:1425.

31. Shu S, Cochran A, Huang RR, Morton DL, et al. Immune response in the draining lymph nodes against cancer: implications for immunotherapy. Cancer Metastasis Rev 2006;25:233.

32. Chapman PB, Einhorn LH, Meyers ML, et al. Phase III multicenter randomized trial of the Dartmouth regimen versus dacarbazine in patients with metastatic melanoma. J Clin Oncol 1999;17:2745.

33. Middleton MR, Grob JJ, Aaronson N, et al. Randomized phase III study of temozolomide versus dacarbazine in the treatment of patients with advanced metastatic malignant melanoma. J Clin Oncol 2000;18:158.

34. Bafaloukos D, Tsoutsos D, Kalofonos H, et al. Temozolomide and cisplatin versus temozolomide in patients with advanced melanoma: a randomized phase II study of the Hellenic Cooperative Oncology Group. Ann Oncol 2005;16:950.

35. Kim KB, Eton O, Davis DW, et al. Phase II trial of imatinib mesylate in patients with metastatic melanoma. Br J Cancer 2008;99:734.

36. Eisen T, Ahmad T, Flaherty KT, et al. Sorafenib in advanced melanoma: a Phase II randomised discontinuation trial analysis. Br J Cancer 2006;95:581.

37. Varker KA, Biber JE, Kefauver C, et al. A randomized phase 2 trial of bevacizumab with or without daily low-dose interferon alfa-2b in metastatic malignant melanoma. Ann Surg Oncol 2007;14:2367.

38. Weber J. Ipilimumab: controversies in its development, utility and autoimmune adverse events. Cancer Immunol Immunother 2009;58:823.

39. Keilholz U, Goey SH, Punt CJ, et al. Interferon alfa-2a and interleukin-2 with or without cisplatin in metastatic melanoma: a randomized trial of the European Organization for Research and Treatment of Cancer Melanoma Cooperative Group. J Clin Oncol 1997;15:2579.
40. Keilholz U, Punt CJ, Gore M, et al. Dacarbazine, cisplatin, and interferon-alfa-2b with or without interleukin-2 in metastatic melanoma: a randomized phase III trial (18951) of the European Organisation for Research and Treatment of Cancer Melanoma Group. J Clin Oncol 2005;23:6747.
41. Sparano JA, Fisher RI, Sunderland M, et al. Randomized phase III trial of treatment with high-dose interleukin-2 either alone or in combination with interferon alfa-2a in patients with advanced melanoma. J Clin Oncol 1969;11:1993.
42. Atkins MB, Hsu J, Lee S, et al. Phase III trial comparing concurrent biochemotherapy with cisplatin, vinblastine, dacarbazine, interleukin-2, and interferon alfa-2b with cisplatin, vinblastine, and dacarbazine alone in patients with metastatic malignant melanoma (E3695): a trial coordinated by the Eastern Cooperative Oncology Group. J Clin Oncol 2008;26:5748.
43. Morton DL, Thompson JF, Cochran AJ, et al. Sentinel-node biopsy or nodal observation in melanoma. N Engl J Med 2006;355(13):1307–17.
44. Hauschild A, Weichenthal M, Balda BR, et al. Prospective randomized trial of interferon alfa-2b and interleukin-2 as adjuvant treatment for resected intermediate- and high-risk primary melanoma without clinically detectable node metastasis. J Clin Oncol 2003;21:2883–8.
45. Sondak VK, Liu PY, Tuthill RJ, et al. Adjuvant immunotherapy of resected, intermediate-thickness, node-negative melanoma with an allogeneic tumor vaccine: overall results of a randomized trial of the Southwest Oncology Group. J Clin Oncol 2002;20:2058–66.

Randomized Clinical Trials in Breast Cancer

Aimee M. Crago, MD, PhD[a], Michelle Azu, MD[b],
Shannon Tierney, MD[b], Monica Morrow, MD[b],*

KEYWORDS

- Breast cancer • Randomized clinical trials
- Literature review • Breast-conserving therapy

Breast cancer remains the most common cancer diagnosed in women and the second leading cause of cancer-related deaths in this group. Significant advances in the treatment of breast cancer and in the ability to screen for the disease mean that it is also one of the most curable forms of cancer. In the previous edition of this article, initial results from trials evaluating breast-conserving therapy (BCT) were presented as well as trials enumerating the benefits of adjuvant radiotherapy (RT), chemotherapy, and endocrine therapy. Long-term updates of these trials have been published in the interim. Results demonstrate that BCT remains a viable option for most patients, and that local control is related to overall survival (OS). New chemotherapeutic options and endocrine therapies are available to select subsets of patients, and the use of endocrine therapy in breast cancer prevention has been shown to be of clear benefit. The sheer number of breast cancer-related randomized, controlled trials makes it impossible to review all level IA evidence in this article but, where possible, extensive referencing and tabular review of related trials are used to provide the reader with a clear outline of the central data dictating current standard of care.

LEVEL IA EVIDENCE: PROSPECTIVE RANDOMIZED SURGICAL TRIALS IN BREAST CANCER

1. Twenty-five-year follow-up of a randomized trial comparing radical mastectomy, total mastectomy, and total mastectomy followed by irradiation. Fisher B, Jeong JH, Anderson S, et al. N Engl J Med 2002;347:567–75.[1]

Disclosure: See last page of article.
[a] Division of Surgical Oncology, Department of Surgery, Memorial Sloan Kettering Cancer Center, 1275 York Avenue, New York, NY 10065, USA
[b] Division of Breast Surgery, Department of Surgery, Memorial Sloan Kettering Cancer Center, 1275 York Avenue, New York, NY 10065, USA
* Corresponding author.
E-mail address: morrowm@mskcc.org (M. Morrow).

Hypothesis: Less radical surgery with or without RT is as effective as the Halstead radical mastectomy (RM) in primary operable breast cancer.

NSABP B-04 Trial Results

No. of Patients Randomized	Study Groups	Stratification	Significance Demonstrated	% Change Identified in Trial
1079 with clinically negative nodes	RM n = 362 TM with axillary RT n = 352 TM observation n = 365	N/A	No, in survival	N/A
586 with clinically palpable nodes	RM n = 292 TM with axillary RT n = 294	N/A	No, in survival	N/A

Abbreviations: N/A, not available; RM, radical mastectomy; TM, total mastectomy.

Published abstract: BACKGROUND: In women with breast cancer, the role of radical mastectomy, as compared with less extensive surgery, has been a matter of debate. We report 25-year findings of a randomized trial initiated in 1971 to determine whether less extensive surgery with or without radiation therapy was as effective as the Halsted radical mastectomy. METHODS: A total of 1079 women with clinically negative axillary nodes underwent radical mastectomy, total mastectomy without axillary dissection but with postoperative irradiation, or total mastectomy plus axillary dissection only if their nodes became positive. A total of 586 women with clinically positive axillary nodes either underwent radical mastectomy or underwent total mastectomy without axillary dissection but with postoperative irradiation. Kaplan-Meier and cumulative-incidence estimates of outcome were obtained. RESULTS: No significant differences were observed among the 3 groups of women with negative nodes or between the 2 groups of women with positive nodes with respect to disease-free survival, relapse-free survival, distant disease-free survival, or overall survival. Among women with negative nodes, the hazard ratio for death among those who were treated with total mastectomy and radiation as compared with those who underwent radical mastectomy was 1.08 (95% confidence interval, 0.91 to 1.28; $P = .38$), and the hazard ratio for death among those who had total mastectomy without radiation as compared with those who underwent radical mastectomy was 1.03 (95% confidence interval, 0.87 to 1.23; $P = .72$). Among women with positive nodes, the hazard ratio for death among those who underwent total mastectomy and radiation as compared with those who underwent radical mastectomy was 1.06 (95% confidence interval, 0.89 to 1.27; $P = .49$). CONCLUSIONS: The findings validate earlier results showing no advantage from radical mastectomy. Although differences of a few percentage points cannot be excluded, the findings fail to show a significant survival advantage from removing occult positive nodes at the time of initial surgery or from radiation therapy. (Copyright 2002, Massachusetts Medical Society. All rights reserved. Reprinted with permission.)

Editor's summary and comments: The NSABP B-04 trial compared less extensive operations (TM) with or without RT to traditional RM in women with primary operable breast cancer, and with long-term follow-up, no differences in any survival outcomes were observed. NSABP B-04 has been fundamental in shaping the approach to breast cancer treatment for the last 35 years as its findings supported the "systemic" disease hypothesis, which proposed that alterations in local therapy were unlikely to impact survival. The proof of principle that more radical treatment did not increase cure rate opened the door for subsequent trials of BCT.

Of note, 40% of the clinically node-negative patients in the RM arm of NSABP B-04 had nodal involvement on final pathology, but only 18% of those in the no axillary lymph node dissection (ALND) arm developed clinical axillary recurrence requiring delayed ALND. This result, coupled with the lack of survival differences observed between arms, led to ALND being regarded as a staging rather than a therapeutic procedure. For this reason, the role of completion dissection after a positive sentinel node biopsy (SLNB) is a source of debate, but when considering the role of B04 in defining appropriate treatment of the axilla, it is important to recall that no systemic therapy was used in the trial, and by modern standards B04 was underpowered to detect a small (less than 10%) benefit in survival related to ALND.

2. Twenty-year follow-up of a randomized trial comparing total mastectomy, lumpectomy, and lumpectomy plus irradiation for the treatment of invasive breast cancer. Fisher B, Anderson S, Bryant J, et al. N Engl J Med 2002; 347:1233–41.[2]

Hypothesis: BCT with RT is equivalent to TM.

NSABP B-06 Trial Results				
No. of Patients Randomized and Analyzed	Study Groups	Stratification	Significance Demonstrated	% Change Identified in Trial
1851	TM n = 589 Lumpectomy n = 634 Lumpectomy with RT n = 628	Nodal status	Yes, IBTR	39.2% vs 14.3% in lumpectomy vs lumpectomy with RT at 20 y

Abbreviation: IBTR, ipsilateral breast tumor recurrence.

Published abstract: BACKGROUND: In 1976, we initiated a randomized trial to determine whether lumpectomy with or without radiation therapy was as effective as total mastectomy for the treatment of invasive breast cancer. METHODS: A total of 1851 women for whom follow-up data were available and nodal status was known underwent randomly assigned treatment consisting of total mastectomy, lumpectomy alone, or lumpectomy and breast irradiation. Kaplan-Meier and cumulative-incidence estimates of the outcome were obtained. RESULTS: The cumulative incidence of recurrent tumor in the ipsilateral breast was 14.3% in the women who underwent lumpectomy and breast irradiation, as compared with 39.2% in the women who underwent lumpectomy without irradiation (P<.001). No significant differences were observed among the 3 groups of women with respect to disease-free survival, distant disease-free survival, or overall survival. The hazard ratio for death among the women who underwent lumpectomy alone, as compared with those who underwent total mastectomy, was 1.05 (95% confidence interval, 0.90 to 1.23; P = .51). The hazard ratio for death among the women who underwent lumpectomy followed by breast irradiation, as compared with those who underwent total mastectomy, was 0.97 (95% confidence interval, 0.83 to 1.14; P = .74). Among the lumpectomy-treated women whose surgical specimens had tumor-free margins, the hazard ratio for death among the women who underwent postoperative breast irradiation, as compared with those who did not, was 0.91 (95% confidence interval, 0.77 to 1.06; $P = .23$). Radiation therapy was associated with a marginally significant decrease in deaths due to breast cancer. This decrease was partially offset by an increase in deaths from other causes. CONCLUSIONS: Lumpectomy followed by breast irradiation continues to be appropriate therapy for women with breast cancer, provided that the margins of resected specimens are free of tumor and an acceptable cosmetic result can be obtained. (Copyright 2002, Massachusetts Medical Society. All rights reserved. Reprinted with permission.)

Editor's summary and comments: NSABP-06 was designed to evaluate the efficacy of BCT with and without RT in women with tumors smaller than 4 cm in diameter. The trial is one of several large studies evaluating the role of BCT and now reporting follow-up at 13 to 20 years after randomization.[3–5] The findings reported here are similar to those previously published; no differences in survival exist between the treatment groups. The use of adjuvant RT did significantly reduce IBTR in both node-positive and node-negative patients undergoing lumpectomy, and recurrence in patients treated without RT occurred earlier (73% within 5 years of surgery) than in those treated with RT (40% within 5 years of surgery). In comparing NSABP B-06 to the Milan, EORTC 10801, and National Cancer Institute (NCI) trials (**Table 1**), it is important to realize that excision to negative margins was not required for the NCI and EORTC 10801 studies, resulting in higher rates of IBTR, and confirming that complete surgical resection with negative (no tumor on ink) margins is an essential component of BCT.

In NSABP B-06, only patients with positive axillary nodes received adjuvant chemotherapy. This treatment combined with RT resulted in 50% fewer IBTRs (8.8%) than seen with RT alone in the lower risk node-negative patients (17%), indicating that chemotherapy can act synergistically with RT to prevent a subset of local recurrences.

3. Effects of radiotherapy and of differences in the extent of surgery for early breast cancer on local recurrence and 15-year survival: an overview of the randomised trials. Early Breast Cancer Trialists' Collaborative Group (EBCTG). Lancet 2006;366:2087–106.[6]

Hypothesis: Differences in local regional recurrence (LRR) resulting from more versus less local therapy result in long-term survival differences.

Published abstract: BACKGROUND: In early breast cancer, variations in local treatment that substantially affect the risk of locoregional recurrence could also affect long-term breast cancer mortality. To examine this relationship, collaborative meta-analyses were undertaken, based on individual patient data, of the relevant randomized trials that began by 1995. METHODS: Information was available on 42,000 women in 78 randomized treatment comparisons (radiotherapy vs no radiotherapy, 23,500; more vs less surgery, 9300; more surgery vs radiotherapy, 9300). Twenty-four types of local treatment comparison were identified. To help relate the effect on local (ie, locoregional) recurrence to that on breast cancer mortality, these were grouped according to whether or not the 5-year local recurrence risk exceeded 10% (<10%, 17,000 women; >10%, 25,000 women). FINDINGS: About three-quarters of the eventual local recurrence risk occurred during the first 5 years. In the comparisons that involved little (<10%) difference in 5-year local recurrence risk there was little difference in 15-year breast cancer mortality. Among the 25,000 women in the comparisons that involved substantial (>10%) differences, however, 5-year local recurrence risks were 7% active versus 26% control (absolute reduction 19%), and

Table 1
RCT comparing breast-conserving therapy and mastectomy

Trial	No. of Patients	Study Groups	Stratification	Follow-up	Significance Demonstrated	% Change Identified in Trial
NSABP B-06[2]	1851	TM n = 589, lumpectomy n = 634, lumpectomy with RT n = 682	Nodal status	20 y	Yes, in local recurrence	39.2% vs 14.3% in lumpectomy vs lumpectomy with RT
Milan I[5]	701	RM, n = 349, BCT and RT n = 352	Menopausal status	20 y	Yes, in local recurrence	2.3% vs 8.8% in RM vs BCT and RT
EORTC 10801[4]	902	MRM n = 420, BCT and RT n = 448	Participating center, stage (I vs II), menopausal status	13.4 y	Yes, in local recurrence	12% vs 20% in MRM vs BCT and RT
NCI[3]	237	MRM n = 116, BCT and RT n = 121	Age and clinical lymph node status	18.4 y	Yes, in local recurrence	0% vs 22.4% in MRM vs BCT and RT

Abbreviations: MRM, modified radical mastectomy; RM, radical mastectomy.

15-year breast cancer mortality risks were 44·6% versus 49·5% (absolute reduction 5·0%, SE 0·8, 2p<.001). These 25,000 women included 7300 with breast-conserving surgery (BCS) in trials of radiotherapy (generally just to the conserved breast), with 5-year local recurrence risks (mainly in the conserved breast, as most had axillary clearance and node-negative disease) 7% versus 26% (reduction 19%), and 15-year breast cancer mortality risks 30.5% versus 35.9% (reduction 5.4%, SE 1.7, 2p = .0002; overall mortality reduction 5.3%, SE 1.8, 2p = .005). They also included 8500 with mastectomy, axillary clearance, and node-positive disease in trials of radiotherapy (generally to the chest wall and regional lymph nodes), with similar absolute gains from radiotherapy; 5-year local recurrence risks (mainly at these sites) 6% versus 23% (reduction 17%), and 15-year breast cancer mortality risks 54.7% versus 60.1% (reduction 5.4%, SE 1.3, 2p = .0002; overall mortality reduction 4.4%, SE 1.2, 2p = .0009). Radiotherapy produced similar *proportional* reductions in local recurrence in all women (irrespective of age or tumor characteristics) and in all major trials of radiotherapy versus not (recent or older; with or without systemic therapy), so large *absolute* reductions in local recurrence were seen only if the control risk was large. To help assess the life-threatening side effects of radiotherapy, the trials of radiotherapy versus not were combined with those of radiotherapy versus more surgery. There was, at least with some of the older radiotherapy regimens, a significant excess incidence of contralateral breast cancer (rate ratio 1.18, SE 0.06, 2p = .002) and a significant excess of non-breast cancer mortality in irradiated women (rate ratio 1.12, SE 0.04, 2p = .001). Both were slight during the first 5 years, but continued after year 15. The excess mortality was mainly from heart disease (rate ratio 1.27, SE 0.07, 2p = .0001) and lung cancer (rate ratio 1.78, SE 0.22, 2p = .0004). INTERPRETATION: In these trials, avoidance of a local recurrence in the conserved breast after BCS and avoidance of a local recurrence elsewhere (eg, the chest wall or regional nodes) after mastectomy were of comparable relevance to 15-year breast cancer mortality. Differences in local treatment that substantially affect local recurrence rates would, in the hypothetical absence of any other causes of death, avoid about one breast cancer death over the next 15 years for every 4 local recurrences avoided, and should reduce 15-year overall mortality. (Copyright 2006, Elsevier. Reprinted with permission.)

Editor's summary and comments: The Early Breast Cancer Trialists' Collaborative Group (EBCTG) has centrally reviewed individual patient data every 5 years since 1985 to study the effects of RT and the extent of surgery on local control and cause-specific mortality in early breast cancer. An important new finding in the 15-year review is that differences in local recurrence of greater than 10% at 5 years result in statistically significant differences in OS at 15 years. The ratio of absolute effect is 4 to 1 (ie, for every 4 local recurrences prevented, 1 life is saved).

This principle is reflected in analyses addressing lumpectomy with or without RT, an adjuvant therapy resulting in an absolute risk reduction (ARR) of 19% in IBTR and 5.4% in breast cancer–specific mortality in this meta-analysis. Node-positive mastectomy patients similarly experienced large risk reductions in 5-year local recurrence with adjuvant RT (23% vs 6%), translating into a 15-year ARR in breast cancer–specific mortality of 5.4%. Survival outcomes in node-negative patients treated with modified radical mastectomy (MRM) were not improved with RT, a reflection of the small difference in local control between groups (ARR 4%). Subgroup analyses did not identify BCT patients who failed to benefit from adjuvant RT.

Another finding of the meta-analysis was that adjuvant RT results in a small increase in long-term mortality related to contralateral breast cancer, heart disease, and lung cancer. The increase in these events was 1.3% at 15 years and did not exceed the benefit of RT on breast cancer-specific survival. The impact of modern chemotherapy and RT regimens on these outcomes requires further study.

LEVEL IA EVIDENCE: PROSPECTIVE RANDOMIZED TRIALS IN EVALUATION AND MANAGEMENT OF THE AXILLA

4. Sentinel-lymph node biopsy as a staging procedure in breast cancer: update of a randomized controlled trial. Veronesi U, Paganelli G, Viale G, et al. Lancet Oncol 2006;6:983–90.[7]

Hypothesis: SLNB is equivalent to ALND in node-negative patients.

Milan Institute Trial Results				
No. of Patients Randomized	Study Groups	Stratification	Significance Demonstrated	% Change Identified in Trial
516	SLNB ± ALND n = 259 ALND n = 257	Randomized patients whose SLN mapped on lymphoscintigraphy	None	N/A

Published abstract: BACKGROUND: In women with breast cancer, sentinel-lymph-node biopsy (SLNB) provides information that allows surgeons to avoid axillary-lymph-node dissection (ALND) if the SLN does not have metastasis, and has a favorable effect on quality of life. Results of our previous trial showed that SLNB accurately screens the ALN for metastasis in breast cancers of diameter 2 mm or less. We aimed to update this trial with results from longer follow-up. METHODS: Women with breast tumors of diameter 2 cm or less were randomly assigned after breast-conserving surgery either to SLNB and total ALND (ALND group), or to SLNB followed by ALND only if the SLN was involved (SLN group). Analysis was restricted to patients whose tumor characteristics met eligibility criteria after treatment. The major end points were the number of axillary metastases in women in the SLN group with negative SLNs, staging power of SLNB, and disease-free and overall survival. FINDINGS: Of the 257 patients in the ALND group, 83 (32%) had a positive SLN and 174 (68%) had a negative SLN; 8 of those with negative SLNs were found to have false-negative SLNs. Of the 259 patients in the SLN group, 92 (36%) had a positive SLN and 167 (65%) had a negative SLN. One case of overt clinical axillary metastasis was seen in the follow-up of the 167 women in the SLN group who did not receive ALND (ie, one false-negative). After a median follow-up of 79 months (range 15–97), 34 events associated with breast cancer occurred: 18 in the ALND group, and 16 in the SLN group (log-rank $p = .6$). The overall 5-year survival of all patients was 96.4% (95% CI 94.1–98.7) in the ALND group and 98.4% (96.9–100) in the SLN group (log-rank $p = .1$). INTERPRETATIONS: SLNB can allow total ALND to be avoided in patients with negative SLNs, while reducing postoperative morbidity and the costs of hospital stay. The findings that only one overt axillary metastasis occurred during follow-up of patients who did not receive ALND (whereas 8 cases were expected) could be explained by various hypotheses, including those from cancer-stem-cell research. (Copyright 2006, Elsevier. Reprinted with permission.)

Editor's summary and comments: SLN mapping in breast cancer was described by Giuliano and colleagues[8] in 1994, and subsequently shown to predict axillary nodal status in 95.6% of patients. In the NSABP B-32 trial of 5611 patients, more than

97% of patients had an SLN detected and removed using lymphoscintigraphy, blue dye, and palpation; accuracy was 97.1%, confirming feasibility of the technique.[9] In the ACOSOG Z10 trial involving a similar number of patients, no difference in SLN detection rate was observed when tracing was performed with blue dye alone, isotope alone, or the combination of blue dye and isotope.[10]

The Milan trial randomized 516 patients with T1 tumors undergoing quadrantectomy with planned adjuvant RT to either SLNB followed by ALND or to SLNB followed by completion ALND (cALND) only if the SLN contained metastases. Concordant with earlier reports, the accuracy of SLN in patients undergoing ALND was 96.9%; in addition, patients in the SLNB group had a decrease in both short- and long-term morbidity. Quality of life benefits have been confirmed in subsequent trials designed to specifically address this question.[11]

To date, oncologic outcomes appear identical in the 2 arms of the Milan Institute trial, although the relatively small size of the patient cohort limits its power to show small differences in survival. Results of NSABP B-32, which enrolled a significantly larger number of patients than the Milan Institute or the underpowered Sentinella/GIVOM study,[12] should, when mature, provide additional data regarding associated disease-free survival (DFS) and OS outcomes.

After a median follow-up of 79 months, only one case of overt clinical axillary metastasis was observed in the SLNB arm of the Italian study, although 8 false negatives would be expected based on technical outcomes. This result demonstrated, as in NSABP-B04, that not all nodal metastases become clinically evident. In addition, a subset analysis of the 60 patients with isolated micrometastatic disease in the SLN showed that only 17% of these patients had other axillary nodal metastases, providing additional evidence that cALND may not be warranted in all such cases. Retrospective studies have been performed to stratify the risk of additional positive lymph nodes in this subgroup of patients, with the goal of identifying a population for whom observation may be appropriate management.[13]

LEVEL IA EVIDENCE: PROSPECTIVE RANDOMIZED TRIALS ADDRESSING ADJUVANT RADIATION OF THE BREAST

5. Prevention of invasive breast cancer in women with ductal carcinoma *in situ*: an update of the National Surgical Adjuvant Breast and Bowel Project experience. Fisher B, Land S, Mamounas E, et al. Semin Oncol 2001;28:400–18.[14]

Hypothesis: RT after excision of ductal carcinoma in situ (DCIS) reduces IBTR.

NSABP B-17 Trial Results				
No. of Patients Randomized	Study Groups	Stratification	Significance Demonstrated	% Change Identified in Trial
818	Excision n = 405 Excision and RT n = 413	Age, presence of LCIS, method of detection, performance of ALND	Yes, in IBTR	31.7% vs 15.7% at 12 y

Abbreviation: LCIS, lobular carcinoma in situ.

Published abstract: The National Surgical Adjuvant Breast and Bowel Project (NSABP) conducted 2 sequential randomized clinical trials to aid in resolving uncertainty about the treatment of women with small, localized, mammographically detected ductal carcinoma in situ (DCIS). After removal of the tumor and normal breast tissue so that specimen margins were histologically tumor-free (lumpectomy), 818 patients in the B-17 trial were randomly assigned to receive either radiation therapy to the ipsilateral breast or no radiation therapy. B-24, the second study, which involved 1804 women, tested the hypothesis that, in DCIS patients with or without positive tumor specimen margins, lumpectomy, radiation, and tamoxifen (TAM) would be more effective than lumpectomy, radiation, and placebo in preventing invasive and noninvasive ipsilateral breast tumor recurrences (IBTRs), contralateral breast tumors (CBTs), and tumors at metastatic sites. The findings in this report continue to demonstrate through 12 years of follow-up that radiation after lumpectomy reduces the incidence rate of all IBTRs by 58%. They also demonstrate that the administration of TAM after lumpectomy and radiation therapy results in a significant decrease in the rate of all breast cancer events, particularly in invasive cancer. The findings from the B-17 and B-24 studies are related to those from the NSABP prevention (P-1) trial, which demonstrated a 50% reduction in the risk of invasive cancer in women with a history of atypical ductal hyperplasia (ADH) or lobular carcinoma in situ (LCIS) and a reduction in the incidence of both DCIS and LCIS in women without a history of those tumors. The B-17 findings demonstrated that patients treated with lumpectomy alone were at greater risk for invasive cancer than were women in P-1 who had a history of ADH or LCIS and who received no radiation therapy or TAM. Although women who received radiation benefited from that therapy, they remained at higher risk for invasive cancer than women in P-1 who had a history of LCIS and who received placebo or TAM. Thus, if it is accepted from the P-1 findings that women at increased risk for invasive cancer are candidates for an intervention such as TAM, then it would seem that women with a history of DCIS should also be considered for such therapy in addition to radiation therapy. That statement does not imply that, as a result of the findings presented here, all DCIS patients should receive radiation and TAM. It does suggest, however, that, in the treatment of DCIS, the appropriate use of current and better therapeutic agents that become available could diminish the significance of breast cancer as a public health problem. (Copyright 2001, Elsevier. Reprinted with permission.)

Editor's summary and comments: NSABP-17 is 1 of 4 major randomized controlled trials that address the role of adjuvant RT in local control of DCIS (**Table 2**). Outcomes after 12 years demonstrated a 55% relative risk reduction in IBTR following RT. Five years after randomization, the benefit of RT appeared greatest in reducing invasive recurrences,[15] but with longer follow-up there was equal reduction in rates of intraductal and invasive cancers. Radiation had no effect on the secondary survival end points in this study, which is not powered to identify such changes.

Similar themes are observed in the SweDCIS, EORTC 10853, and the UK-ANZ trials,[16–18] also examining adjuvant RT in DCIS treatment. All studies reported significant radiation-associated benefits on local control, and no subset analysis has been able to identify patients in whom RT does not affect rates of local recurrence. Patient subsets were extensively evaluated in the EORTC trial, which looked at subgroups of patients younger than 40 years, high-grade tumors, patients with symptoms at presentation, cribriform and solid growth patterns, and doubtful margin status; benefit from RT was seen in each subgroup.[17] Adjuvant tamoxifen does not obviate the need for RT as evidenced in the UK-ANZ study, a 2 × 2 trial, which randomized patients not only to RT but also to adjuvant tamoxifen or placebo groups.[18]

This article by Fisher and colleagues[14] also reviews most recent outcomes analysis from NSABP B-24, which sought to examine the role of adjuvant tamoxifen in patients with DCIS treated by lumpectomy and RT. Patients were not required to have histologically negative margins to enroll in NSABP B-24. After a mean follow-up of almost 7 years, event-free survival was 83% in patients treated with tamoxifen and only

Table 2
Adjuvant radiation following BCT for DCIS

Trial	No. of Patients Randomized	Study Groups	Stratification	Significance Demonstrated	% Change Identified in Trial
NSABP B-17[14]	818	Excision n = 405, Excision and RT n = 413	Age, presence of LCIS, method of detection, performance of ALND	Yes, in IBTR	31.7% vs 15.7% at 12 y
SweDCIS[16]	1046	Excision n = 520, Excision and RT n = 526	Health care region	Yes, in IBTR	22% vs 7% at mean 5.4 y
EORTC 10853[17]	1010	Excision n = 503, Excision and RT n = 507	Institution	Yes, in IBTR	26% vs 15% at median 10.5 y
UK-ANZ[18]	1030	Excision n = 508, Excision and RT n = 522	Tamoxifen prescription	Yes, in IBTR	16% vs 7% at median 52.6 mo

Abbreviations: ALND, axillary lymph node dissection; IBTR, ipsilateral breast tumor recurrence; LCIS, lobular carcinoma in situ; RT, radiotherapy.

77% in those treated with placebo. Tamoxifen treatment resulted in a relative risk reduction of 47% in IBTR, but no effect of tamoxifen on OS was observed. The benefit for tamoxifen was seen in all subgroups analyzed; however, in NSABP B-24, patients were not selected for tamoxifen treatment on the basis of estrogen receptor (ER) status. A subsequent subset analysis by Allred and colleagues[19] did report a 59% reduction in breast cancer events among patients with ER-positive tumors taking tamoxifen, but no significant effect was observed on ER-negative DCIS.

Tamoxifen is an option for patients with DCIS, but is not mandatory; the most favorable risk-benefit ratio is seen in premenopausal women with both breasts at risk and those with hormone receptor–positive lesions. Of note, in patients with positive margins, the use of tamoxifen was not able to reduce IBTR rates to the level seen with excision to negative margins and placebo, confirming that adjuvant endocrine therapy is not a substitute for adequate surgical resection.

6. Locoregional radiation therapy in patients with high-risk breast cancer receiving adjuvant chemotherapy: 20-year results of the British Columbia randomized trial. Ragaz J, Spinelli JJ, Phillips N, et al. J Natl Cancer Inst 2005;97:116–26.[20]

Hypothesis: Postoperative RT improves locoregional recurrence, DFS, and OS in premenopausal patients with high risk breast cancer.

British Columbia Trial Results				
No. of Patients Randomized	Study Groups	Stratification	Significance Demonstrated	% Change Identified in Trial
318	Adjuvant RT n = 164 Observation n = 154	N/A	Yes, in DFS Yes, in OS	52% vs 70% at 20 years 37% vs 47% at 20 years

Published abstract: BACKGROUND: The British Columbia randomized radiation trial was designed to determine the survival impact of locoregional radiation therapy in premenopausal patients with lymph node-positive breast cancer treated by modified radical mastectomy and adjuvant chemotherapy. Three hundred eighteen patients were assigned to receive no further therapy or radiation therapy (37.5 Gy in 16 fractions). Previous analysis at the 15-year follow-up showed that radiation therapy was associated with a statistically significant improvement in breast cancer survival but that improvement in overall survival was of only borderline statistical significance. We report the analysis of data from the 20-year follow-up. METHODS: Survival was analyzed by the Kaplan-Meier method. Relative risk estimates were calculated by the Wald test from the proportional hazards regression model. All statistical tests were 2-sided. RESULTS: At the 20 year follow up (median follow up for live patients: 249 months) chemotherapy and radiation therapy, compared with chemotherapy alone, were associated with a statistically significant improvement in all end points analyzed, including survival free of isolated locoregional recurrences (74% versus 90%, respectively; relative risk [RR] = 0.36, 95% confidence interval [CI] = 0.18 to 0.71; P = .002), systemic relapse-free survival (31% versus 48%; RR = 0.66, 95% CI = 0.49 to 0.88; P = .004), breast cancer-free survival (48% versus 30%; RR = 0.63, 95% CI = 0.47 to 0.83; P = .001), event-free survival (35% versus 25%; RR = 0.70, 95% CI = 0.54 to 0.92; P = .009), breast cancer-specific survival (53% versus 38%; RR = 0.67, 95% CI = 0.49 to 0.90; P = .008), and, in contrast to the 15-year follow-up results, overall survival (47% versus 37%; RR = 0.73, 95% CI = 0.55 to 0.98; P = .03). Long-term toxicities, including cardiac deaths (1.8% versus 0.6%), were minimal for both arms. CONCLUSION: For patients with high-risk breast cancer treated with modified radical mastectomy, treatment with radiation therapy (schedule of 16 fractions) and adjuvant chemotherapy leads to better survival outcomes than chemotherapy alone, and it is well tolerated, with acceptable long-term toxicity. (Copyright 2005, Oxford University Press. Reprinted with permission.)

Editor's summary and comments: Twenty-year follow-up of the British Columbia trial confirmed the benefit of RT on locoregional disease but demonstrated a statistically significant difference in overall and disease-specific survival as well. These results are comparable with those reported by the Danish Breast Cancer Cooperative Group.[21,22] In these studies, evaluating postmenopausal patients with positive axillary lymph nodes, tumors greater than 5 cm in diameter and lesions invading the skin and pectoralis fascia, neither CMF (cyclophosphamide, methotrexate, fluorouracil) nor tamoxifen alone were as effective at controlling local or systemic disease as the drugs when administered in conjunction with chest wall irradiation. Interpretation of these studies is complicated, in part, by newer methods of RT delivery and the development of anthracycline-based regimens, aromatase inhibitors, and trastuzumab, which could possibly reduce the ARR that these trials report. The importance of these studies lies, however, in that they were the first to clearly document that improvements in local control translate to improved survival even in patients with high risk of systemic recurrence.

Much attention has been paid to the Danish and British Columbia trial subgroup analyses, based on small groups of patients, in an attempt to determine if involvement of 1 to 3 axillary nodes is an indication for adjuvant RT. In the British Columbia trial, patients with 1 to 3 positive nodes had an improvement in DFS from 32% to 44% and in OS from 50% to 57% when treated with postmastectomy RT. The Danish trials also observed a survival benefit in this subset. The absolute and relative risk reductions were similar in patients with greater than 4 positive lymph nodes. Due to limited axillary surgery in these studies, rates of local recurrence were higher than those observed in the United States, raising questions about whether the findings could be generalized. Until further data addressing the questions of risk stratification in a prospective manner are available, postmastectomy RT in the moderate risk patients must be considered in the context of individual patient risk and comorbidity.

LEVEL IA EVIDENCE: META-ANALYSIS ANALYZING USE OF POLYCHEMOTHERAPY IN OPERABLE BREAST CANCER

7. Effects of chemotherapy and hormonal therapy for early breast cancer on recurrence and 15-year survival: and overview of the randomised trials. Early Breast Cancer Trialists' Collaborative Group. Lancet 2005;365:1687–717.[23]

Hypothesis: Adjuvant chemotherapy and endocrine therapy improve survival in patients with breast cancer.

Published abstract: BACKGROUND: Quinquennial overviews (1985–2000) of the randomized trials in early breast cancer have assessed the 5-year and 10-year effects of various systemic adjuvant therapies on breast cancer recurrence and survival. Here, we report the 10-year and 15-year effects. METHODS: Collaborative meta-analyses were undertaken of 194 unconfounded randomized trials of adjuvant chemotherapy or hormonal therapy that began by 1995. Many trials involved CMF (cyclophosphamide, methotrexate, fluorouracil), anthracycline-based combinations such as FAC (fluorouracil, doxorubicin, cyclophosphamide) or FEC (fluorouracil, epirubicin, cyclophosphamide), tamoxifen, or ovarian suppression: none involved taxanes, trastuzumab, raloxifene, or modern aromatase inhibitors. FINDINGS: Allocation to about 6 months of anthracycline-based polychemotherapy (eg, with FAC or FEC) reduces the annual breast cancer death rate by about 38% (SE 5) for women younger than 50 years of age when diagnosed and by about 20% (SE 4) for those of age 50 to 69 years when diagnosed, largely irrespective of the use of tamoxifen and of estrogen receptor (ER) status, nodal status, or other tumor characteristics. Such regimens are significantly ($2p = .0001$ for recurrence, $2p<.00001$ for breast cancer mortality) more effective than CMF chemotherapy. Few women of age 70 years or older entered these chemotherapy trials. For ER-positive disease only, allocation to about 5 years of adjuvant tamoxifen reduces the annual breast cancer death rate by 31% (SE 3), largely irrespective of the use of chemotherapy and of age (<50, 50–69, $>$ or $= 70$ years), progesterone receptor status, or other tumor characteristics. 5 years is significantly ($2p<.00001$ for recurrence, $2p = .01$ for breast cancer mortality) more effective than just 1 to 2 years of tamoxifen. For ER-positive tumors, the annual breast cancer mortality rates are similar during years 0 to 4 and 5 to 14, as are the proportional reductions in them by 5 years of tamoxifen, so the cumulative reduction in mortality is more than twice as big at 15 years as at 5 years after diagnosis. These results combine 6 meta-analyses: anthracycline-based versus no chemotherapy (8000 women); CMF-based versus no chemotherapy (14,000); anthracycline-based versus CMF-based chemotherapy (14,000); about 5 years of tamoxifen versus none (15,000); about 1 to 2 years of tamoxifen versus none (33,000); and about 5 years versus 1 to 2 years of tamoxifen (18,000). Finally, allocation to ovarian ablation or suppression (8000 women) also significantly reduces breast cancer mortality, but appears to do so only in the absence of other systemic treatments. For middle-aged women with ER-positive disease (the commonest type of breast cancer), the breast cancer mortality rate throughout the next 15 years would be approximately halved by 6 months of anthracycline-based chemotherapy (with a combination such as FAC or FEC) followed by 5 years of adjuvant tamoxifen. For, if mortality reductions of 38% (age <50 years) and 20% (age 50–69 years) from such chemotherapy were followed by a further reduction of 31% from tamoxifen in the risks that remain, the final mortality reductions would be 57% and 45%, respectively (and, the trial results could well have been somewhat stronger if there had been full compliance with the allocated treatments). Overall survival would be comparably improved, since these treatments have relatively small effects on mortality from the aggregate of all other causes. INTERPRETATION: Some of the widely practicable adjuvant drug treatments that were being tested in the 1980s, which substantially reduced 5-year recurrence rates (but had somewhat less effect on 5-year mortality rates), also substantially reduce 15-year mortality rates. Further improvements in long-term survival could well be available from newer drugs, or better use of older drugs. (Copyright 2005, Elsevier. Reprinted with permission.)

Editor's summary and comments: The EBCTCG meta-analysis of trials examining adjuvant chemotherapy and endocrine treatment in patients with early breast cancer was initiated in 1985 and reviews primary data collected in eligible randomized controlled trials. Among 29,000 patients enrolled in trials examining the impact of polychemotherapy on outcomes, clear benefit was observed with the addition of adjuvant anthracycline- or cyclophosphamide-based therapy. Of note, the ARR seen for OS continued to increase between 5 and 15 years post therapy in at least a subset of patients. For example, patients younger than 50 years had breast cancer–specific mortality of 20% versus 15.7% at 5 years (ARR 4.3%) and 42.4% versus 32.4% at 15 years of follow-up (ARR 10%). These benefits may actually be greater in the context of modern chemotherapy that incorporates the use of taxanes, as more than a dozen trials published since the inception of the meta-analysis have now shown additional small increases in survival when these drugs are added to adjuvant treatment regimens.[24]

Little, if any, gain was seen with prolonged courses of chemotherapy in this meta-analysis, but anthracycline-based regimens had a slight advantage over cyclophosphamide, methotrexate and fluorouracil (CMF). The benefit of doxorubicin is not consistently seen across randomized controlled trials, however, and remains controversial. Results presented in EBCTG also indicate that chemotherapy is effective even in the setting of subsequent tamoxifen use among patients with estrogen receptor (ER)-positive tumors.

The data reported in this meta-analysis also specifically address the role of postoperative endocrine therapy in early breast cancer. Whereas no effect on 5-year recurrence and survival was seen in patients with ER-negative tumors, significant reduction in 5-year breast cancer recurrence and breast cancer mortality were reported for those with tumors expressing hormone receptors, regardless of menopausal status. The magnitude of effect was dependent on the length of time endocrine therapy was administered. After 2 years of endocrine therapy, patient outcomes including recurrence, contralateral breast cancer, and survival showed improvement, but the magnitude of benefit increased with 5 years of therapy. Treatment was discontinued at this point in most cohorts. Despite cessation of therapy, however, the relative risk for yearly recurrence continued to be approximately two-thirds between years 5 and 10, suggesting persistent effects of tamoxifen after discontinuation of treatment. In fact, the ARR in breast cancer mortality at 15 years is increased to 9.2% versus the benefit of only 3.6% at 5 years among ER-positive patients who completed the recommended course of endocrine therapy.

8. Preoperative chemotherapy in patients with operable breast cancer: nine-year results from National Surgical Adjuvant Breast and Bowel Project B-18. Wolmark N, Wang J, Mamounas E, et al. J Natl Inst Canc Monogr 2001;30:96–102.[25]

Hypothesis: Neoadjuvant chemotherapy improves survival in patients with operable breast cancer as compared with adjuvant treatment.

NSABP B-18 Trial Results				
No. of Patients Randomized	Study Groups	Stratification	Significance Demonstrated	% Change Identified in Trial
1523	Neoadjuvant $n = 763$ Adjuvant $n = 760$	Age, tumor size, lymph node status	Yes, in rates of BCT	67.8% vs 59.8% in neoadjuvant vs adjuvant arms

Published abstract: National Surgical Adjuvant Breast and Bowel Project (NSABP) Protocol B-18 was initiated in 1988 to determine whether 4 cycles of doxorubicin/cyclophosphamide given preoperatively improve survival and disease-free survival (DFS) when compared with the same chemotherapy given postoperatively. Secondary aims included the evaluation of preoperative chemotherapy in downstaging the primary breast tumor and involved axillary lymph nodes, the comparison of lumpectomy rates and rates of ipsilateral breast tumor recurrence (IBTR) in the 2 treatment groups, and the assessment of the correlation between primary tumor response and outcome. Initially published findings were based on a follow-up of 5 years; this report updates results through 9 years of follow-up. There continue to be no statistically significant overall differences in survival or DFS between the 2 treatment groups. Survival at 9 years is 70% in the postoperative group and 69% in the preoperative group ($P = .80$). DFS is 53% in postoperative patients and 55% in preoperative patients ($P = .50$). A statistically significant correlation persists between primary tumor response and outcome, and this correlation has become statistically stronger with longer follow-up. Patients assigned to preoperative chemotherapy received notably more lumpectomies than postoperative patients, especially among patients with tumors greater than 5 cm at study entry. Although the rate of IBTR was slightly higher in the preoperative group (10.7% versus 7.6%), this difference was not statistically significant. Marginally statistically significant treatment-by-age interactions appear to be emerging for survival and DFS, suggesting that younger patients may benefit from preoperative therapy, whereas the reverse may be true for older patients. (Copyright 2001, Oxford University Press. Reprinted with permission.)

Editor's summary and comments: Although no differences in OS or DFS were observed between pre- and postoperative chemotherapy regimens, patients had higher rates of lumpectomy if randomized to the neoadjuvant treatment.[26] Of concern, however, was a trend toward higher rates of locoregional recurrence in the subset of patients requiring chemotherapy to downstage and permit BCT in lieu of mastectomy. The effect of neoadjuvant therapy on cell death is often patchy, and it is uncertain whether a negative margin definition of tumor not touching ink is adequate following neoadjuvant therapy. Although the difference in local recurrence did not translate into survival effects here, locoregional recurrence is associated with small increases in long-term mortality in large meta-analyses of breast cancer patients.[6]

The secondary analysis of outcomes related to pathologic complete response is important in our understanding of breast cancer biology. Patients with complete pathologic response had better outcomes than did patients with lesser responses. Response to neoadjuvant therapy is clearly a marker for good outcomes, a fact that likely reflects favorable tumor biology and response to therapy, not improved treatment delivery in the neoadjuvant setting. Data supporting this assertion have been presented in NSABP B-27, where comparison of neoadjuvant adriamycin and Cytoxan (AC) and docetaxel compared with AC alone resulted in an increased pathologic complete response rate but did not translate to improved survival.[27]

9. Neoadjuvant versus adjuvant systemic treatment in breast cancer: a meta-analysis. Mauri D, Pavlidis N, and Ioannidis JP. J Natl Cancer Inst 2005;97:188–94.[28]

Hypothesis: Survival outcomes are equivalent in patients with operable breast cancer whether chemotherapy is administered before or after surgery.

Published abstract: BACKGROUND: Interest in the use of preoperative systemic treatment in the management of breast cancer has increased because such neoadjuvant therapy appears to reduce the extent of local surgery required. We compared the clinical end points of patients with breast cancer treated preoperatively with systemic therapy (neoadjuvant therapy) and of those treated postoperatively with the same regimen (adjuvant therapy) in a meta-analysis of randomized trials. METHODS: We evaluated 9 randomized studies, including a total of 3946 patients with breast cancer, that compared neoadjuvant therapy with adjuvant therapy regardless of what additional surgery or radiation treatment was used. Fixed and random effects methods were used to combine data. Primary outcomes were death, disease progression, distant disease recurrence, and loco-regional disease recurrence. Secondary outcomes were local response and conservative local treatment. All statistical tests were 2-sided. RESULTS: We found no statistically or clinically significant difference between neoadjuvant therapy and adjuvant therapy arms associated with death (summary risk ratio [RR] = 1.00, 95% confidence interval [CI] = 0.90 to 1.12), disease progression (summary RR = 0.99, 95% CI = 0.91 to 1.07), or distant disease recurrence (summary RR = 0.94, 95% CI = 0.83 to 1.06). However, neoadjuvant therapy was statistically significantly associated with an increased risk of loco-regional disease recurrences (RR = 1.22, 95% CI = 1.04 to 1.43), compared with adjuvant therapy, especially in trials where more patients in the neoadjuvant, than the adjuvant, arm received radiation therapy without surgery (RR = 1.53, 95% CI = 1.11 to 2.10). Across trials, we observed heterogeneity in the rates of complete clinical response (range = 7%–65%; P for heterogeneity of <.001), pathologic response (range = 4%–29%; P for heterogeneity of <.001), and adoption of conservative local treatment (range = 28%–89% in neoadjuvant arms, P for heterogeneity of <.001). CONCLUSIONS: Neoadjuvant therapy was apparently equivalent to adjuvant therapy in terms of survival and overall disease progression. Neoadjuvant therapy, compared with adjuvant therapy, was associated with a statistically significant increased risk of loco-regional recurrence when radiotherapy without surgery was adopted. (Copyright 2005, Oxford University Press. Reprinted with permission.)

Editor's summary and comments: In this meta-analysis, 9 studies were identified that randomized operable patients to pre- or postoperative chemotherapy. Although the included studies differed somewhat in median patient age and average tumor size, primary results were similar. Timing of chemotherapy did not alter rates of OS, DFS, or distant disease recurrence. There was, however, an increase in relative risk of locoregional disease recurrence if patients received neoadjuvant therapy. This finding may be related to the fact that in 4 of the trials, patients with complete clinical response received RT instead of surgery. It is impossible at this point to identify the subset of patients who have complete pathologic response without microscopic examination of the treated tissue, and radiation of residual tumor without surgical excision is known to result in higher rates of local recurrence. Until a reliable means of identifying pathologic complete response is available, surgical excision of the tumor bed will remain an essential component in minimizing the risk of IBTR.

10. Trastuzumab plus adjuvant chemotherapy for operable HER2-positive breast cancer. Romond, E.H., Perez EA, Bryant J, et al. N Engl J Med 2005;353(16):1673–84.[29]

Hypothesis: Trastuzumab given concurrently with adjuvant chemotherapy improves DFS in patients with operable breast cancer overexpressing HER2.

NASABP B-31 and NCCTG N9831 Trial Results				
No. of Patients Randomized	Study Groups	Stratification	Significance Demonstrated	% Change Identified in Trial
3351	Trastuzumab $n = 1672$ Control $n = 1679$	Study, paclitaxel schedule, nodal status, hormone receptor status	Yes, in DFS Yes, in OS	87.1% vs 75.4% 91.4% vs 86.6%

Published abstract: We present the combined results of 2 trials that compared adjuvant chemotherapy with or without concurrent trastuzumab in women with surgically removed HER2-positive breast cancer. METHODS: The National Surgical Adjuvant Breast and Bowel Project trial B-31 compared doxorubicin and cyclophosphamide followed by paclitaxel every 3 weeks (group 1) with the same regimen plus 52 weeks of trastuzumab beginning with the first dose of paclitaxel (group 2). The North Central Cancer Treatment Group trial N9831 compared 3 regimens: doxorubicin and cyclophosphamide followed by weekly paclitaxel (group A), the same regimen followed by 52 weeks of trastuzumab after paclitaxel (group B), and the same regimen plus 52 weeks of trastuzumab initiated concomitantly with paclitaxel (group C). The studies were amended to include a joint analysis comparing groups 1 and A (the control group) with groups 2 and C (the trastuzumab group). Group B was excluded because trastuzumab was not given concurrently with paclitaxel. RESULTS: By March 15, 2005, 394 events (recurrent, second primary cancer, or death before recurrence) had been reported, triggering the first scheduled interim analysis. Of these, 133 were in the trastuzumab group and 261 in the control group (hazard ratio, 0.48; $P<.0001$). This result crossed the early stopping boundary. The absolute difference in disease-free survival between the trastuzumab group and the control group was 12% at 3 years. Trastuzumab therapy was associated with a 33% reduction in the risk of death ($P = .015$). The 3-year cumulative incidence of class III or IV congestive heart failure or death from cardiac causes in the trastuzumab group was 4.1% in trial B-31 and 2.9% in trial N9831. CONCLUSIONS: Trastuzumab combined with paclitaxel after doxorubicin and cyclophosphamide improves outcomes among women with surgically removed HER2-positive breast cancer. (Copyright 2005, Massachusetts Medical Society. All rights reserved. Reprinted with permission.)

Editor's summary and comments: This article combines results obtained through analysis of both the NSABP B-31 and North Central Cancer Treatment Group N9831 trials examining the role of trastuzumab in addition to chemotherapy. After only 3 years, significant improvements in both DFS and OS were observed in cohorts treated with trastuzumab. The drug reduces risk of recurrence by half, a finding that has led to the routine adjuvant use of trastuzumab in patients with HER2 amplified cancer. Similar results were reported from the HERA trial, an international, multicenter trial that examined 5102 patients with HER2-positive tumors who, after completion of standard chemotherapy, were randomized to observation, for 1 or 2 years of traztuzumab.[30] The 1- versus 2-year comparison is not yet mature, but these results are awaited with great interest.

Significant risk of cardiac complications was seen with administration of trastuzimab in all reports; 4.1% of patients in NSABP B-31 developed congestive heart failure or died of cardiac disease while enrolled in the study. Cardiotoxicity caused 4.3% of patients in the HERA trial to discontinue the drug during trial despite stringent entry requirements. Drug reduction schemes such as that presented in the FinHer trial seem to reduce this risk without compromising efficacy.[31]

LEVEL IA EVIDENCE: PROSPECTIVE RANDOMIZED TRIALS ADDRESSING THE ROLE OF ENDOCRINE THERAPY IN BREAST CANCER PREVENTION AND TREATMENT

11. Tamoxifen for the prevention of breast cancer: current status of the National Surgical Adjuvant Breast and Bowel Project P-1 study. Fisher B, Costantino JP, Wickerman DL, et al. J Natl Cancer Inst 2005;97(22): 1652–62.[32]

Hypothesis: Tamoxifen, prescribed for 5 years, reduces the risk of breast cancer in high-risk populations.

NSABP P-1 Trial Results				
No. of Patients Randomized	Study Groups	Stratification	Significance Demonstrated	% Change Identified in Trial
13207	Tamoxifen n = 6610 Placebo n = 6597	Age, race, history of LCIS, 5-year predicted risk of breast cancer	Yes, in number of new breast cancers	5.8% vs 3.4%

Published abstract: Initial findings from the National Surgical Adjuvant Breast and Bowel Project Breast Cancer Prevention Trial (P-1) demonstrated that tamoxifen reduced the risk of estrogen receptor positive tumors and osteoporotic fractures in women at increased risk for breast cancer. Side effects of varying clinical significance were observed. The trial was unblinded because of the positive results, and follow-up continued. This report updates our initial findings. METHODS: Women (n = 13,388) were randomly assigned to receive placebo or tamoxifen for 5 years. Rates of breast cancer and other events were compared by the use of risk ratios (RRs) and 95% confidence intervals (CIs). Estimates of the net benefit from 5 years of tamoxifen therapy were compared by age, race, and categories of predicted breast cancer risk. Statistical tests were 2-sided. RESULTS: After 7 years of follow-up, the cumulative rate of invasive breast cancer was reduced from 42.5 per 1000 women in the placebo group to 24.8 per 1000 women in the tamoxifen group (RR = 0.57, 95% CI = 0.46 to 0.70) and the cumulative rate of noninvasive breast cancer was reduced from 15.8 per 1000 women in the placebo group to 10.2 per 1000 women in the tamoxifen group (RR = 0.63, 95% CI = 0.45 to 0.89). These reductions were similar to those seen in the initial report. Tamoxifen led to a 32% reduction in osteoporotic fractures (RR = 0.68, 95% CI = 0.51 to 0.92). Relative risks of stroke, deep-vein thrombosis, and cataracts (which increased with tamoxifen) and of ischemic heart disease and death (which were not changed with tamoxifen) were also similar to those initially reported. Risks of pulmonary embolism were approximately 11% lower than in the original report, and risks of endometrial cancer were about 29% higher, but these differences were not statistically significant. The net benefit achieved with tamoxifen varied according to age, race, and level of breast cancer risk. CONCLUSIONS: Despite the potential bias caused by the unblinding of the P-1 trial, the magnitudes of all beneficial and undesirable treatment effects of tamoxifen were similar to those initially reported, with notable reductions in breast cancer and increased risks of thromboembolic events and endometrial cancer. Readily identifiable sub sets of individuals comprising 2.5 million women could derive a net benefit from the drug. (Copyright 2005, Oxford University Press. Reprinted with permission.)

Editor's summary and comments: NSABP P-1 is the largest of 4 trials examining the role of tamoxifen in breast cancer prevention (**Table 3**).[33–35] Patients at increased risk of developing breast cancer (defined by age, history of LCIS, or atypical hyperplasia, and estimated 5-year risk) were randomized to receive 5 years of tamoxifen therapy or placebo. After 7 years, the trial was unblinded due to a clear benefit for tamoxifen, and one-third of patients in the placebo group crossed over to tamoxifen. Data was censored at this point, but the cross-over diminished the differences observed between groups. Tamoxifen was found to significantly decrease the incidence of both invasive and noninvasive breast cancers. All of the effect was observed in hormone receptor–positive tumors; tamoxifen had no effect on the incidence of hormone receptor–negative breast cancer.

Table 3
Randomized controlled trials in breast cancer prevention

Trial	No. of Patients	Risk Factors Considered	Follow-up	Significant Difference in Invasive Breast Cancer	RR
NSABP P-1[32]	13388	Age, estimated 5-y risk, LCIS, atypical hyperplasia	7 y	Yes	0.57
CONSORT (Royal Marsden)[33]	2471	Family history	20 y	No	0.78
IBIS-1[34]	7145	Age, family history, parity, atypical hyperplasia, LCIS	8 y	Yes	0.74
Italian chemoprevention[35]	5408	Hysterectomy (53% of whom had bilateral oopherectomy)	11 y	No	0.84

Abbreviation: RR, relative risk.

The results of P-1 are similar to those published in an earlier analysis of this patient group as well as updates of the CONSORT, Italian chemoprevention trial, and the IBIS-1 study (see **Table 3**). Although significance was not demonstrated in the CONSORT trial or the Italian chemoprevention trial (in which patients were not uniformly at elevated risk), trends in each case were consistent with those reported in NSABP P-1 and IBIS-1. A meta-analysis based on the combined patient data from these 4 trials showed overall relative risk reduction of 38%.[36] No difference in survival was noted, but these trials were not powered to detect differences in these outcomes.

Side effect profiles for the drug were identical across trials; increases in endometrial cancer (most commonly International Federation of Gynecology and Obstetrics stage I tumors) and thromboembolic disease (venous thromboembolism; VTE) were observed with tamoxifen therapy. These complications were statistically increased in patients older than 50 years, but still affected far less than 1% of women, and should therefore not generally be considered prohibitive. Results of the NSABP P-2 (STAR) trial, addressing the relative efficacy and side effect profiles of tamoxifen and the selective estrogen receptor modulator (SERM) raloxifene in postmenopausal patients at high risk for breast cancer, have subsequently been reported.[37] Raloxifene provided no improvement over tamoxifen in reducing rates of invasive breast cancer, and appeared slightly inferior to tamoxifen in prevention of DCIS. Rates of VTE, cataract formation, and endometrial cancer were reduced in patients taking raloxifene, however, and both groups showed equivalent benefits related to osteoporotic bone fractures. Raloxifene is a reasonable alternative to tamoxifen for postmenopausal women, and drug choice can be made based, at least in part, on patient risk factors and comorbidities.

12. Five versus more than five years of tamoxifen for lymph node-negative breast cancer: updated findings from the National Surgical Adjuvant Breast and Bowel Project B-14 randomized trial. Fisher B, Dignam J, Bryant J, et al. J Natl Cancer Inst 2001;93:684–90.[38]

Hypothesis: More than 5 years of adjuvant tamoxifen therapy does not improve outcomes when compared with 5 years of therapy.

NSABP B-14 Trial Results				
No. of Patients Randomized	Study Groups	Stratification	Significance Demonstrated	% Change Identified in Trial
1172	Prolonged tamoxifen n = 583 5 years tamoxifen n = 569	Age, tumor size, type of surgery, expression levels of ER	Yes, in DFS	78% in 5-year treatment group vs 82% in prolonged treatment group

Published abstract: BACKGROUND: Previously reported information from B-14, a national Surgical Adjuvant Breast and Bowel Project (NSABP) randomized, placebo-controlled clinical trial, demonstrated that patients with estrogen receptor (ER)-positive breast cancer and negative axillary lymph nodes experienced a prolonged benefit from 5 years of tamoxifen therapy. When these women were rerandomized to receive either placebo or more prolonged tamoxifen therapy, they obtained no additional advantage from tamoxifen through 4 years of follow-up. Because the optimal duration of tamoxifen administration continues to be controversial and because there have been 3 more years of follow-up and a substantial increase in the number of events since our last report, an update of the B-14 study is appropriate. METHODS: Patients (n = 1172) who had completed 5 years of tamoxifen therapy and who were disease free were rerandomized to receive placebo (n = 579) or tamoxifen (n = 593). Survival, disease-free survival (DFS), and relapse-free survival (RFS) were estimated by the Kaplan-Meier method; the differences between the treatment groups were assessed by the log-rank test. Relative risks of failure (with 95% confidence intervals) were determined by the Cox proportional hazards model. *P* values were 2-sided. RESULTS: Through 7 years after reassignment of tamoxifen-treated patients to either placebo or continued tamoxifen therapy, a slight advantage was observed in patients who discontinued tamoxifen relative to those who continued to receive it: DFS = 82% versus 78% (*P* = .03), RFS = 94% versus 92% (*P* = .13), and survival = 94% versus 91% (*P* = .07), respectively. The lack of benefit from additional tamoxifen therapy was independent of age or other characteristics. CONCLUSION: Through 7 years of follow-up after rerandomization, there continues to be no additional benefit from tamoxifen administered beyond 5 years in women with ER-positive breast cancer and negative axillary lymph nodes. (Copyright 2001, Oxford University Press. Reprinted with permission.)

Editor's summary and comments: NSABP B-14 demonstrated a significant improvement in DFS and OS in node-negative, ER-positive breast cancer patients receiving 5 years of tamoxifen. After 5 years of therapy, patients who remained disease free were randomized to receive further treatment with the tamoxifen versus administration of placebo in an attempt to determine the optimal duration of tamoxifen therapy. Seven years following rerandomization, the group receiving further tamoxifen therapy actually did slightly worse than those receiving placebo. The results of this study established 5 years as the standard duration of tamoxifen treatment. More recent recognition of the extremely prolonged hazard of death in hormone receptor–positive breast cancer has led to a reevaluation of the optimal duration of tamoxifen treatment in the ATLAS trial.[39]

13. Effect of anastrozole and tamoxifen as adjuvant treatment for early-stage breast cancer: 100-month analysis of the ATAC trial. Arimidex, Tamoxifen, Alone or in Combination (ATAC) Trialists' Group, Forbes JF, Cusick J, Budzar A, et al. Lancet Oncol 2008;9:45–53.[40]

Hypothesis: Five years of adjuvant anastrozole treatment improves survival compared with tamoxifen therapy, and has an improved side effect profile.

ATAC Trial Results				
No. of Patients Randomized	Study Groups	Stratification	Significance Demonstrated	% Change Identified in Trial
6241	Anastrazole n = 3125 Tamoxifen n = 3116	Hormone receptor status	Yes, in DFS	21.8% vs 17% in anastrozole vs tamoxifen at 100 months

Published abstract: BACKGROUND: Little data exist on whether efficacy benefits or side-effects persist after 5 years of adjuvant treatment with an aromatase inhibitor. We aimed to study long-term outcomes in the Arimidex, Tamoxifen, Alone or in Combination (ATAC) trial that compares anastrozole with tamoxifen after a median follow-up of 100 months. METHODS: We analyzed postmenopausal women with localized invasive breast cancer. The primary endpoint disease-free survival (DFS), and the secondary endpoints time to recurrence (TTR), incidence of new contralateral breast cancer (CLBC), time to distant recurrence (TTDR), overall survival (OS), and death after recurrence were assessed in the total population (intention to treat; ITT: anastrozole, n = 3125; tamoxifen, n = 3116; total 6241) and the hormone-receptor-positive subpopulation, the clinically important subgroup for which endocrine treatment is now known to be effective (84% of ITT: anastrozole, n = 2618; tamoxifen, n = 2598; total 5216). After treatment completion, fractures and serious adverse events continued to be collected blindly (safety population: anastrozole, n = 3092; tamoxifen, n = 3094; total 6186). This study is registered as an International Standard Randomized Controlled Trial, number ISRCTN18233230. FINDINGS: At a median follow-up of 100 months (range 0–126), DFS, TTR, TTDR, and CLBC were improved significantly in the ITT and hormone-receptor-positive populations. For hormone-receptor-positive patients: DFS hazard ratio (HR) 0.85 (95% CI 0.76–0.94), $P = .003$; TTR HR 0.76 (0.67–0.87), $P = .0001$; TTDR HR 0.84 (0.72–0.97), $P = .022$; and CLBC HR 0.60 (0.42–0.85), $P = .004$. Absolute differences in time to recurrence increased over time (TTR 2.8% [anastrozole 9.7% vs tamoxifen 12.5%] at 5 years and 4.8% [anastrozole 17.0% vs tamoxifen 21.8%] at 9 years) and recurrence rates remained significantly lower on anastrozole compared with tamoxifen after treatment completion (HR 0.75 [0.61–0.94], $P = .01$). The fewer deaths after recurrence (anastrozole 245 vs tamoxifen 269) was not significant (HR 0.90 [0.75–1.07], $P = .2$), and no effect was noted for OS (anastrozole 472 vs tamoxifen 477) HR 0.97 [0.86–1.11], $P = .7$. Fracture rates were higher in patients receiving anastrozole than in those receiving tamoxifen during active treatment (number [annual rate]: 375 [2.93%] vs 234 [1.90%]; incidence rate ratio [IRR] 1.55 [1.31–1.83], $P<.0001$), but were not different after treatment was completed (off treatment: 146 [1.56%] vs 143 [1.51%]; IRR 1.03 [0.81–1.31], $P = .79$). We did not note any significant difference in risk of cardiovascular morbidity or mortality between anastrozole and tamoxifen treatment groups. INTERPRETATION: These data show long-term safety findings and establish clearly the long-term efficacy of anastrozole compared with tamoxifen as initial adjuvant treatment for postmenopausal women with hormone-sensitive, early breast cancer, and provide statistically significant evidence of a larger carryover effect after 5 years of adjuvant treatment with anastrozole compared with tamoxifen. (Copyright 2008, Elsevier. Reprinted with permission.)

Editor's summary and comments: The ATAC trial sought to examine the efficacy of adjuvant anastrozole in preventing recurrence of invasive breast cancer. It was anticipated that the drug, which lacks the weak estrogenicity of tamoxifen, would potentially improve breast cancer outcomes, and would have an improved side effect profile compared with tamoxifen. At 5 years, a 2% reduction in the ARR of recurrence was seen with anastrozole. No benefit in OS was demonstrated in this study, but time to recurrence, risk of new contralateral breast cancer, and time to distal recurrence were all significantly impacted by randomization to anastrozole versus tamoxifen. Nearly identical outcomes were observed in the BIG 1-98 trial, which randomized postmenopausal patients with hormone-responsive, localized breast cancers to receive 5 years of therapy with tamoxifen or 5 years of treatment with the aromatase inhibitor (AI) letrozole.[41]

Several studies have addressed the question of transitioning postmenopausal patients already receiving tamoxifen to AIs for the balance of the 5 years of adjuvant treatment, and analysis of these patient groups demonstrates that in this case as well patients show significant improvement in disease control when treated with a transition to an aromatase inhibitor compared with completing tamoxifen therapy (**Table 4**).[42,43] Three large trials have also defined a role for aromatase inhibitor therapy after

Table 4
Randomized controlled trials addressing adjuvant aromatase inhibitor therapy

Trial	No. of Patients	Prior Tamoxifen	Aromatase Inhibitor	Follow-up	Affect on DFS	Affect on OS
ATAC[40]	6241	No	Anastrazole (vs tamoxifen)	Median 100 mo	ARR 4.1%	No
BIG 1-98[41]	4922	No	Letrozole (vs tamoxifen)	Median 51 mo	ARR 2.9%	No
Intergroup Exemestane Study[42]	4742	Yes, 2–3 y	Exemestane (vs tamoxifen)	Median 30.6 mo	ARR 4.7%	No
ABCSG trial 8 & ARNO 95[43]	3224	Yes, 2–3 y	Anastrazole (vs tamoxifen)	Median 28 mo	ARR 3.1% (at 3 y)	No
NSABP B-33[44]	1598	Yes, 5 y	Exemestane (vs placebo)	Median 30 mo	ARR 2% (P = .07)	No
NCIC CTG intergroup MA.17[45]	5169	Yes, 5 y	Letrozole (vs placebo)	Median 30 mo	ARR 4.3–5.3% (at 4 y, varies by age)	No
Goss et al[46]	5187	Yes, 5 y	Letrozole (vs placebo)	Median 2.4 y	ARR 6% (at 4 y)	No

Abbreviation: ARR, absolute risk reduction.

completing a 5-year course of tamoxifen therapy,[44–46] again demonstrating an improvement in DFS. In the NCIC CTG Intergroup MA.17 study, high-risk, node-positive patients also had a significant improvement in OS. Initial observations that AIs were particularly beneficial in progesterone receptor-negative or HER2-overexpressing tumors have not been consistently reproduced. In aggregate, these studies demonstrate a small but real benefit for an AI (compared with SERM) as a part of adjuvant therapy. Tamoxifen remains a reasonable alternative for patients who cannot tolerate the side effects of AIs or have contraindications to their use.

In fact, there are multiple complications related to AIs that should be taken into account by the prescribing clinician. Patients have higher rates of osteoporosis-related fractures while taking AIs versus SERMs (2.93% vs 1.90% in the ATAC trial). Also, a small but insignificant increase in overall deaths was noted in ATAC as well as increases in nonbreast and endometrial cancer. It is expected that with longer follow-up the potential implications of these data will be elucidated. In all studies, there did seem to be a small reduction in endometrial cancer rates among patients receiving AI therapy versus tamoxifen. In general, high-risk patients are thought to benefit most from the improved efficacy of adjuvant treatment with AIs, whereas comorbidities and side effect profiles are of much more importance in choosing appropriate treatment for those with low-risk tumors.

DISCLOSURE

Authors have nothing to disclose.

REFERENCES

1. Fisher B, Jeong JH, Anderson S, et al. Twenty-five-year follow-up of a randomized trial comparing radical mastectomy, total mastectomy, and total mastectomy followed by irradiation. N Engl J Med 2002;347:567–75.
2. Fisher B, Anderson S, Bryant J, et al. Twenty-year follow-up of a randomized trial comparing total mastectomy, lumpectomy, and lumpectomy plus irradiation for the treatment of invasive breast cancer. N Engl J Med 2002;347:1233–41.
3. Poggi MM, Danforth DN, Sciuto LC, et al. Eighteen-year results in the treatment of early breast carcinoma with mastectomy versus breast conservation therapy: the National Cancer Institute Randomized Trial. Cancer 2003;98:697–702.
4. van Dongen JA, Voogd AC, Fentiman IS, et al. Long-term results of a randomized trial comparing breast-conserving therapy with mastectomy: European Organization for Research and Treatment of Cancer 10801 trial. J Natl Cancer Inst 2000;92:1143–50.
5. Veronesi U, Cascinelli N, Mariani L, et al. Twenty-year follow-up of a randomized study comparing breast-conserving surgery with radical mastectomy for early breast cancer. N Engl J Med 2002;347:1227–32.
6. Clarke M, Collins R, Darby S, et al. Early Breast Cancer Trialists' Collaborative Group (EBCTG). Effects of radiotherapy and of differences in the extent of surgery for early breast cancer on local recurrence and 15-year survival: an overview of the randomised trials. Lancet 2006;366:2087–106.
7. Veronesi U, Paganelli G, Viale G, et al. Sentinel-lymph node biopsy as a staging procedure in breast cancer: update of a randomized controlled trial. Lancet Oncol 2006;6:983–90.
8. Giuliano A, Kirgan D, Guenther J, et al. Lymphatic mapping and sentinel lymphadenectomy for breast cancer. Ann Surg 1994;220:391–401.
9. Krag DN, Anderson SJ, Julian TB, et al. Technical outcomes of sentinel-lymph-node resection and conventional axillary-lymph-node dissection in patients with

clinically node-negative breast cancer: results from the NSABP B-32 randomised phase III trial. Lancet Oncol 2007;8:881–8.

10. Posther KE, McCall LM, Blumencranz PW, et al. Sentinel node skills verification and surgeon performance: data from a multicenter clinical trial for early-stage breast cancer. Ann Surg 2005;242:593–9.

11. Mansel RE, Fallowfield L, Kissin M, et al. Randomized multicenter trial of sentinel node biopsy versus standard axillary treatment in operable breast cancer: the ALMANAC Trial. J Natl Cancer Inst 2006;98:599–609.

12. Zavagno G, De Salvo GL, Scalco G, et al. A randomized clinical trial on sentinel lymph node biopsy versus axillary lymph node dissection in breast cancer: results of the Sentinella/GIVOM trial. Ann Surg 2008;247:207–13.

13. Van Zee KJ, Manasseh DM, Bevilacqua JL, et al. A nomogram for predicting the likelihood of additional nodal metastases in breast cancer patients with a positive sentinel node biopsy. Ann Surg Oncol 2003;10:1140–51.

14. Fisher B, Land S, Mamounas E, et al. Prevention of invasive breast cancer in women with ductal carcinoma in situ: an update of the National Surgical Adjuvant Breast and Bowel Project experience. Semin Oncol 2001;28:400–18.

15. Fisher B, Costantino J, Redmond C, et al. Lumpectomy compared with lumpectomy and radiation therapy for the treatment of intraductal breast cancer. N Engl J Med 1993;328:1581–6.

16. Emdin SO, Granstrand B, Ringberg A, et al. SweDCIS: Radiotherapy after sector resection for ductal carcinoma in situ of the breast. Results of a randomised trial in a population offered mammography screening. Acta Oncol 2006;45:536–43.

17. Bijker N, Meijnen P, Peterse JL, et al. Breast-conserving treatment with or without radiotherapy in ductal carcinoma-in-situ: ten-year results of European Organisation for Research and Treatment of Cancer randomized phase III trial 10853—a study by the EORTC Breast Cancer Cooperative Group and EORTC Radiotherapy Group. J Clin Oncol 2006;24:3381–7.

18. Houghton J, George WD, Cuzick J, et al. Radiotherapy and tamoxifen in women with completely excised ductal carcinoma in situ of the breast in the UK, Australia, and New Zealand: randomised controlled trial. Lancet 2003;362:95–102.

19. Allred DC, Bryant J, Land S, et al. Estrogen expression as a predictive marker of the effectiveness of tamoxifen in the treatment of intraductal breast cancer: findings of the NSABP Protocol B-24 [abstract]. Breast Cancer Res Treat 2002;76:S36.

20. Ragaz J, Ollivotto IA, Spinelli JJ, et al. Locoregional radiation therapy in patients with high-risk breast cancer receiving adjuvant chemotherapy: 20-year results of the British Columbia randomized trial. J Natl Cancer Inst 2005;97:116–26.

21. Overgaard M, Hansen PS, Overgaard J, et al. Postoperative radiotherapy in high-risk premenopausal women with breast cancer who receive adjuvant chemotherapy. Danish Breast Cancer Cooperative Group 82b Trial. N Engl J Med 1997;337:949–55.

22. Overgaard M, Jensen MB, Overgaard J, et al. Postoperative radiotherapy in high-risk postmenopausal breast-cancer patients given adjuvant tamoxifen: Danish Breast Cancer Cooperative Group DBCG 82c randomised trial. Lancet 1999;353:1641–8.

23. Early Breast Cancer Trialists' Collaborative Group. Effects of chemotherapy and hormonal therapy for early breast cancer on recurrence and 15-year survival: and overview of the randomised trials. Lancet 2005;365:1687–717.

24. Henderson IC, Berry DA, Demetri GD, et al. Improved outcomes from adding sequential Paclitaxel but not from escalating Doxorubicin dose in an adjuvant

chemotherapy regimen for patients with node-positive primary breast cancer. J Clin Oncol 2003;21:976.

25. Wolmark N, Wang J, Mamounas E, et al. Preoperative chemotherapy in patients with operable breast cancer: nine-year results from National Surgical Adjuvant Breast and Bowel Project B-18. J Natl Cancer Inst Monogr 2001;30:96–102.

26. Fisher B, Brown A, Mamounas E, et al. Effect of preoperative chemotherapy on local-regional disease in women with operable breast cancer: findings from National Surgical Adjuvant Breast and Bowel Project B-18. J Clin Oncol 1997;15:2483.

27. Rastogi P, Anderson SJ, Bear HD, et al. Preoperative chemotherapy: updates of National Surgical Adjuvant Breast and Bowel Project Protocols B-18 and B-27. J Clin Oncol 2008;26:778–85.

28. Mauri DN, Pavlidis N, Ioannidis JP. Neoadjuvant versus adjuvant systemic treatment in breast cancer: a meta-analysis. J Natl Cancer Inst 2005;97:188–94.

29. Romond EH, Perez EA, Bryant J, et al. Trastuzumab plus adjuvant chemotherapy for operable HER2-positive breast cancer. N Engl J Med 2005; 353(16):1673–84.

30. Smith I, Procter M, Gelber RD, et al. 2-year follow-up of trastuzumab after adjuvant chemotherapy in HER2-positive breast cancer: a randomised controlled trial. Lancet 2007;369:29–36.

31. Joensuu H, Kellokumpu-Lehtinen PL, Bono P, et al. Adjuvant docetaxel or vinorelbine with or without trastuzumab for breast cancer. N Engl J Med 2006;354:809.

32. Fisher B, Costantino JP, Wickerham DL, et al. Tamoxifen for the prevention of breast cancer: current status of the National Surgical Adjuvant Breast and Bowel Project P-1 study. J Natl Cancer Inst 2005;97(22):1652–62.

33. Powles TJ, Ashley S, Tidy A, et al. Twenty-year follow-up of the Royal Marsden randomized, double-blinded tamoxifen breast cancer prevention trial. J Natl Cancer Inst 2007;99:283–90.

34. Cuzick J, Forbes JF, Sestak I, et al. Long-term results of tamoxifen prophylaxis for breast cancer—96-month follow-up of the randomized IBIS-I trial. J Natl Cancer Inst 2007;99:272–82.

35. Veronesi U, Maisonneuve P, Rotmensz N, et al. Tamoxifen for the prevention of breast cancer: late results of the Italian Randomized Tamoxifen Prevention Trial among women with hysterectomy. J Natl Cancer Inst 2007;99:727–37.

36. Cuzick J. A brief review of the current breast cancer prevention trials and proposals for future trials. Eur J Cancer 2000;36:1298.

37. Vogel VG, Costantino JP, Wickerham DL, et al. Effects of tamoxifen vs raloxifene on the risk of developing invasive breast cancer and other disease outcomes: the NSABP Study of Tamoxifen and Raloxifene (STAR) P-2 trial. JAMA 2006;295: 2727.

38. Fisher B, Dignam J, Bryant J, et al. Five versus more than five years of tamoxifen for lymph node-negative breast cancer: updated findings from the National Surgical Adjuvant Breast and Bowel Project B-14 randomized trial. J Natl Cancer Inst 2001;93:684–90.

39. Peto R. The worldwide overview: new results for systemic adjuvant therapies. Breast Cancer Res 2007;106:S5.

40. Forbes JF, Cuzick J, Buzdar A, et al. Effect of anastrozole and tamoxifen as adjuvant treatment for early-stage breast cancer: 100-month analysis of the ATAC trial. Lancet Oncol 2008;9:45–53.

41. Crivellari D, Sun Z, Coates AS, et al. Letrozole compared with tamoxifen for elderly patients with endocrine-responsive early breast cancer: the BIG 1–98 trial. J Clin Oncol 2008;26:1972–9.

42. Coombes RC, Hall E, Gibson LJ, et al. A randomized trial of exemestane after two to three years of tamoxifen therapy in postmenopausal women with primary breast cancer. N Engl J Med 2004;350:1081–92.

43. Jakesz R, Jonat W, Gnant M, et al. Switching of postmenopausal women with endocrine-responsive early breast cancer to anastrozole after 2 years' adjuvant tamoxifen: combined results of ABCSG trial 8 and ARNO 95 trial. Lancet 2005; 366:455.

44. Mamounas EP, Jeong JH, Wickerham DL, et al. Benefit from exemestane as extended adjuvant therapy after 5 years of adjuvant tamoxifen: intention-to-treat analysis of the National Surgical Adjuvant Breast And Bowel Project B-33 trial. J Clin Oncol 2008;26:1965–71.

45. Muss HB, Tu D, Ingle JN, et al. Efficacy, toxicity, and quality of life in older women with early-stage breast cancer treated with letrozole or placebo after 5 years of tamoxifen: NCIC CTG intergroup trial MA.17. J Clin Oncol 2008;26:1956.

46. Goss PE, Ingle JN, Martino S, et al. A randomized trial of letrozole in postmeno-pausal women after five years of tamoxifen therapy for early-stage breast cancer. N Engl J Med 2003;349:1793–802.

Randomized Clinical Trials in Esophageal Carcinoma

Stephen A. Barnett, MD, Nabil P. Rizk, MD, MS*

KEYWORDS

- Esophageal cancer • Prospective randomized controlled trials
- Level Ia evidence • Literature review

The treatment of esophageal cancer with curative intent remains highly controversial, with advocates of surgery alone, chemoradiotherapy (CRT) alone, surgery with adjuvant therapy (including neoadjuvant and postoperative), and trimodality therapy each contributing prospective randomized controlled trials (PRCTs) to the body of scientific publications between 2000 and 2008. Any improvements in survival have been small in absolute percentage terms, and as such PRCTs published over the last decade have met the same primary obstacle encountered by the studies from the two decades prior and reviewed in the previous summary article, namely lack of power to detect small differences in outcome. Many of the best trials in attempting to address this issue by careful power calculations have been thwarted by lack of accrual due largely to patient and physician preference for a particular treatment modality.

Attempts have been made to address this deficiency by the publication of 8 meta-analyses[1–8]; these in turn are limited by: the *heterogeneity of patients* included with respect to clinical stage, methods used to assess clinical stage (ranging from upper gastrointestinal endoscopy [UGIE], abdominal ultrasound [US], and chest radiography (CXR) alone, through to high-resolution computed tomography [CT], positron emission tomography [PET]-CT, endoscopic ultrasound [EUS], staging laparoscopy, and thoracoscopy), performance status of patients, and histology of tumor; the *heterogeneity of treatment* with respect to anesthetic and perioperative care, surgery (including operative approach, conduit used and technique of reconstruction), radiotherapy (RT) including planning (hardware, software, and extent of treatment) and delivery (hardware, software, fractionation, and total dose), chemotherapy varying in agent, dose, and number and timing (induction, postoperative, or both) of cycles, and CRT varying with respect to the factors already mentioned, as well as whether administered concurrently or sequentially; and *publication bias*.

Disclosure: See last page of article.
Department of Surgery, Memorial Sloan-Kettering Cancer Center, 1275 York Avenue, New York, NY 10021, USA
* Corresponding author.
E-mail address: rizkn@mskcc.org (N.P. Rizk).

These limitations remain despite sophisticated statistical methods employed to address said limitations. These deficiencies are seemingly intuitively apparent to clinicians working in the area and make the conclusions of the meta-analyses (which themselves vary) difficult to confidently and broadly apply. In any case, meta-analyses do not represent level Ia evidence and are not the subject of this review.

These variations in staging methods, surgical technique, RT technique, and chemotherapy regime have in turn been the subject of PRCTs over the last nine years. In many cases primary end points have not been survival but rather rates of complication or response.

CURATIVE INTENT: SURGERY VERSUS CHEMORADIOTHERAPY

The only PRCT published in the last nine years comparing surgery alone to definitive CRT was conducted in Hong Kong.[9] This multicenter trial enrolled biopsy-proven squamous cell carcinoma (SCC) of the mid and lower esophagus with preoperative stage T_{1-3}, N_{0-1}, M_{0-1a}, and had 80% power to discern a doubling in median survival from 15 to 30 months. Such an expectation was perhaps overly optimistic, and despite near equivalence in two-year survival (58% vs 55%, $P = .45$) and a nonsignificant risk ratio (0.89 confidence interval [CI] 0.37–2.17), a smaller but clinically relevant improvement in overall survival (OS) has not been discounted. The secondary end point of median hospital stay was longer in the CRT group (41 vs 27 days, $P = .022$). Despite stated analysis on an intention-to-treat basis, one patient randomized to esophagectomy was removed from analysis after failing to undergo planned treatment. This trial has much to commend it: extensive staging of patients with modalities including EUS, CT, and neck US; modern RT techniques including concurrent CRT and 3D conformal delivery; and inclusion of patients with clinically advanced disease (ie, M_{1a}, a group often included in studies of CRT but excluded from surgical trials); however, it remains underpowered to confirm a clinically relevant superiority of one treatment over the other.

CURATIVE INTENT: SURGERY ALONE VERSUS NEOADJUVANT THERAPY

If from the aforementioned PRCT[9] one accepts surgery as a standard of care, it is reasonable to include it as the control arm of further PRCTs of adjuvant therapy (including neoadjuvant and postoperative). Ten such trials employing neoadjuvant therapy have been published in the last nine years,[10–19] including two previously reported trials with updated follow-up (**Table 1**).[13,19–21]

Of the six PRCTs employing neoadjuvant CRT, two showed improvement in OS[17,19,20] and four did not.[11,14,16,18] All trials used concurrent CRT, with total doses ranging from 35 to 50.4 Gy. Chemotherapy consisted of cisplatin at total doses of 60 to 100 mg/m^2 per cycle and 5-flourouracil (5-FU).

Of the four PRCTs employing neoadjuvant chemotherapy, two showed improvement in OS[12,15] and two did not.[10,13,21] Three of four trials employed cisplatin and 5-FU,[10,13,15,21] whereas one employed epirubicin, cisplatin, and 5-FU.[12]

Of note, each of the negative trials either did not report a power calculation,[16] failed to accrue the calculated sample size,[10] or had only 80% power to detect 50% or more improvement in survival.[11,14,18] In this context the implication from these non significant trials is that there remains a 20% chance that at least a 50% improvement in survival exists but was not detected, or indeed that there is an even greater chance of a real difference in survival of less than 50% being present but undetected.

The notable exception to this implication is the North American Intergroup trial (INT113)[13,21] which, despite power of 90% to detect a 38% increase in median survival, showed no difference in survival. The integration of the results of this trial

Table 1
Prospective randomized trials of induction chemotherapy or chemoradiotherapy versus surgery alone

Authors (Institution, Region)	Accrual	Power Calculation	n	Induction Regime	Survival, Induction & S vs S	Significance	Hazard Ratio
Walsh et al (single, Ireland)[19,20]	1990–1995	80%, 2 y from 23% to 43% required 190 pts	113	C, 5-FU (×2) 2.5 Gy × 16 (40 Gy)	Median: 17 vs 12 mo; 5 y: 32% vs 6%	0.002	
Urba et al (single, North America)[18]	1989–1994	80%, Median from 1 to 2.2 y	100	C, 5-FU, V (×2) 1.5 Gy BD ×15 (45 Gy)	Median: 16.9 vs 17.6 mo	NS	0.73
Burmeister et al AGITG (multi, Australasia)[11]	1994–2000	80%, 3 y PFS from 20% to 35%	256	C, 5-FU (×1) 15 Gy ×1.3 (35 Gy)	Median: 16 vs 12[b] mo	NS	0.82
Tepper et al CALGB 9781 (multi, North America)[17]	1997–2000	90%, 5 y from 20% to 32% required 500 pts	56	C, 5-FU (×2) 1.8 Gy ×28 (50.4 Gy)	Median: 54 vs 21 mo; 5 y: 39% vs 16%	0.002	
Natsugoe et al (single, Japan)[16]	1997–2001	None reported	45	C, 5-FU (continuous) 2 Gy ×20 (40 Gy)	5 y: 57% vs 41%	NS	
Lee et al (single, South Korea)[14]	1999–2002	80%, 2 y from 20% to 30%	101	C, 5-FU (×2, S, ± ×3) 1.2 Gy BD ×19 (45.6 Gy)	Median: 27.3 vs 28.2 mo	NS	
Kelsen et al Intergroup 113 (multi, North America)[13,21]	1990–1995	90%, 38% improvement in median	443	C, 5-FU (×3, S ± ×2)	Median: 14.9 vs 16.1 mo	NS	
Ancona et al (single, Italy)[10]	1992–1997	80%, 2 y improved 20% required 240 pts	94	C, 5-FU (×2–3)	Median: 25 vs 24 mo; 5 y: 34% vs 22%	NS	
Girling et al MRC (multi, Europe)[15]	1992–1998	90%, 2 y from 20% to 30%	802	C, 5-FU (×2)	Median: 16.8 vs 13.3 mo	0.004	0.79
Cunningham et al "MAGIC", MRC (multi, Europe)[12]	1994–2002	90%, 5 y from 23% to 38%	503[a]	C, 5-FU, E (×3, S, ×3)	5 y: 36% vs 23%	0.009	0.75

Abbreviations: C, cisplatin; E, epirubicin; 5-FU, 5-flourouracil; NS, not significant; pts, patients; S, surgery; V, vinblastine.
[a] 131 patients esophageal or gastroesophageal junction.
[b] Progression-free survival.

to clinical practice has remained problematic for advocates of neoadjuvant chemotherapy alone. The larger MRC trial (OEO2)[15] and INT113 are often compared as the accrual of demographically similar patients with seemingly similar treatment regimes resulting in disparate outcomes. Some differences between the two trials may explain the conflicting results. The OEO2 stratified patients, according to treatment center and surgeon, had a shorter time from randomization to surgery (63 vs 93 days), had a higher percentage of patients in the induction arm proceed to surgery (92% vs 80%), and used a less toxic cisplatin regimen (160 vs 450 mg/m^2). This last point is perhaps most salient. The inability of North American patients to tolerate the higher doses of cisplatin (71% completed planned preoperative chemotherapy compared with 90%, and only 38% completed planned postoperative treatment whereas OEO2 did not include postoperative chemotherapy) may imply that any benefit in terms of eradication of micrometastases was counterbalanced by side effects and toxicities resulting in no net change in survival. Finally, the negative result of INT113 may simply represent the 10% chance of a trial with 90% power not detecting a real difference in survival.

The observed magnitude of improvement in survival with CRT has been similar to that of chemotherapy alone, with median survival after neoadjuvant CRT improving from 12 to 17 months[19] and after neoadjuvant chemotherapy improving from 13 to 17 months.[15]

CURATIVE INTENT: SURGERY ALONE VERSUS ADJUVANT THERAPY

Four PRCTs have addressed the use of adjuvant therapy with curative intent after resection.[22–25]

Adjuvant RT was tested at multiple institutions in China between 1986 and 1997 in 495 patients with SCC of the thoracic esophagus more than 4 cm in length randomized to 60 Gy external beam RT versus surgery alone.[25] Five-year survival was 41.3% in the treatment group compared with 31.7% in the surgery alone group ($P = .45$). Subgroup analysis showed 5-year survival to be better after adjuvant RT in stage III patients (35.1 vs 13.1%, $P = .0027$). The impact of this trial has been limited, as no power calculation was undertaken, groups were not well balanced with respect to sex and nodal status, and intention-to-treat principles were not applied.

Adjuvant chemotherapy was tested at multiple institutions in Japan by the Japanese Clinical Oncology Group (JCOG) between 1992 and 1997 in 242 patients with completely resected SCC randomized to two cycles of cisplatin and 5-FU versus surgery alone.[22] Patients were stratified according to institution and pathologic nodal status. The primary end point of disease-free survival (DFS) favored the adjuvant treatment arm (55 vs 45%, $P = .037$). In subgroup analysis 5-year DFS in pN_0 patients showed no difference (70 vs 76%, $P = .4$), but was enhanced in pN_1 patients (52 vs 38%, $P = .04$). Of note, no significant difference was seen in OS.

Adjuvant chemotherapy was compared with adjuvant concurrent CRT at a single institution in Japan between 1991 and 2000 in 45 patients with completely resected SCC and pathologic stage I_b to III tumors randomized to adjuvant CRT (cisplatin 50 mg/m^2 days 1, 15, 5-FU 300 mg/m^2 days 1–35, and concurrent external beam RT 45–50 Gy) versus chemotherapy alone (cisplatin 50 mg/m^2 days 1, 15, and 5-FU 300 mg/m^2 days 1–35).[24] Patients with postoperative complication were not eligible. No power calculation was reported and no difference was found in median survival (31 vs 28 months, not significant).

Adjuvant CRT (leucovorin 20 mg/m^2 and 5-FU 450 mg/m^2 days 1–5, 28–31, 58–60, 90–94, 120–124, plus external beam RT of 45 Gy in divided doses 5 times per week days 28–60) was compared with surgery alone at multiple institutions in North America between 1991 and 1998 in 556 patients with completely resected adenocarcinoma

(AC) of the stomach or gastroesophageal junction, and including approximately 20% with tumors of the cardia.[23] Median OS was improved in patients receiving adjuvant therapy (36 vs 27 months, P = .005). Hazard ratio (HR) of death was 1.35 (CI = 1.09–1.66).

In summary, RT alone or in addition to chemotherapy did not improve primary end points. Adjuvant chemotherapy alone and CRT showed improvement compared with surgery alone.

CURATIVE INTENT: DEFINITIVE CHEMORADIOTHERAPY VERSUS TRIMODALITY THERAPY

If from the aforementioned PRCT[9] one accepts definitive CRT as a standard of care, it is reasonable to include it as the control arm of further PRCTs of trimodality therapy. Two such trials have been undertaken.[26–28]

The first trial to be published is perhaps the most significant to be discussed in the context of this review. Stahl and colleagues[28] randomized 172 patients from 11 institutions in Germany with SCC of the upper and mid esophagus to trimodality therapy versus definitive CRT. After induction chemotherapy with cisplatin, 5-FU, etoposide, and leucovorin patients were randomized to either concurrent CRT with cisplatin, etoposide, and 40 Gy RT then transthoracic esophagectomy or definitive concurrent CRT with cisplatin, etoposide, and 60 to 65 Gy RT. The patients were staged with EUS (though the details are not reported) and CT scan, but not PET. T_{3-4} (excluding airway invasion) and N_{1-0} patients were stratified by: center, TNM, completeness of EUS, sex, and weight loss.

Of interest, the trial was designed to assess equivalence of treatments; as such a reduction in two-year survival of greater than 15% in the definitive CRT arm from the expected 35% in the surgery arm would have resulted in a negative trial. In fact two-year survival was 39.9% in the trimodality arm and 35.4% in the definitive CRT arm (P = .007). Thus the trial was positive, implying there is only a 5% chance of a greater than 15% absolute difference in two-year OS between the two groups. Of note, if the more usual design attempting to discern a survival advantage had been employed one would be discussing an adequately powered (80%) trial that was negative, that is, had failed to show improvement in two-year survival from 20% to 35%, and likely questioning the overly optimistic expectation of a 75% improvement in survival.

When treatments are equivalent in terms of OS, attention logically turns to other measures of outcome. Secondary end points included progression-free survival (PFS), which at two years was 64.3% versus 40.7% (P = .003) favoring the trimodality arm; and treatment-related deaths, which clearly favored the definitive CRT arm: 11 of 86 (12.8%) versus three of 85 (3.5%) (P = .03) including two deaths due to complications of induction chemotherapy in each arm. Finally, a regression analysis revealed response to initial induction chemotherapy to be the only significant predictor of survival.

In summary, there was no difference in OS, progression was less common, and treatment-related death more common in the trimodality arm, and response to induction chemotherapy (regardless of other treatments) was the only significant predictor of survival.

A second European multi-institution trial undertaken in France has resulted in two publications. The first article addressed quality of life (which was a secondary end point of the trial and not the focus of a power analysis), and found a short-term reduction in the trimodality arm but no difference between arms beyond six months.[27] The second[26] reported the trial in detail, and is notable (particularly after the findings of the regression analysis in the first trimodality trial) in that only patients with esophageal SCC responding to induction therapy (259/444) were subsequently randomized to surgery versus continued CRT. Sequential or concurrent CRT was allowed in both arms and surgical approach was not mandated. The trial was again designed to assess equivalence and (despite planned accrual of 500 patients to provide 80% power to confirm <10% difference in OS between the arms) was ceased after interim analysis showed no chance of rejecting the hypothesis of equivalence with further enrollments. Two-year survival was 34% in the trimodality arm and 40% in the definitive CRT arm ($P = .03$), implying equivalence of the 2 treatments.

Secondary end points included locoregional relapse (HR = 1.63, CI 1.04–2.55, $P = .03$) and treatment for dysphagia (24% vs 46%, $P = .001$), which both favored the trimodality arm, whereas 3-month mortality (9.3% vs 0.8%, $P = .002$) and length of stay (68 vs 52 days, $P = .02$) favored the definitive CRT arm.

CURATIVE INTENT: SURGICAL TECHNIQUE

Two PRCTs of surgical approach comparing esophageal resection with and without thoracotomy have been reported. The first,[29] undertaken at two centers in the Netherlands and accruing between 1994 and 2000, compared transhiatal esophagectomy to transthoracic esophagectomy in 220 patients with T_{1-3}, N_{0-1}, M_0 AC of the mid esophagus to gastric cardia. The trial was powered to detect a 50% improvement in median survival from 14 to 22 months in the transthoracic arm. There was no such improvement, with median survival in the transhiatal compared with transthoracic arm 1.8 versus 2.0 years ($P = .38$), 5-year survival 29% versus 38% (CI −3% to 23%), and median DFS 1.4 versus 1.7 years ($P = .15$). Of note, transhiatal esophagectomy was associated with significantly less blood loss, pulmonary complication, chyle leak, and ventilated days. Despite this higher rate of complications there was no significant increase in perioperative mortality in the transthoracic arm. Thus this trial implies there is less than a 50% improvement in survival and no increased perioperative mortality when transthoracic esophagectomy is undertaken, despite an increase in perioperative morbidity. A second publication[30] was generated based on this trial, and reported actual five-year survival of 34% versus 36% ($P = .71$). Subgroup analysis of patients found to have 1 to 8 malignant lymph nodes had OS of 19% versus 39% ($P = .05$) and DFS of 23% versus 64% ($P = .02$). This retrospective analysis, while of interest, was based on pathologic results and excluded patients undergoing exploratory surgery (though R1 resections were included). As such, intention-to-treat principles were not adhered to, postoperative stage migration is likely, and the report at best represents a level "1c" PRCT.

The second trial,[31] undertaken at 27 Japanese hospitals under the auspices of the JCOG and accruing between 1995 and 2003, compared left thoracoabdominal to transhiatal resection in 167 patients with T_{2-4}, M_0 gastric AC with 3 cm or less esophageal involvement. The trial was designed with 80% power to detect a 10.5% improvement in five-year survival with thoracoabdominal resection, and initially planned enrollment of 302 patients over 4 years. After eight years and accrual of 167 patients, interim statistical analysis showed less than a 3.65% chance of proving thoracoabdominal resection superior with completion of accrual, thus the trial was closed. The investigators conclude that thoracoabdominal resection does not offer a survival advantage compared with transhiatal resection in Siewert II and III tumors.

Three single-institution PRCTs have compared hand-sewn to stapled anastomosis after esophagectomy.[32–34] Rate of anastomotic leak, perioperative morbidity and mortality, dysphagia, anastomotic diameter, stricture rate, and quality of life were not different between the two approaches.

Further variations of reconstructive technique have been addressed by three PRCTs. Gupta and colleagues[35] found a lower leak rate of 4.3% versus 20.8% ($P = .03$) and stricture rate of 8.5% versus 29.2% (P = .02) after a "novel" hand-sewn esophagogastric anastomosis compared with a standard hand-sewn anastomosis. Bhat and colleagues[36] found anastomotic leak dramatically reduced after omental wrap of the esophagogastric anastomosis versus standard anastomosis (3.09% versus 14.43%, P = .005). Tabira and colleagues[37] found no difference in anastomotic leak or postoperative nutritional status at 6 and 12 months after use of a slender gastric tube for reconstruction after esophagectomy when compared with a more generous gastric tube.

Shackcloth and colleagues[38] completed a well-planned and executed study addressing the most appropriate use of nasogastric tubes (NGT) in the first 48 hours post esophagectomy. Thirty-four patients were randomized to NGT with continuous sump suction, single-lumen NGT with 4-hourly aspirations or no NGT. The patients receiving continuous suction via the sump system spent significantly less time with pH less than 5.5 than either of the other two groups (4.3% vs 39.7% vs 40.3% [P = .007]). Patients randomized to no NGT had significantly more pulmonary complications, 7 of 12 versus 4 of 22 (P = .02), and required an NGT to be inserted in 7 of 12 cases. This simple study argues strongly for the use of sump NGT in all patients in the immediate perioperative period.

Method of endoscopic resectional technique,[39] extent of lymph node resection,[40] thoracotomy versus thoracoscopy,[41] antibiotic bowel decontamination,[42] and PGE1 infusion[43] have been reported in "1c" trials without difference in primary end points.

CURATIVE INTENT: RADIOTHERAPY TECHNIQUE

Before 2002, primarily based on evidence from two phase three trials and one phase II trial, and as reviewed more recently in a Cochrane review of randomized clinical trials (all but one trial completed before 2003), the standard of care for the nonsurgical management of locally advanced esophageal cancer consisted of concurrent CRT.[44] RTOG 8501, initially published in 1992,[45] was a randomized trial evaluating concurrent CRT (cisplatin 75 mg/m^2 and 5-FU 1000 mg/m^2 in weeks one and five, concurrent with 50 Gy given as daily 2-Gy fractions and followed by 2 additional chemotherapy cycles, compared with 64 Gy of RT alone), which definitively showed that combined modality therapy achieves significantly better OS and disease control, with acceptable increased toxicity. RTOG 9207, a phase I to II trial published in 1997,[46] evaluated the addition of brachytherapy administered with the first of two planned chemotherapy cycles following the completion of 50 Gy concurrent with cisplatin, 75 mg/m^2 and 5-FU, 1000 mg/m^2. There was an 8% treatment-related mortality rate, as well as 12% esophageal fistula rate. This result established that brachytherapy causes potentially more harm than good. Lastly, RTOG 9405[47] was a randomized trial that compared concurrent CRT, combining four cycles of cisplatin 75 mg/m^2, 5-FU 1000 mg/m^2 either with 50.4 Gy (1.8 Gy/d) or with 64.8 Gy (1.8 Gy/d). This study was stopped early due to an interim analysis showing an excessive number of treatment-related deaths in the high dose arm, albeit 7 of the 11 deaths occurred before surpassing 50 Gy. Overall results showed no differences in local/regional disease control or in survival, and the conclusion was that a higher dose of RT does not improve outcome. Finally, a Cochrane review of randomized trials[44] concluded that there is a 12% one-year and a 4% two-year survival benefit of CRT, and an absolute decrease in local recurrence of 12% compared with RT alone.

In this context, there are only four randomized trials published in the literature since 2001 evaluating the nonsurgical management of esophageal cancer using variations of the most accepted RT techniques as listed in the RTOG trials.[48–51] The techniques evaluated included split-course RT (1 week, a break, then 1 week),[50] hyperfractionated

RT (RT twice a day),[49,51] and the addition of brachytherapy following standard RT.[48] All these studies are underpowered. Furthermore, given that the accepted standard of care at the time of patient accrual for these studies was CRT, it is difficult to justify the presence of an RT-only arm in three of the four studies. Likewise, when chemotherapy was included it was either as single agent[48,50] or the doses were too low.[51] In none of theses studies did the clinical staging include a PET scan or EUS, making comparisons between groups and studies difficult. Post-therapy follow-up was likewise inadequate in these studies, with most not even including routine CT scan as a means to evaluate for disease recurrence. Despite these caveats, the studies that evaluated late-course accelerated hyperfractionated RT (LCAF) do show some impressive local control and long-term survival results, yet due to methodological issues better studies are needed to compare this modality with standard RT techniques.

STAGING

Designing randomized clinical trials for staging of esophageal cancer is difficult, and as such the standards of care have primarily evolved as technologies have been adopted, using retrospective studies and prospective case series to support "standards" of care. At present, most clinicians would agree that the standard staging workup for esophageal cancer should include a PET scan,[52] an EUS,[53] and CT scan.[54] Less well characterized are the use of laparoscopy and thoracoscopy.[55] Of the randomized staging studies reviewed for this article, none can be described as a true phase III trial. Two of the studies compared the accuracy of different EUS scopes[56,57] and two evaluated the added "impact" to patient management when an EUS is added to preoperative staging.[58,59] None of these trials is truly randomized. The fundamental problem with the "impact" studies is that the same physicians reviewed patient clinical staging histories both with and without the benefit of the EUS result to evaluate the independent impact of EUS to clinical management; it is not credible to believe that the clinicians were capable of being blinded in this study. In both these studies the conclusion was that EUS had an impact in deciding whether surgery was appropriate.[58,59] Regarding the studies that compared two EUS techniques, one compared transverse-array EUS (TA-EUS) to linear array EUS (L-EUS),[56] whereas the other compared curved array EUS (CAE) and radial EUS (RE).[57] In one study,[56] the conclusion of which was that TA-EUS should be the primary method of staging esophageal cancer, fewer than 50% of patients underwent surgical resection for pathologic correlation to EUS findings. Furthermore, of those who did undergo resection, two-thirds received preoperative therapy, making comparisons to pretreatment EUS dubious. Similarly in the article by Siemsen and colleagues,[57] the conclusion of which was that there was no difference between CAE and RE, 26 of the 62 patients explored were not resected yet these patients were still used as pathologic correlates to the EUS findings.

PALLIATIVE INTENT: ADJUVANT CHEMOTHERAPY

Although there was no one standard of care in the treatment of advanced stage gastroesophageal cancer before 2002, there were some general guidelines that were recently summarized in a meta-analysis of randomized phase II and phase III trials.[60] This meta- analysis noted that in the management of advanced gastric and gastroesophageal cancers: (1) chemotherapy is better than best supportive care (HR 0.39), (2) combination chemotherapy is better than single-agent chemotherapy (HR 0.74), (3) a 5-FU/cisplatin/anthracycline combination is better than a 5-FU/cisplatin combination (HR 0.62), and (4) a 5-FU/cisplatin/anthracycline combination is better than an 5-FU/anthracycline combination (HR 0.76). Most of the trials included in this meta-analysis were published in the 1990s and are not reviewed for this publication. In general, however, many of the trials were poorly designed, raising some concern about the validity of any conclusions drawn from a meta-analysis. Some common problems included small sample size and inappropriate primary end points (ie, other than survival). Furthermore, many of these trials did not distinguish patients with locally advanced unresectable disease from patients who had true metastatic disease; clearly different subsets that could have created significant unrecognized biases. Most importantly, most of these studies consisted primarily of gastric tumors, and whereas some included a proportion of gastroesophageal tumors, none of them treated exclusively esophageal tumors. It is consequently questionable whether the findings from this meta-analysis can be extrapolated to the management of advanced stage esophageal and gastroesophageal junction cancers.

There has been significant progress since 2001, with several well-designed clinical trials published contributing significantly to the management of advanced stage gastro-esophageal cancer.[61–69] Although these contemporary studies should be viewed to be primarily gastric cancer oriented, they all contain a sizeable proportion of gastroesophageal junction tumors, and two also contain true esophageal ACs as well as SCCs. Furthermore, whereas each of these individual trials has faults, as a group they tend to build on previously available results in a logical, stepwise fashion. Combining the findings of the 2006 meta-analysis[84] with the publications reviewed in this section, one can ultimately conclude the following: first-line chemotherapy for advanced stage esophageal and gastroesophageal cancer should be either docetaxel/cisplatin/5-FU (DCF) or epirubi-cin/cisplatin/5-FU (ECF), and that within the latter regimen oxaliplatin can be substituted for cisplatin, and capecitabine can be substituted for 5-FU. Furthermore, there is also supporting data for the use of irinotecan in combination with 5-FU and folinic acid. The basis for these conclusions is based primarily on the studies from this section considered "Ia" and reviewed in detail at the end of the article.[64,65,69,70]

SUMMARY OF LEVEL IA EVIDENCE

1. Medical Research Council Esophageal Cancer Working Group. Surgical resection with or without preoperative chemotherapy in esophageal cancer: a randomized controlled trial. Lancet 2002;359:1727–33.[15]

Hypothesis: Induction chemotherapy before surgery improves OS compared with surgery alone in resectable esophageal cancer of any cell type.

Outcome: Hypothesis supported.

No. of Patients Randomized	Study Groups	Stratification	Significance	% Change P value
802	Two cycles cisplatin 80 mg/m² plus 5-FU 4000 mg/m² followed by surgery N=402 Surgery alone N=400	Surgeon, tumor site, WHO performance status, histology	OS improved DFS improved	16.8 vs 13.3 months median survival; HR=0.79; P = .004. HR = 0.74, P = .0014

Published abstract: BACKGROUND: The outlook for patients with esophageal cancer undergoing surgical resection with curative intent is poor. We aimed to assess the effects of preoperative chemotherapy on survival, dysphagia, and performance status in this group of patients. METHODS: 802 previously untreated patients with resectable esophageal cancer of any cell type were randomly allocated either two 4-day cycles, three weeks apart, of cisplatin 80 mg/m^2 by infusion over 4 h plus 5-FU 1000 mg/m^2 daily by continuous infusion for four days followed by surgical resection (CS group, n = 400), or resection alone (S group, 402). Clinicians could choose to give preoperative RT to all their patients irrespective of randomization. Primary outcome measure was survival time. Analysis was by intention to treat. FINDINGS: No patients dropped out of the study. Resection was microscopically complete in 233 (60%) of 390 assessable CS patients and 215 (54%) of 397 S patients (P<.0001). Postoperative complications were reported in 146 (41%) CS and 161 (42%) S patients. OS was better in the CS group (hazard ratio 0.79; 95% CI 0.67–0.93; P = .004). Median survival was 512 days (16.8 months) in the CS group compared with 405 days (13.3 months) in the S group (difference 107 days; 95% CI 30–196), and two-year survival rates were 43% and 34% (difference 9%; 3–14). INTERPRETATION: Two cycles of preoperative cisplatin and 5-FU improve survival without additional serious adverse events in the treatment of patients with resectable esophageal cancer. (Copyright © 2002, Elsevier. Reprinted with permission.)

Editor's comments: This large trial changed practice throughout Europe when first published. It remains strong evidence in favor of induction chemotherapy before surgery. R0 resection rate was improved (60% vs 54%, P<.0001) and increased postoperative complication rates were not observed. Detractors have criticized its minimal preoperative staging (consisting in some cases of no more than a CXR and liver ultrasound) and clinical follow-up; however, the pragmatic design allowed enrollment of the largest cohort of patients to date and allows the results to be applied to patients in the general community with confidence.

2. Tepper J, Krasna MJ, Niedzwiecki D, et al. Phase III trial of trimodality therapy with cisplatin, fluorouracil, radiotherapy, and surgery compared with surgery alone for esophageal cancer: CALGB 9781. J Clin Oncol 2008;26:1086–92.[17]

Hypothesis: Induction CRT before surgery improves OS compared with surgery alone in resectable esophageal cancer of any cell type.

No. of Patients Randomized	Study Groups	Stratification	Significance	% Change P value
56	Two cycles cisplatin 100 mg/m^2, 5-FU 4000 mg/m^2, plus 50.4 Gy concurrent RT followed by surgery N = 30 Surgery alone N=26	CT N$_1$ nodes, clinical stage, histology	OS improved	4.48 vs 1.78 y median survival; P = .002

Outcome: Hypothesis supported.

Published abstract: PURPOSE: The primary treatment modality for patients with carcinoma of the esophagus or gastroesophageal junction has been surgery, although primary RT with concurrent chemotherapy produces similar results. As both have curative potential, there has been great interest in the use of trimodality therapy. To this end, we compared survival, response, and patterns of failure of trimodality therapy to esophagectomy alone in patients with nonmetastatic esophageal cancer. PATIENTS AND METHODS: Four hundred seventy-five eligible patients were planned for enrollment. Patients were randomly assigned to either esophagectomy with node dissection alone or cisplatin 100 mg/m^2 and fluorouracil 1000 mg/m^2/d for 4 days on weeks 1 and 5 concurrent with radiation therapy (50.4 Gy total: 1.8 Gy/fraction over 5.6 weeks) followed by esophagectomy with node dissection. RESULTS: Fifty-six patients were enrolled between October 1997 and March 2000, when the trial was closed due to poor accrual. Thirty patients were randomly assigned to trimodality therapy and 26 were assigned to surgery alone. Patient and tumor characteristics were similar between groups. Treatment was generally well tolerated. Median follow-up was six years. An intent-to-treat analysis showed a median survival of 4.48 vs 1.79 years in favor of trimodality therapy (exact stratified log-rank, $P = .002$). Five-year survival was 39% (95% CI, 21%–57%) vs 16% (95% CI, 5%–33%) in favor of trimodality therapy. CONCLUSION: The results from this trial reflect a long-term survival advantage with the use of CRT followed by surgery in the treatment of esophageal cancer, and support trimodality therapy as a standard of care for patients with this disease. (Copyright © 2008, American Society of Clinical Oncology. Reprinted with permission.)

Editor's comments: Despite poor accrual (<12% of planned enrolment was achieved) and a relatively small sample size, the reported clear survival advantage of preoperative CRT over surgery alone lends support to advocates of this approach. There is intellectual danger and little scientific merit in the comparison of results between trials; even so the superlative result of this trial (4.48 vs 1.79 years, $P = .002$) compared with previous trials in improvement in and absolute median survival can perhaps be explained by two factors: first, thorough staging including CT, EUS, laparoscopy, and thoracoscopy confirmed only 25% of patients with clinical N1 disease, much less than the usual clinical population of whom around 80% can be expected to present with T_3N_1 disease; second, modern RT planning and concurrent delivery with chemotherapy were employed, resulting in complete pathologic response in 10 of 26 patients. Of concern, 3.3% (1/30) patients died during induction and of interest, the 95% CIs of five-year survival overlap (21%–57% vs 5%–33%). These two factors could be further evaluated in an appropriately powered trial; however, given the authors' advocacy of trimodality therapy as a "standard of care," such a trial is unlikely to ever be mounted in North America.

3. Stahl M, Stuschke M, Lehmann N, et al. Chemoradiation with and without surgery in patients with locally advanced squamous cell carcinoma of the esophagus. J Clin Oncol 2005;23:2310-7.[28]

Hypothesis: High-dose CRT with curative intent will have equivalent OS to induction CRT and surgery in resectable SCCs of the upper two-thirds of the esophagus.

No. of Patients Randomized	Study Groups	Stratification	Significance	% Change P value
172	Three cycles cisplatin, leucovorin, 5-FU, and etoposide Cisplatin, etoposide plus 40 Gy concurrent RT Surgery N=86	Center, TNM, EUS, sex, weight loss	OS equivalent	16.4 vs 14.9 months median survival; $P = .02$ (ie, implying no significant difference in survival)
	Three cycles cisplatin, leucovorin, 5-FU, and etoposide Cisplatin, etoposide plus 65 Gy concurrent RT N=86			

Outcome: Hypothesis supported.

Published abstract: PURPOSE: Combined CRT with and without surgery are widely accepted alternatives for the curative treatment of patients with locally advanced esophageal cancer. The value of adding surgery to chemotherapy and RT is unknown. PATIENTS AND METHODS: Patients with locally advanced SCC (SCC) of the esophagus were randomly allocated to either induction chemotherapy followed by CRT (40 Gy) followed by surgery (arm A), or the same induction chemotherapy followed by CRT (at least 65 Gy) without surgery (arm B). Primary outcome was OS time. RESULTS: The median observation time was six years. The analysis of 172 eligible, randomized patients (86 patients per arm) showed OS to be equivalent between the two treatment groups (log-rank test for equivalence, $P<.05$). Local PFS was better in the surgery group (two-year PFS, 64.3%; 95% CI, 52.1%–76.5%) than in the CRT group (two-year PFS, 40.7%; 95% CI, 28.9%–52.5%; hazard ratio [HR] for arm B vs arm A, 2.1; 95% CI, 1.3–3.5; $P = .003$). Treatment-related mortality was significantly increased in the surgery group than in the CRT group (12.8% vs 3.5%, respectively; $P = .03$). Cox regression analysis revealed clinical tumor response to induction chemotherapy to be the single independent prognostic factor for OS (HR, 0.30; 95% CI, 0.19–0.47; $P<.0001$). CONCLUSION: Adding surgery to CRT improves local tumor control but does not increase survival of patients with locally advanced esophageal SCC. Tumor response to induction chemotherapy identifies a favorable prognostic group within these high-risk patients, regardless of the treatment group. (Copyright © 2005, American Society of Clinical Oncology. Reprinted with permission.)

Editor's comments: The design and outcome of this trial imply that definitive CRT of SCC of the upper two-thirds of the esophagus is equivalent to induction CRT and surgery in terms of OS. "Equivalence" was defined statistically as a less than 43% reduction in two-year survival (from an expected 35% two-year survival in the trimodality arm to 20% in the definitive CRT arm). When treatments are equivalent in terms of OS, attention logically turns to other measures of outcome. Excellent rates of freedom from progression at two years (64.3% vs 40.7%, $P = .003$) imply superior oncological outcome, whereas excessive treatment-related deaths in the trimodality arm (11/86 [12.8%] vs 3/85 [3.5%], $P = .03$) may explain why OS was not significantly different between the two arms. Regression analysis revealed response to initial induction chemotherapy to be the only significant predictor of survival. In summary, there was no difference in OS, progression was less common, and treatment-related death more common in the trimodality arm, while response to induction chemotherapy (regardless of other treatments) was the only significant predictor of survival.

4. Hulscher JBF, van Sandick JW, de Boer AGEM, et al. Extended transthoracic resection compared with limited transhiatal resection for adenocarcinoma of the esophagus. N Engl J Med 2002;347:1662–9.[29]

Hypothesis: OS and DFS will be superior after transthoracic esophagectomy with extended lymphadenectomy compared with transhiatal esophagectomy.

No. of Patients Randomized	Study Groups	Stratification	Significance	% Change P value
220	Transhiatal esophagectomy N=106	Tumor, center	No difference in OS	1.8 vs 2 years median survival;
			No difference in DFS	$P = .38$
	Transthoracic esophagectomy with lymph node dissection N=114			29% vs 38% 5 year survival (CI of difference −3% to 23%)

Outcome: Hypothesis not supported.

Published abstract: BACKGROUND: Controversy exists about the best surgical treatment for esophageal carcinoma. METHODS: We randomly assigned 220 patients with adenocarcinoma of the mid-to-distal esophagus or adenocarcinoma of the gastric cardia involving the distal esophagus either to transhiatal esophagectomy or to trans-thoracic esophagectomy with extended en bloc lymphadenectomy. Principal end points were OS and disease-free survival. Early morbidity and mortality, the number of quality-adjusted life-years gained, and cost effectiveness were also determined. RESULTS: A total of 106 patients were assigned to undergo transhiatal esophagec-tomy, and 114 to undergo transthoracic esophagectomy. Demographic characteristics and characteristics of the tumor were similar in the two groups. Perioperative morbidity was higher after transthoracic esophagectomy, but there was no significant difference in in-hospital mortality ($P = .45$). After a median follow-up of 4.7 years, 142 patients had died—74 (70%) after transhiatal resection and 68 (60%) after transthoracic resection ($P = .12$). Although the difference in survival was not statistically significant, there was a trend toward a survival benefit with the extended approach at five years: disease-free survival was 27% in the transhiatal-esophagectomy group, as compared with 39% in the transthoracic-esophagectomy group (95% confidence interval for the difference, -1% to 24% [the negative value indicates better survival with transhiatal resection]), whereas OS was 29% as compared with 39% (95% confidence interval for the difference, -3% to 23%). CONCLUSIONS: Transhiatal esophagectomy was associ-ated with lower morbidity than transthoracic esophagectomy with extended en bloc lymphadenectomy. Although median overall, disease-free, and quality-adjusted survival did not differ statistically between the groups, there was a trend toward improved long-term survival at five years with the extended transthoracic approach. (Copyright © 2002, Massachusetts Medical Society. All rights reserved.)

Editor's comments: This trial reached its planned enrollment of 220 patients providing 90% power to detect a 50% improvement in OS. Although a clinically mean-ingful 31% improvement in actuarial five-year survival from 29% to 38% was observed, favoring the transthoracic group, this difference was not statistically signif-icant. Thus the major shortcoming of the trial was planning for such an optimistic improvement in OS. Pulmonary complications, chyle leak, ventilator-dependent days, and days in intensive care unit were all significantly reduced in the transhiatal group, although perioperative mortality was no different. Therefore, transthoracic esophagectomy increased major nonfatal complications without either associated increased perioperative mortality or improved OS.

5. Cunningham D, Starling N, Rao S, et al. Capecitabine and oxaliplatin for advanced esophagogastric cancer. N Engl J Med 2008;358:36–46.[64]

Hypothesis: In patients with advanced esophagogastric cancer, chemotherapeutic triplets containing capecitabine versus fluorouracil and oxaliplatin versus cisplatin will not have inferior OS.

No. of Patients Randomized	Study Groups	Stratification	Significance	% Change *P* value
1002	ECF N= 263 ECX N=250 EOF N= 245 EOX N=244	Performance, center, extent of disease	n.b. CI did not cross 1.23 and as such, treatments considered not different in terms of OS	Capecitabine HR for death 0.86 95% CI = 0.80–0.99 Oxaliplatin HR for death 0.92 95% CI = 0.80–1.10

Abbreviations: E, epirubicin; C, cisplatin; F, fluorouracil; X, capecitabine; O, oxaliplatin.

Outcome: Hypothesis supported.

Published abstract: BACKGROUND: We evaluated capecitabine (an oral fluoropyri-midine) and oxaliplatin (a platinum compound) as alternatives to infused fluorouracil and cisplatin, respectively, for untreated advanced esophagogastric cancer. METHODS: In a 2-by-2 design, we randomly assigned 1002 patients to receive triplet therapy with epirubicin and cisplatin plus either fluorouracil (ECF) or capecitabine (ECX), or triplet therapy with epirubicin and oxaliplatin plus either fluorouracil (EOF) or capecitabine (EOX). The primary end point was noninferiority in overall survival for the triplet therapies containing capecitabine as compared with fluorouracil and for those containing oxaliplatin as compared with cisplatin. RESULTS: For the capecitabine-fluorouracil comparison, the hazard ratio for death in the capecitabine group was 0.86 (95% confidence interval [CI], 0.80–0.99); for the oxaliplatin-cisplatin comparison, the hazard ratio for the oxaliplatin group was 0.92 (95% CI, 0.80–1.10). The upper limit of the confidence intervals for both hazard ratios excluded the predefined noninferiority margin of 1.23. Median survival times in the ECF, ECX, EOF, and EOX groups were 9.9 months, 9.9 months, 9.3 months, and 11.2 months, respectively; survival rates at one year were 37.7%, 40.8%, 40.4%, and 46.8%, respectively. In the secondary analysis, overall survival was longer with EOX than with ECF, with a hazard ratio for death of 0.80 in the EOX group (95% CI, 0.66–0.97; $P = .02$). Progression-free survival and response rates did not differ significantly among the regimens. Toxic effects of capecitabine and fluorouracil were similar. As compared with cisplatin, oxaliplatin was associated with lower incidences of grade III or IV neutropenia, alopecia, renal toxicity, and thromboembolism but with slightly higher incidences of grade III or IV diarrhea and neuropathy. CONCLUSIONS: Capecitabine and oxaliplatin are as effective as fluorouracil and cisplatin, respectively, in patients with previously untreated esophagogastric cancer. (Copyright © 2008, Massachusetts Medical Society. All rights reserved.)

Editor's comments: This study was a follow-up to the group's previous study,[71] which had established ECF as a standard regimen. The REAL 2 study was designed to see if O could replace C and if X could replace F. The potential benefit of these replacements was decreased toxicity and ease of administration. Patients with locally advanced (inoperable) or metastatic adenocarcinoma and SCC of the esophagus, gastroesophageal junction, and stomach were randomized to four groups: ECF, ECX, EOF, or EOX. The primary end point was noninferiority of OS. Secondary end points included PFS, response rate (RR), toxicity, and quality of life (QOL). 1002 patients were accrued from 2000 to 2005. Groups were well balanced. EOX appeared to have the best OS. PFS, and RR appeared to be similar between the groups. In addition, O had less toxicity than C. QOL was poorly documented. The overall conclusion from this study was that EOX was at least as efficacious as any other regimen, but less toxic and easier to administer.

6. Van Cutsem E, Moiseyenko VM, Tjulandin S, et al. Phase III study of docetaxel and cisplatin plus fluorouracil compared with cisplatin and fluorouracil as first-line therapy for advanced gastric cancer: a report of the V325 Study Group. J Clin Oncol 2006;24:4991–7.[69]

Hypothesis: In patients with advanced gastric cancer, time to progression will be prolonged after treatment with DCF compared with CF.

No. of Patients Randomized	Study Groups	Stratification	Significance	% Change P value
445	DCF N = 221 CF N = 224	Center Liver metastases Measurable disease Weight loss	TTP improved OS improved	DCF vs CF 32% risk reduction P = .02 DCF vs CF 23% risk reduction P<.001

Abbreviations: D, docetaxel; C, cisplatin; F, fluorouracil; TTP, Time to progression.

Outcome: Hypothesis supported.

Published abstract: PURPOSE: In the randomized, multinational phase II/III trial (V325) of untreated advanced gastric cancer patients, the phase II part selected docetaxel, cisplatin, and fluorouracil (DCF) over docetaxel and cisplatin for comparison against cisplatin and fluorouracil (CF; reference regimen) in the phase III part. PATIENTS AND METHODS: Advanced gastric cancer patients were randomly assigned to docetaxel 75 mg/m^2 and cisplatin 75 mg/m^2 (day 1) plus fluorouracil 750 mg/m^2/d (days 1 to 5) every three weeks or cisplatin 100 mg/m^2 (day 1) plus fluorouracil 1,000 mg/m^2/d (days 1 to 5) every four weeks. The primary end point was time-to-progression (TTP). RESULTS: In 445 randomly assigned and treated patients (DCF = 221; CF = 224); TTP was longer with DCF versus CF (32% risk reduction; log-rank $P<.001$). Overall survival was longer with DCF versus CF (23% risk reduction; log-rank $P = .02$). Two-year survival rate was 18% with DCF and 9% with CF. Overall response rate was higher with DCF (chi2 $P = .01$). Grade III to IV treatment-related adverse events occurred in 69% (DCF) v 59% (CF) of patients. Frequent grade III to IV toxicities for DCF v CF were: neutropenia (82% v 57%), stomatitis (21% v 27%), diarrhea (19% v 8%), lethargy (19% v 14%). Complicated neutropenia was more frequent with DCF than CF (29% v 12%). CONCLUSION: Adding docetaxel to CF significantly improved TTP, survival, and response rate in gastric cancer patients, but resulted in some increase in toxicity. Incorporation of docetaxel, as in DCF or with other active drug(s), is a new therapy option for patients with untreated advanced gastric cancer. (Copyright © 2006, American Society of Clinical Oncology. Reprinted with permission.)

Editor's comments: This study evaluated whether adding D to CF, one standard regimen for advanced gastric and GE junction cancers, results in better disease control. The V-325 study also resulted in two additional publications regarding the clinical benefits and QOL of the two regimens. Patients with metastatic or locally recurrent disease secondary to gastric or gastroesophageal AC were randomized to either to DCF or to CF. The primary end point was TTP. Secondary end points were OS, overall response rate (ORR), safety, QOL, and clinical benefit. Four hundred and fifty seven patients were randomized. The two groups were well balanced. TTP was longer in DCF (5.6 mo vs 3.7 m, $P<.001$, respectively). Likewise, OS was longer, ORR was higher, and QOL was better in the DCF arm. DCF had more treatment related neutropenic complications. This study clearly shows the superiority of DCF over CF. Two subsequent publications also showed that DCF resulted in better QOL[61] and clinical benefit.[62]

7. Dank M, Zaluski J, Barone C, et al. Randomized phase III study comparing irinotecan combined with 5-fluorouracil and folinic acid to cisplatin combined with 5-fluorouracil in chemotherapy naïve patients with advanced adenocarcinoma of the stomach or esophagogastric junction. Ann Oncol 2008;19:1450–7.[65]

Hypothesis: In patients with chemonaïve gastric or esophagogastric AC, time to progression will be prolonged after treatment with IF compared with CF.

No. of Patients Randomized	Study Groups	Stratification	Significance	% Change P value
333	IF N= 170 CF N= 163	Center, prior surgery, weight loss, liver metastases	TTP no difference OS improved TTF improved	5.0 vs 4.2 months median, $P = .088$ 9.0 vs 8.7 months median, $P<.001$ 4.0 vs 3.4 months median, $P = .018$

Abbreviations: IF, irinotecan/5-fluorouracil; CF, cisplatin/5-fluorouracil; TTP, time to progression; TTF, time to treatment failure.

Outcome: Hypothesis not supported.

Published abstract: BACKGROUND: We aimed to establish the superiority (or noninferiority if superiority was not achieved) in terms of time to progression (TTP) of irinotecan/5-fluorouracil (IF) over cisplatin/5-fluorouracil (CF) in chemonaïve patients with adenocarcinoma of the stomach/esophagogastric junction. PATIENTS AND METHODS: Patients received either IF: i.v. irinotecan 80 mg/m^2 30 min, folinic acid 500 mg/m^2 2 h, 5-fluorouracil (5-FU) 2000 mg/m^2 22 h, for 6/7 weeks or CF: cisplatin 100 mg/m^2 1–3 h, with 5-FU 1000 mg/m^2/day 24 h, days 1–5, every 4 weeks. RESULTS: In all, 333 patients were randomized and treated (IF 170, CF 163). Patient characteristics were balanced except more IF patients had Karnofsky performance status 100%. TTP for IF was 5.0 months (95% confidence interval [CI] 3.8–5.8) and 4.2 months (95% CI 3.7–5.5) for CF (*P* = .088). Overall survival (OS) was 9.0 versus 8.7 months, response rate 31.8% versus 25.8%, time to treatment failure (TTF) 4.0 versus 3.4 months for IF and CF, respectively. The difference in TTF was statistically significant (*P* = .018). IF was better in terms of toxic deaths (0.6% vs 3%), discontinuation for toxicity (10.0% vs 21.5%), severe neutropenia, thrombocytopenia, and stomatitis, but not diarrhea. CONCLUSION: IF did not yield a significant TTP or OS superiority over CF, and the results of noninferiority of IF were borderline. However, IF may provide a viable, platinum-free front-line treatment alternative for metastatic gastric cancer. (Copyright © 2008, Oxford University Press. Reprinted with permission.)

Editor's comments: This study evaluated whether CPT11/F/FA was better than CF. The combination of CPT11/F/FA was chosen based on a previous trial by Pozzo and colleagues[67] comparing CPT11/5-FU/FA to CPT 11/C, in which the two regimens were equally effective but the former was better tolerated. Patients with metastatic or locally recurrent adenocarcinoma of the stomach and GE junction were randomized to either CPT11/F/FA or CF. The primary end point was TTP. Secondary end points included RR, duration of response, TTF, and OS. Three hundred and thirty-seven patients were randomized. The two groups were imbalanced with respect to data regarding response evaluation as well as the initial Karnofsky Performance Status score. TTP and OS were the same. TTF was better in CPT11/F/FA (4 months vs 3.4 months, *P* = .018). This study showed that CPT11/F/FA was at least as effective as CF, and perhaps that it was better tolerated.

8. Ross P, Nicolson M, Cunningham D, et al. Prospective randomized trial comparing mitomycin, cisplatin, and protracted venous-infusion fluorouracil (PVI 5-FU) with epirubicin, cisplatin, and PVI 5-FU in advanced esophagogastric cancer. J Clin Oncol 2002;20:1996–2004.[70]

Hypothesis: In previously untreated patients with advanced esophagogastric cancer, survival, response, toxicity, and QOL will be improved after treatment with ECF compared with MCF.

No. of Patients Randomized	Study Groups	Stratification	Significance	% Change *P* value
580	ECF N= 289 MCF N= 285	Center	ORR no difference OS no different Global QOL scores were better with ECF at 3 and 6 months	42.4% vs 44.1%, *P* = .692 9.4 vs 8.7 months median, *P* = .315

Abbreviations: ECF, epirubicin, cisplatin, and protracted venous-infusion fluorouracil (PVI 5-FU); MCF, mitomycin, cisplatin, and PVI 5-FU; ORR, overall response rate.

Outcome: Hypothesis not supported.

Published abstract: PURPOSE: We report the results of a prospectively randomized study that compared the combination of epirubicin, cisplatin, and protracted venous-infusion fluorouracil (PVI 5-FU) (ECF) with the combination of mitomycin, cisplatin, and PVI 5-FU (MCF) in previously untreated patients with advanced esophagogastric cancer. PATIENTS AND METHODS: Five hundred eighty patients with adenocarcinoma, squamous carcinoma, or undifferentiated carcinoma were randomized to receive either ECF (epirubicin 50 mg/m^2 every three weeks, cisplatin 60 mg/m^2 every three weeks, and PVI 5-FU 200 mg/m^2/d) or MCF (mitomycin 7 mg/m^2 every six weeks, cisplatin 60 mg/m^2 every three weeks, and PVI 5-FU 300 mg/m^2/d) and analyzed for survival, response, toxicity, and quality of life (QOL). RESULTS: The overall response rate was 42.4% (95% confidence interval [CI], 37%–48%) with ECF and 44.1% (95% CI, 38%–50%) with MCF ($P = .692$). Toxicity was tolerable, and there were only two toxic deaths. ECF resulted in more grade III/IV neutropenia and grade II alopecia, but MCF caused more thrombocytopenia and plantar-palmar erythema. Median survival was 9.4 months with ECF and 8.7 months with MCF ($P = .315$); at one year, 40.2% (95% CI, 34%–46%) of ECF and 32.7% (95% CI, 27%–38%) of MCF patients were alive. Median failure-free survival was seven months with both regimens. Global QOL scores were better with ECF at three and six months. CONCLUSION: This study confirms response, survival, and QOL benefits of ECF observed in a previous randomized study. The equivalent efficacy of MCF was demonstrated, but QOL was superior with ECF. ECF remains one of the reference treatments for advanced esophagogastric cancer. (Copyright © 2002, American Society of Clinical Oncology. Reprinted with permission.)

Editor's comments: This study was a follow-up on a prior study that had established that ECF was better than the then standard of care, FAMTX (fluorouracil, doxorubicin, methotrexate).[71] The impetus for this current study was to see if mitomycin could be substituted for epirubicin to allow higher dosing of the 5-FU. The primary end point was OS and the secondary end points included toxicity, OR, and QOL. Patients with inoperable AC and SCC of the esophagus, GE junction, and stomach were randomized to either ECF or MCF. Five hundred and eighty patients were randomized. The groups were not balanced regarding locally advanced versus metastatic disease. OS, OR, and toxicity were similar both on univariate and multivariate analysis. QOL was better in the ECF group, albeit this was a poorly documented end point. The conclusion from this study was that whereas the efficacy was equivalent, QOL was better with ECF.

DISCLOSURE

Authors have nothing to disclose.

REFERENCES

1. Fiorica F, Di Bona D, Schepis F, et al. Preoperative chemoradiotherapy for oesophageal cancer: a systematic review and meta-analysis. Gut 2004;53:925.
2. Gebski V, Burmeister B, Smithers BM, et al. Survival benefits from neoadjuvant chemoradiotherapy or chemotherapy in oesophageal carcinoma: a meta-analysis. Lancet Oncol 2007;8:226.
3. Greer SE, Goodney PP, Sutton JE, et al. Neoadjuvant chemoradiotherapy for esophageal carcinoma: a meta-analysis. Surgery 2005;137:172.

4. Kaklamanos IG, Walker GR, Ferry K, et al. Neoadjuvant treatment for resectable cancer of the esophagus and the gastroesophageal junction: a meta-analysis of randomized clinical trials. Ann Surg Oncol 2003;10:754.

5. Malthaner RA, Collin S, Fenlon D. Preoperative chemotherapy for resectable thoracic esophageal cancer. Cochrane Database Syst Rev 2006;(3):CD001556.

6. Malthaner RA, Wong RK, Rumble RB, et al. Neoadjuvant or adjuvant therapy for resectable esophageal cancer: a systematic review and meta-analysis. BMC Med 2004;2:35.

7. Urschel JD, Vasan H. A meta-analysis of randomized controlled trials that compared neoadjuvant chemoradiation and surgery to surgery alone for resectable esophageal cancer. Am J Surg 2003;185:538.

8. Wong R, Malthaner R. Esophageal cancer: a systematic review. Curr Probl Cancer 2000;24:297.

9. Chiu PWY, Chan ACW, Leung SF, et al. Multicenter prospective randomized trial comparing standard esophagectomy with chemoradiotherapy for treatment of squamous esophageal cancer: early results from the Chinese University Research Group for Esophageal Cancer (CURE). J Gastrointest Surg 2005;9:794.

10. Ancona E, Ruol A, Santi S, et al. Only pathologic complete response to neoadjuvant chemotherapy improves significantly the long term survival of patients with resectable esophageal squamous cell carcinoma: final report of a randomized, controlled trial of preoperative chemotherapy versus surgery alone. Cancer 2001;91:2165.

11. Burmeister BH, Smithers BM, Gebski V, et al. Surgery alone versus chemoradiotherapy followed by surgery for resectable cancer of the oesophagus: a randomised controlled phase III trial. Lancet Oncol 2005;6:659.

12. Cunningham D, Allum WH, Stenning SP, et al. Perioperative chemotherapy versus surgery alone for resectable gastroesophageal cancer. N Engl J Med 2006;355:11.

13. Kelsen DP, Winter KA, Gunderson LL, et al. Long-term results of RTOG trial 8911 (USA Intergroup 113): a random assignment trial comparison of chemotherapy followed by surgery compared with surgery alone for esophageal cancer. J Clin Oncol 2007;25:3719.

14. Lee JL, Park SI, Kim SB, et al. A single institutional phase III trial of preoperative chemotherapy with hyperfractionation radiotherapy plus surgery versus surgery alone for resectable esophageal squamous cell carcinoma. Ann Oncol 2004; 15:947.

15. Medical Research Council Oesophageal Cancer Working Group. Surgical resection with or without preoperative chemotherapy in oesophageal cancer: a randomised controlled trial. Lancet 2002;359:1727.

16. Natsugoe S, Okumura H, Matsumoto M, et al. Randomized controlled study on preoperative chemoradiotherapy followed by surgery versus surgery alone for esophageal squamous cell cancer in a single institution. Dis Esophagus 2006;19:468.

17. Tepper J, Krasna MJ, Niedzwiecki D, et al. Phase III trial of trimodality therapy with cisplatin, fluorouracil, radiotherapy, and surgery compared with surgery alone for esophageal cancer: CALGB 9781. J Clin Oncol 2008;26:1086.

18. Urba SG, Orringer MB, Turrisi A, et al. Randomized trial of preoperative chemoradiation versus surgery alone in patients with locoregional esophageal carcinoma. J Clin Oncol 2001;19:305.

19. Walsh TN, Grennell M, Mansoor S, et al. Neoadjuvant treatment of advanced stage esophageal adenocarcinoma increases survival. Dis Esophagus 2002; 15:121.

20. Walsh TN, Noonan N, Hollywood D, et al. A comparison of multimodal therapy and surgery for esophageal adenocarcinoma. N Engl J Med 1996;335:462.
21. Kelsen DP, Ginsberg R, Pajak TF, et al. Chemotherapy followed by surgery compared with surgery alone for localized esophageal cancer. N Engl J Med 1998;339:1979.
22. Ando N, Iizuka T, Ide H, et al. Surgery plus chemotherapy compared with surgery alone for localized squamous cell carcinoma of the thoracic esophagus: a Japan Clinical Oncology Group Study—JCOG9204. J Clin Oncol 2003;21:4592.
23. Macdonald JS, Smalley SR, Benedetti J, et al. Chemoradiotherapy after surgery compared with surgery alone for adenocarcinoma of the stomach or gastro-esophageal junction. N Engl J Med 2001;345:725.
24. Tachibana M, Yoshimura H, Kinugasa S, et al. Postoperative chemotherapy vs chemoradiotherapy for thoracic esophageal cancer: a prospective randomized clinical trial. Eur J Surg Oncol 2003;29:580.
25. Xiao ZF, Yang ZY, Liang J, et al. Value of radiotherapy after radical surgery for esophageal carcinoma: a report of 495 patients. Ann Thorac Surg 2003;75:331.
26. Bedenne L, Michel P, Bouche O, et al. Chemoradiation followed by surgery compared with chemoradiation alone in squamous cancer of the esophagus: FFCD 9102. J Clin Oncol 2007;25:1160.
27. Bonnetain F, Bouche O, Michel P, et al. A comparative longitudinal quality of life study using the Spitzer quality of life index in a randomized multicenter phase III trial (FFCD 9102): chemoradiation followed by surgery compared with chemora-diation alone in locally advanced squamous resectable thoracic esophageal cancer. Ann Oncol 2006;17:827.
28. Stahl M, Stuschke M, Lehmann N, et al. Chemoradiation with and without surgery in patients with locally advanced squamous cell carcinoma of the esophagus. J Clin Oncol 2005;23:2310.
29. Hulscher JB, van Sandick JW, de Boer AG, et al. Extended transthoracic resec-tion compared with limited transhiatal resection for adenocarcinoma of the esophagus. N Engl J Med 2002;347:1662.
30. Omloo JMT, Lagarde SM, Hulscher JBF, et al. Extended transthoracic resection compared with limited transhiatal resection for adenocarcinoma of the mid/distal esophagus: five-year survival of a randomized clinical trial. Ann Surg 2007;246:992.
31. Sasako M, Sano T, Yamamoto S, et al. Left thoracoabdominal approach versus abdominal-transhiatal approach for gastric cancer of the cardia or subcardia: a randomised controlled trial. Lancet Oncol 2006;7:644.
32. Hsu H-H, Chen J-S, Huang P-M, et al. Comparison of manual and mechanical cervical esophagogastric anastomosis after esophageal resection for squamous cell carcinoma: a prospective randomized controlled trial. Eur J Cardiothorac Surg 2004;25:1097.
33. Okuyama M, Motoyama S, Suzuki H, et al. Hand-sewn cervical anastomosis versus stapled intrathoracic anastomosis after esophagectomy for middle or lower thoracic esophageal cancer: a prospective randomized controlled study. Surg Today 2007;37:947.
34. Walther B, Johansson J, Johnsson F, et al. Cervical or thoracic anastomosis after esophageal resection and gastric tube reconstruction: a prospective randomized trial comparing sutured neck anastomosis with stapled intrathoracic anasto-mosis. Ann Surg 2003;238:803.
35. Gupta NM, Gupta R, Rao MS, et al. Minimizing cervical esophageal anastomotic complications by a modified technique. Am J Surg 2001;181:534.

36. Bhat MA, Dar MA, Lone GN, et al. Use of pedicled omentum in esophagogastric anastomosis for prevention of anastomotic leak. Ann Thorac Surg 2006;82:1857.
37. Tabira Y, Sakaguchi T, Kuhara H, et al. The width of a gastric tube has no impact on outcome after esophagectomy. Am J Surg 2004;187:417.
38. Shackcloth MJ, McCarron E, Kendall J, et al. Randomized clinical trial to determine the effect of nasogastric drainage on tracheal acid aspiration following oesophagectomy. Br J Surg 2006;93:547.
39. May A, Gossner L, Behrens A, et al. A prospective randomized trial of two different endoscopic resection techniques for early stage cancer of the esophagus. Gastrointest Endosc 2003;58:167.
40. Nagatani S, Shimada Y, Kondo M, et al. A strategy for determining which thoracic esophageal cancer patients should undergo cervical lymph node dissection. Ann Thorac Surg 1881;80:2005.
41. Nakatsuchi T, Otani M, Osugi H, et al. The necessity of chest physical therapy for thoracoscopic oesophagectomy. J Int Med Res 2005;33:434.
42. Farran L, Llop J, Sans M, et al. Efficacy of enteral decontamination in the prevention of anastomotic dehiscence and pulmonary infection in esophagogastric surgery. Dis Esophagus 2008;21:159.
43. Miyazaki T, Kuwano H, Kato H, et al. Predictive value of blood flow in the gastric tube in anastomotic insufficiency after thoracic esophagectomy. World J Surg 2002;26:1319.
44. Wong R, Malthaner R. Combined chemotherapy and radiotherapy (without surgery) compared with radiotherapy alone in localized carcinoma of the esophagus. Cochrane Database Syst Rev 2006;(1):Art. No:CD002092.
45. Herskovic A, Martz K, al-Sarraf M, et al. Combined chemotherapy and radiotherapy compared with radiotherapy alone in patients with cancer of the esophagus. N Engl J Med 1992;326:1593.
46. Gaspar LE, Winter K, Kocha WI, et al. A phase I/II study of external beam radiation, brachytherapy, and concurrent chemotherapy for patients with localized carcinoma of the esophagus (Radiation Therapy Oncology Group Study 9207): final report. Cancer 2000;88:988.
47. Minsky BD, Pajak TF, Ginsberg RJ, et al. INT 0123 (Radiation Therapy Oncology Group 94-05) phase III trial of combined-modality therapy for esophageal cancer: high-dose versus standard-dose radiation therapy. J Clin Oncol 2002;20:1167.
48. Kumar S, Dimri K, Khurana R, et al. A randomised trial of radiotherapy compared with cisplatin chemo-radiotherapy in patients with unresectable squamous cell cancer of the esophagus. Radiother Oncol 2007;83:139.
49. Wang Y, Shi X-H, He S-Q, et al. Comparison between continuous accelerated hyperfractionated and late-course accelerated hyperfractionated radiotherapy for esophageal carcinoma. Int J Radiat Oncol Biol Phys 2002;54:131.
50. Wobbes T, Baron B, Paillot B, et al. Prospective randomised study of split-course radiotherapy versus cisplatin plus split-course radiotherapy in inoperable squamous cell carcinoma of the oesophagus. Eur J Cancer 2001;37:470.
51. Zhao KL, Shi XH, Jiang GL, et al. Late course accelerated hyperfractionated radiotherapy plus concurrent chemotherapy for squamous cell carcinoma of the esophagus: a phase III randomized study. Int J Radiat Oncol Biol Phys 2005;62:1014.
52. Meyers BF, Downey RJ, Decker PA, et al. The utility of positron emission tomography in staging of potentially operable carcinoma of the thoracic esophagus: results of the American College of Surgeons Oncology Group Z0060 trial. J Thorac Cardiovasc Surg 2007;133:738.

53. Puli SR, Reddy JB, Bechtold ML, et al. Staging accuracy of esophageal cancer by endoscopic ultrasound: a meta-analysis and systematic review. World J Gastroenterol 2008;14:1479.
54. Patel AN, Buenaventura PO. Current staging of esophageal carcinoma. Surg Clin North Am 2005;85:555.
55. Krasna MJ, Reed CE, Nedzwiecki D, et al. CALGB 9380: a prospective trial of the feasibility of thoracoscopy/laparoscopy in staging esophageal cancer. Ann Thorac Surg 2001;71:1073.
56. Matthes K, Bounds BC, Collier K, et al. EUS staging of upper GI malignancies: results of a prospective randomized trial. Gastrointest Endosc 2006;64: 496.
57. Siemsen M, Svendsen LB, Knigge U, et al. A prospective randomized comparison of curved array and radial echoendoscopy in patients with esophageal cancer. Gastrointest Endosc 2003;58:671.
58. Mortensen MB, Edwin B, Hunerbein M, et al. Impact of endoscopic ultrasonography (EUS) on surgical decision-making in upper gastrointestinal tract cancer: an international multicenter study. Surg Endosc 2007;21:431.
59. Preston SR, Clark GWB, Martin IG, et al. Effect of endoscopic ultrasonography on the management of 100 consecutive patients with oesophageal and junctional carcinoma. Br J Surg 2003;90:1220.
60. Wagner AD, Grothe W, Haerting J, et al. Chemotherapy in advanced gastric cancer: a systematic review and meta-analysis based on aggregate data. J Clin Oncol 2006;24:2903.
61. Ajani JA, Moiseyenko VM, Tjulandin S, et al. Quality of life with docetaxel plus cisplatin and fluorouracil compared with cisplatin and fluorouracil from a phase III trial for advanced gastric or gastroesophageal adenocarcinoma: the V-325 Study Group. J Clin Oncol 2007;25:3210.
62. Ajani JA, Moiseyenko VM, Tjulandin S, et al. Clinical benefit with docetaxel plus fluorouracil and cisplatin compared with cisplatin and fluorouracil in a phase III trial of advanced gastric or gastroesophageal cancer adenocarcinoma: the V-325 Study Group. J Clin Oncol 2007;25:3205.
63. Al-Batran S-E, Hartmann JT, Probst S, et al. Phase III trial in metastatic gastro-esophageal adenocarcinoma with fluorouracil, leucovorin plus either oxaliplatin or cisplatin: a study of the Arbeitsgemeinschaft Internistische Onkologie. J Clin Oncol 2008;26:1435.
64. Cunningham D, Starling N, Rao S, et al. Capecitabine and oxaliplatin for advanced esophagogastric cancer. N Engl J Med 2008;358:36.
65. Dank M, Zaluski J, Barone C, et al. Randomized phase III study comparing irinotecan combined with 5-fluorouracil and folinic acid to cisplatin combined with 5-fluorouracil in chemotherapy naïve patients with advanced adenocarcinoma of the stomach or esophagogastric junction. Ann Oncol 2008;19:1450.
66. Moehler M, Eimermacher A, Siebler J, et al. Randomised phase II evaluation of irinotecan plus high-dose 5-fluorouracil and leucovorin (ILF) vs 5-fluorouracil, leucovorin, and etoposide (ELF) in untreated metastatic gastric cancer. Br J Cancer 2005;92:2122.
67. Pozzo C, Barone C, Szanto J, et al. Irinotecan in combination with 5-fluorouracil and folinic acid or with cisplatin in patients with advanced gastric or esophageal-gastric junction adenocarcinoma: results of a randomized phase II study. Ann Oncol 2004;15:1773.
68. Tebbutt NC, Norman A, Cunningham D, et al. A multicentre, randomised phase III trial comparing protracted venous infusion (PVI) 5-fluorouracil (5-FU) with PVI

5-FU plus mitomycin C in patients with inoperable oesophago-gastric cancer. Ann Oncol 2002;13:1568.

69. Van Cutsem E, Moiseyenko VM, Tjulandin S, et al. Phase III study of docetaxel and cisplatin plus fluorouracil compared with cisplatin and fluorouracil as first-line therapy for advanced gastric cancer: a report of the V325 Study Group. J Clin Oncol 2006;24:4991.

70. Ross P, Nicolson M, Cunningham D, et al. Prospective randomized trial comparing mitomycin, cisplatin, and protracted venous-infusion fluorouracil (PVI 5-FU) With epirubicin, cisplatin, and PVI 5-FU in advanced esophagogastric cancer. J Clin Oncol 2002;20:1996.

71. Webb A, Cunningham D, Scarffe JH, et al. Randomized trial comparing epirubicin, cisplatin, and fluorouracil versus fluorouracil, doxorubicin, and methotrexate in advanced esophagogastric cancer. J Clin Oncol 1997;15:261.

Randomized Clinical Trials in Gastric Cancer

James J. Mezhir, MD[a], Venu G. Pillarisetty, MD[a],
Manish A. Shah, MD[b], Daniel G. Coit, MD[a],*

KEYWORDS

- Gastric cancer • Randomized clinical trial • Surgery
- Chemotherapy • Neoadjuvant therapy • Adjuvant therapy

In the prior manuscript summarizing randomized clinical trials (RCT) in gastric cancer, 52 trials were reviewed from 1975 to 2000.[1] Of these 52 trials, 23 were designed to study chemotherapy in treating metastatic disease whereas only six trials evaluated surgical technique. In the present article, 64 RCTs published from January 2000 to January 2009 were published for gastric cancer. In contrast to the prior review, only 12 trials focused on the treatment of metastatic disease. Minimally invasive resection has emerged, and there has been continued investigation to determine the appropriate extent of lymphadenectomy in gastric cancer patients. There has also been significant progress in evaluating the role of chemotherapeutic regimens used in the neoadjuvant and adjuvant settings for patients with resectable disease. We also summarize a selection of RCT trials focused on the perioperative care of the gastric cancer patient.

SURGERY
Extent of Lymphadenectomy

The two major lymphadenectomy (LND) trials from the Netherlands[2] and the United Kingdom[3] highlighted in the prior review showed no difference in survival and an increase in complications in patients undergoing D2 compared with D1 dissection.[1] Although well designed and executed, both studies were criticized for methodological flaws with respect to actual extent of LND, which left this crucial question seemingly unanswered. Hartgrink and colleagues[4] reported the final results of the Dutch Gastric

Disclosure: See last page of article.
[a] Department of Surgery, Memorial Sloan-Kettering Cancer Center, 1275 York Avenue, New York, NY 10065, USA
[b] Department of Medicine, Memorial Sloan-Kettering Cancer Center, 1275 York Avenue, New York, NY 10065, USA
* Corresponding author.
E-mail address: coitd@mskcc.org (D.G. Coit).

Surg Oncol Clin N Am 19 (2010) 81–100
doi:10.1016/j.soc.2009.09.011 surgonc.theclinics.com

Cancer Trial with a median follow up of 11 years. The authors defined D1 LND as removal of perigastric lymph nodes along the greater and lesser curvature. A dissection qualified as D2 when the nodal stations of the left gastric, common hepatic, celiac, and splenic arteries were removed. As in the earlier analysis, there was no difference in overall or disease-specific survival between D1 and D2 LND groups. In-hospital mortality, however, was significantly higher in patients randomized to D2 LND. Subset analyses suggested a possible benefit for patients with advanced nodal disease; however, this was not a planned analysis of the trial and therefore the possibility of random significance does exist.

The only study to demonstrate a difference in survival for D1 versus D2 LND was published in 2006.[5] From a single institution in Japan, 221 patients were randomized to D1 or D2 dissection to be performed by surgeons well trained in the technique of extended LND; all specimens were examined by one pathologist. Five-year survival for D2 patients was significantly higher than for D1 patients; however, the absolute increase in survival was small (59.5% versus. 53.6% 5-year survival, $P = .04$). Additionally, there was no statistically significant difference in recurrence between treatment groups among patients who underwent an R0 resection. Perioperative morbidity and mortality were not reported in this study.

Two RCTs have been performed to evaluate the value of para-aortic nodal dissection (PAND), also known as a D4 dissection, in addition to D2 LND. The Japan Clinical Oncology Group (JCOG) randomized 523 patients from 24 centers to D2 LND with or without PAND.[6] There was a trend toward an increase in operative morbidity in patients undergoing PAND (28.1%) compared with D2 LND alone (20.9%; $P = .07$), but no significant difference in overall or recurrence-free survival. Yonemura and colleagues[7] evaluated 269 eligible patients randomized to D2 or D4 dissection and similarly found no difference in overall survival between treatment groups.

To evaluate the extent of LND for proximal lesions, the Japanese Cancer Oncology Group (JCOG) initiated an RCT comparing a left thoracoabdominal (LTA) approach to transhiatal (TH) approach for treatment of Siewert type 2 and 3 lesions.[8] This study was halted at the first interim analysis owing to the unlikely probability of LTA having a survival advantage over TH. There was no statistically significant difference in 5-year overall survival between groups, however there were more complications observed in patients who had LTA.

Splenectomy and pancreatectomy are notable risk factors for complications associated with extensive LND.[3] Two studies have focused on whether or not splenic preservation compromises oncologic outcome in patients undergoing at least a D2 LND.[9,10] Csendes and colleagues[9] randomized 187 patients to D2 LND with or without splenectomy. There was no difference in overall survival but a significant increase in the rate of subphrenic abscess, postoperative fever, or pulmonary complications in patients undergoing splenectomy. A similar and well-designed study by Yu and colleagues[10] was unable to demonstrate a survival benefit from splenectomy and there was no difference in perioperative complications.

In summary, a D2 LND has not been consistently shown to improve overall survival over D1 LND and is associated with an increase in perioperative complications and mortality. Trials to date have not been designed to assess the impact of extended LND on specific subsets of gastric cancer patients. One single-institution study with very high quality control for surgeons and pathologists has shown a small survival benefit to extended LND, but these findings have not been replicated. Furthermore, data do not support a more extensive (D4) LND, as it is associated with more complications without conferring a survival benefit. Preservation of the spleen during D2 LND does not compromise overall survival and may reduce operative complications.

Minimally Invasive Resection

Minimally invasive approaches in surgical oncology are gaining popularity and several trials were performed to evaluate laparoscopic distal gastrectomy; no RCT to date has applied this technique to total gastrectomy. Despite the efforts to study laparoscopic resection, none of the studies met level 1a evidence criteria because of the small numbers of patients and relatively short follow-up. The largest study performed with long-term follow-up is reported by Huscher and colleagues[11] in which patients were randomized to open (N = 29) or laparoscopic (N = 30) subtotal gastrectomy performed by a single surgeon. Perioperative morbidity and mortality were equivalent, although patients who had laparoscopic resection had less blood loss, were started on oral intake earlier, and had a shorter hospital stay than patients treated with open gastrectomy. There was no difference in the number of lymph nodes harvested between the open (33.4 ± 17.4) and laparoscopic (30.0 ± 14.9) groups. Overall 5-year and disease-specific survival were equivalent. The short-term benefits of laparoscopic resection (blood loss, analgesic use, hospital stay) were also reported in other studies with small numbers of patients.[12,13] As expected, the laparoscopic approach was associated with longer operative times in each of the studies performed.

Kim and colleagues[14] initiated the largest RCT to date of 164 patients with early gastric cancer, and recently reported their interim analysis. This is a noninferiority trial with a primary end point of disease-free survival at 5 years. Consistent with earlier studies, patients who underwent laparoscopic resection had less blood loss and required less postoperative analgesia. Pathologic analysis revealed that patients who underwent laparoscopic resection had significantly fewer lymph nodes harvested than did those who had open gastrectomy (39 ± 11.0 versus 45 ± 13.8, $P < .05$). The proximal resection margin was also an average of 1 cm shorter in the laparoscopic group, but this did not reach statistical significance. The authors also studied several quality of life (QOL) measures and patients randomized to laparoscopic resection had significantly better QOL scores up to 3 months after resection. Similar findings came out of a trial from Korea in which 47 patients were randomized to open or laparoscopic distal gastrectomy.[15] In summary, despite the obvious short-term benefits of the laparoscopic approach to gastric resection, the long-term oncologic outcomes remain unknown.

Surgical Site Infection Prophylaxis

There is one large RCT from Japan addressing antibiotic prophylaxis in gastric cancer surgery. Ten centers randomized 501 patients to single-dose cefazolin or ampicillin-sulbactam 30 minutes before surgery or to a multiple dose regimen of the same antibiotic for 3 days. The surgical site infection rate was equivalent between groups and there was no difference in complications.[16]

Reconstruction After Gastrectomy

Several RCTs evaluated reconstruction techniques after gastrectomy. One study compared Billroth I and Roux-en-Y reconstruction after distal gastrectomy in 50 randomized patients.[17] Patients with Roux-en-Y reconstruction had significantly less bile reflux and inflammatory changes in the remnant stomach on endoscopic examination 5 months postoperatively, but equivalent rates of esophagitis. Because patients in the Roux-en-Y group had a significant increase in hospital stay attributed to gastrojejunal stasis, the authors conclude that Roux-en-Y reconstruction is of limited value. Two RCTs compared Roux-en-Y with or without jejunal pouch reconstruction after total gastrectomy.[18,19] Iivonen and colleagues[18] randomized patients

49 patients and found a decrease in dumping syndrome and early satiety but showed equivalent weight gain and nutritional status to those without pouches 15 months after resection. A larger RCT with long-term follow-up showed that quality of life was similar at 1 year, but was significantly improved at 3, 4, and 5 years after surgery in patients with pouch reconstruction.[19] It appears that there may be some long-term benefits to pouch reconstruction, although larger studies with long-term follow-up are necessary before this can be recommended as a standard reconstruction option.

Intraperitoneal Drainage After Gastrectomy

This highly debated topic has been studied in numerous tumor types across many different centers. Two RCTs address the question of the value of intraperitoneal drainage following gastrectomy for cancer.[20,21] One single-surgeon study randomized 170 patients undergoing gastrectomy with at least a D2 dissection and evaluated the impact of drain placement based on the operation performed (subtotal gastrectomy N = 118, total gastrectomy N = 52).[20] There was no difference in postoperative complications between groups, although the incidence of postoperative abscess in this study was only 2% (3/170). A study from Chile randomized 60 patients after total gastrectomy to no drain or placement of two drains surrounding the gastrojejunostomy.[21] There was a statistically significant increase in hospital stay, morbidity, and need for reexploration in patients with intraperitoneal drains. These studies suggest that there is minimal value to and may be harmful consequences of routine intraperitoneal drainage following gastrectomy.

Nasojejunal Decompression After Total Gastrectomy

The largest RCT was from the Italian Total Gastrectomy Study group who evaluated routine nasojejunal tube placement after total gastrectomy with Roux-en-Y reconstruction.[22] A total of 237 patients were randomized to NJT placement or not. All patients underwent radiographic examination with water-soluble contrast on postoperative day 7, and if no leak was detected, a diet was initiated. There was no difference in postoperative morbidity, anastomotic leak, hospital stay, or time to initiate diet between groups. The results of this study and others with similar results, which have been reported in a recent meta-analysis, obviate the need for routine placement of nasojejunal tubes following total gastrectomy.[23–25]

CHEMOTHERAPY WITH AND WITHOUT RADIATION THERAPY
Neoadjuvant Therapy

Four studies investigated the role for neoadjuvant chemotherapy in resectable gastric cancer. The most notable is the Medical Research Council Adjuvant Gastric Infusional Chemotherapy (MAGIC) Trial published in 2006.[26] This study has had a significant impact on the management of resectable gastric cancer. Patients were randomized to surgery alone or to three preoperative plus three postoperative cycles of epirubicin, cisplatin, and 5-fluorouracil (5-FU). The perioperative chemotherapy group seemed to have been down-staged by neoadjuvant chemotherapy, manifest by smaller tumor size and fewer positive nodes than the surgery-only group. At a median follow-up of 4 years, there was a significant improvement in 5-year overall and progression-free survival in patients treated with perioperative chemotherapy, although only 42% of patients in that group completed protocol therapy. Two smaller studies using different regimens were unable to demonstrate a survival benefit of neoadjuvant chemotherapy over surgery alone.[27,28]

One RCT investigated neoadjuvant chemotherapy with or without radiation in locally advanced gastroesophageal (GE) junction tumors (55% Type I, 45% Type II/III) across 15 centers in Germany.[29] The study was closed early because of poor accrual. Patients (N = 126) were randomized to chemotherapy followed by surgery or chemotherapy followed by chemoradiotherapy before surgery. Patients who had chemoradiation had a significantly higher complete pathologic response rate (15.6% versus 2.0%) and more often had tumor-free lymph nodes compared with patients treated with chemotherapy alone. There was no difference in operative complications or survival at 3 years, although there was a trend toward better survival in patients treated with chemoradiation (47.4% versus 27.7%, log rank $P = .07$). In sum, neoadjuvant therapy has become a standard approach in many centers for patients with locally advanced gastric cancer (T3, N any) who are fit to tolerate treatment. Radiation therapy in the neoadjuvant setting should be reserved for appropriately staged distal esophageal and proximal GE junction tumors.

Adjuvant Chemoradiation

One study has been performed during the period of this review that meets level 1a criteria. The Southwest Oncology Group published an RCT (Intergroup 0116) of surgery alone compared with surgery plus adjuvant chemoradiotherapy (CRT).[30] Following R0 resection of gastric or gastroesophageal junction tumors, 556 well-selected patients were randomized to observation or adjuvant CRT. Of note, 54% of patients underwent a D0 lymphadenectomy. Although there was significant toxicity, overall and disease-specific survival were significantly improved in patients treated with adjuvant CRT.

Adjuvant Chemotherapy

There were 16 randomized adjuvant trials of chemotherapy without radiation performed during the period of this review. Numerous attempts to demonstrate a survival advantage to adjuvant systemic chemotherapy have failed, summarized by the prior review and multiple meta-analyses.[1,31] Critical problems associated with these trials include the lack of surgical standardization and the heterogeneity of patient populations being studied. One trial demonstrating a survival benefit from adjuvant therapy was from Japan where patients were randomized to surgery alone or adjuvant S-1, an oral fluoropyrimidine.[32] Surgical quality control was superior to that of the Intergroup 0116 trial, as all patients received D2 or more LND and were staged with peritoneal cytology. The trial was stopped after the first interim analysis at 1 year because of significantly better survival in patients treated with adjuvant S-1.

The remaining trials of adjuvant chemotherapy have demonstrated no benefit over surgery alone. Di Costanzo and colleagues[33] randomized 258 patients to surgery alone or adjuvant chemotherapy with four cycles of cisplatin, epirubicin, 5-FU, and leucovorin (LV) (PELF). Of note, 47% of the patients in the study had fewer than 15 lymph nodes examined on pathologic analysis. At a median follow-up of 73 months, the rate of recurrence and overall and disease-free survival were similar between groups. Similar findings were reported by De Vita and colleagues[34] who randomized 228 patients to adjuvant 5-FU, LV, epirubicin, and etoposide or to surgery alone. In a study to evaluate the addition of epirubicin and cisplatin to 5-FU, Cascinu and colleagues[35] randomized patients to adjuvant PELF versus adjuvant 5-FU/LV; there was no measurable survival benefit. These studies also demonstrated that chemotherapy, when administered in the adjuvant setting, can impose significant toxicity.

The current evidence to date demonstrates that adjuvant therapy is beneficial in most patients. In Western patients, the standard options supported by level 1a studies are perioperative chemotherapy or adjuvant chemoradiotherapy. No study to date has demonstrated a survival benefit to adjuvant chemotherapy alone in a Western population.

Intraperitoneal Therapy

The largest RCT to date investigating intraperitoneal (IP) chemotherapy was published by Yu and colleagues,[36] who randomized 248 patients to surgery alone or early adjuvant IP mitomycin-C (MMC) and 5-FU. All patients underwent D2 LND and chemotherapy patients received a Tenckhoff catheter for delivery starting on the first postoperative day. Patients treated with chemotherapy had a significant increase in intra-abdominal hemorrhage and abscess formation compared with controls; 24% of patients treated with chemotherapy had mild to moderate abdominal pain during treatment. Eight patients (6.4%) in the chemotherapy group died in the perioperative period compared with two (1.6%) in the control group. Despite the significant increase in perioperative morbidity and mortality, treated patients experienced a significant increase in survival and a decrease in peritoneal recurrence. On subgroup analysis, patients with stage I and II disease did not benefit from IP chemotherapy advocating for a better selection algorithm in these patients.

Intraperitoneal chemotherapy has not gained acceptance as a standard adjuvant therapy for gastric cancer in many centers because of the significant potential for perioperative morbidity. Moreover, there exists the potential to over treat patients with early stage disease. With the development of newer systemic agents, IP chemotherapy is unlikely to become a standard modality in the treatment of gastric cancer.

Helicobacter Pylori Eradication

One trial investigated the role for *Helicobacter pylori* eradication following endoscopic mucosal resection (EMR) in patients with early gastric cancer.[37] This was a multicenter RCT from Japan in which 544 patients with documented *H pylori* infection were randomized to treatment or not following EMR. Patients were evaluated for metachronous cancer up to 36 months following resection and it was found that those who underwent treatment for *H pylori* had a significant reduction in the incidence of metachronous cancer (9 new cancers in treated patients versus 24 controls; odds ratio = 0.35).

METASTATIC DISEASE

Prior phase III studies have demonstrated a benefit to chemotherapy over best supportive care for patients with metastatic disease.[1] None of the trials conducted during the time of this review compared chemotherapy to best supportive care; only different chemotherapy regimens. Of note, several of the trials included patients with esophageal and GE junction tumors.

The V325 Study Group compared cisplatin and 5-FU with or without docetaxel (DCF).[38] The addition of docetaxel slightly increased toxicity but resulted in improved response rates, time to progression, and survival (18% versus 9% at 2 years). Two subsequent analyses reported by this group reported significant improvement in "clinical benefit" measured by performance status[39] and quality of life[40] in patients treated with DCF chemotherapy.

Cunningham and colleagues[41] set out to demonstrate noninferiority of capecitabine to 5-FU and oxaliplatin to cisplatin in patients with advanced gastric and esophageal cancer. More than 1000 patients were randomized in a two-by-two design to epirubicin and cisplatin with either 5-FU (ECF) or capecitabine (ECX) or epirubicin and oxaliplatin plus either 5-FU (EOF) or capecitabine (EOX). There was no difference in response rates or overall or progression-free survival among the different combinations. However, on secondary analysis there was a small benefit to EOX over ECF (median survival of 11.2 months versus 9.9 months, hazard ratio for death 0.8, $P =$ .02). Toxicity differences between the regimens were variable and approximately 40% of patients in each treatment group required dose reduction. One study that compared cisplatin and 5-FU with either MMC or epirubicin showed an equivalent response to therapy but a significant improvement in quality of life with epirubicin.[42]

Koizumi and colleagues[43] randomized patients to S-1 with or without cisplatin and reported a significant improvement in time to progression and median survival for patients with two-drug therapy. Another trial compared PELF to FAMTX showed no difference in survival between treatments but a significant increase in complete clinical response to PELF therapy (13% versus 2% for FAMTX).[44] Oxaliplatin and irinotecan have also been studied in recent trials, but survival outcomes were similar with variable improvements in toxicity.[45,46]

Compared with the prior review, there have clearly been some advances in the chemotherapy available for patients with advanced disease. For metastatic disease, chemotherapy provides a survival advantage over best supportive care. However, the impact on survival has been modest with the currently available drugs. Phase III trials are under way evaluating the addition of biologic agents to chemotherapy for this patient population.

LEVEL 1A EVIDENCE: PROSPECTIVE RANDOMIZED CLINICAL TRIALS IN GASTRIC CANCER

(1) Extended Lymph Node Dissection for Gastric Cancer: Who May Benefit? Final Results of the Randomized Dutch Gastric Cancer Group Trial. Hartgrink H, van de Velde C, Putter H, et al. J Clin Oncol 2004;22:2069–77.[4]

Hypothesis: D2 lymphadenectomy improves outcome over D1 lymphadenectomy in patients with resectable gastric cancer.

No. Patients Randomized	Study Groups	Stratification	Significance Demonstrated	% Change Identified in Trial
711	D1 lymphadenectomy N = 380 D2 lymphadenectomy N = 331	Institution	No Survival	30% (D1) versus 35% (D2) 11-year survival

Published Abstract: PURPOSE: The extent of lymph node dissection appropriate for gastric cancer is still under debate. We have conducted a randomized trial to compare the results of a limited (D1) and extended (D2) lymph node dissection in terms of morbidity, mortality, long-term survival, and cumulative risk of relapse. We have reviewed the results of our trial after follow-up of more than 10 years. PATIENTS AND METHODS: Between August 1989 and June 1993, 1078 patients with gastric adenocarcinoma were randomly assigned to undergo a D1 or D2 lymph node dissection. Data were collected prospectively, and patients were followed for more than 10 years. RESULTS: A total of 711 patients (380 in the D1 group and 331 in the D2 group) were treated with curative intent. Morbidity (25% versus 43%; $P < .001$) and mortality (4% versus 10%; $P = .004$) were significantly higher in the D2 dissection group. After 11 years there is no overall difference in survival (30% versus 35%; $P = .53$). Of all subgroups analyzed, only patients with N2 disease may benefit of a D2 dissection. The relative risk ratio for morbidity and mortality is significantly higher than one for D2 dissections, splenectomy, pancreatectomy, and age older than 70 years. CONCLUSION: Overall, extended lymph node dissection as defined in this study generated no long-term survival benefit. The associated higher postoperative mortality offsets its long-term effect in survival. For patients with N2 disease, an extended lymph node dissection may offer cure, but it remains difficult to identify patients who have N2 disease. Morbidity and mortality are greatly influenced by the extent of lymph node dissection, pancreatectomy, splenectomy, and age. Extended lymph node dissections may be of benefit if morbidity and mortality can be avoided. (Copyright 2004 American Society of Clinical Oncology. Reprinted with permission.)

Editors' Summary and Comments: This well-designed multicenter trial after 11 years of follow-up confirms what was in the initial report: extended lymphadenectomy confers no survival benefit and imposes a significant risk for morbidity and mortality. Subgroup analysis did demonstrate that patients with N2 disease may benefit from the extended dissection (21% of N2 patients who had a D2 LND were alive compared with 0% of D1 patients at the conclusion of the study). However, it is impossible to identify these patients before lymphadenectomy and this was not a preplanned stratified subset analysis. The relative risk for morbidity and mortality was significantly higher when splenectomy or pancreatectomy were performed; these procedures are no longer routinely undertaken as a consequence the findings of this trial and others.

(2) Nodal dissection for patients with gastric cancer: a randomized controlled trial. Wu C, Hsiung C, Lo S, et al. Lancet Oncol 2006;7:309–15.[5]

Hypothesis: D3 (classically D2) lymphadenectomy improves outcome over D1 lymphadenectomy in patients with resectable gastric cancer.

No. Patients Randomized	Study Groups	Stratification	Significance Demonstrated	% Change Identified in Trial
221	D1 lymphadenectomy N = 110 D3 lymphadenectomy N = 111	None	Yes Survival	59.5% D3 versus 53.6% D1 5-year survival

Published Abstract: BACKGROUND: The survival benefit and morbidity after nodal dissection for gastric cancer remains controversial. We aimed to do a single-institution randomized trial to compare D1 (ie, level 1) lymphadenectomy with that of D3 (ie, levels 1, 2, and 3) dissection for gastric cancer in terms of overall survival and disease-free survival. METHODS: From October 7, 1993, to August 12, 1999, 335 patients were registered; 221 patients were eligible, 110 of whom were randomly assigned D1 surgery and 111 of whom were randomly assigned D3 surgery, both with curative intent. Three participating surgeons had done at least 25 independent D3 dissections before the start of the trial, and every procedure was verified by pathologic analyses. The primary end points were 5-year overall survival and 5-year disease-free survival. We also analyzed risk of recurrence. Main analyses were done by intention to treat. This trial is registered at the US National Institutes of Health Web site. FINDINGS: Median follow-up for the 110 (50%) survivors was 94.5 months (range 62.9–135.1). Overall 5-year survival was significantly higher in patients assigned D3 surgery than in those assigned D1 surgery (59.5% [95% CI 50.3–68.7] versus 53.6% [44.2–63.0]; difference between groups 5.9% [−7.3 to 19.1], log-rank $P = .041$). A total of 215 patients who had R0 resection (ie, no microscopic evidence of residual disease) had recurrence at 5 years of 50.6% [41.1–60.2] for D1 surgery and 40.3%

[30.9–49.7] for D3 surgery (difference between groups 10.3% [–3.2 to 23.7], log-rank $P = .197$). INTERPRETATION: D3 nodal dissection, compared with that of D1, offers a survival benefit for patients with gastric cancer when done by well-trained, experienced surgeons. (Copyright Elsevier 2006. Reprinted with permission.)

Editor's Summary and Comments: This is the only RCT to demonstrate an overall survival benefit for patients treated with extended lymphadenectomy. Surgical quality control, which has been a significant criticism of prior LND studies, was excellent. However, there are several points to make regarding this study. First, this is a single-institution study, which makes the findings difficult to generalize. Preoperative staging was not uniform and potentially unreliable in that 114 (34%) of the patients were excluded at laparotomy. Of note, 64 of these patients did not meet histologic criteria for the study protocol (ie, early cancer, positive resection margin), but were included in the intention to treat analysis. *Per protocol analysis* of the 156 eligible patients demonstrated a trend toward improved survival for D3 LND, but the differences were small (difference between groups 6.3% [–6.4 to 22.0], log rank $P = .056$). This small difference may be offset by the morbidity and mortality associated with a D3 LND, although this information was not reported. Despite the excellent effort by the investigators in this study the value of extended lymphadenectomy will continue to be debated.

(3) D2 lymphadenectomy alone or with para-aortic nodal dissection for gastric cancer. Sasako M, Sano T, Yamamoto S, et al. N Engl J Med 2008;359:453–62.[6]

Hypothesis: Para-aortic nodal dissection (PAND) in addition to D2 lymphadenectomy improves outcomes in patients with resectable gastric cancer.

No. Patients Randomized	Study Groups	Stratification	Significance Demonstrated	% Change Identified in Trial
523	D2 lymphadenectomy N = 263 D2 lymphadenectomy plus PAND N = 260	Clinical T stage Borrmann type Institution	No Survival	69.2% (D2) versus 70.3% (D2 + PAND) 5-year survival

Published Abstract: BACKGROUND: Gastrectomy with D2 lymphadenectomy is the standard treatment for curable gastric cancer in eastern Asia. Whether the addition of para-aortic nodal dissection (PAND) to D2 lymphadenectomy for stage T2, T3, or T4 tumors improves survival is controversial. We conducted a randomized, controlled trial at 24 hospitals in Japan to compare D2 lymphadenectomy alone with D2 lymphadenectomy plus PAND in patients undergoing gastrectomy for curable gastric cancer. METHODS: Between July 1995 and April 2001, 523 patients with curable stage T2b, T3, or T4 gastric cancer were randomly assigned during surgery to D2 lymphadenectomy alone (263 patients) or to D2 lymphadenectomy plus PAND (260 patients). We did not permit any adjuvant therapy before the recurrence of cancer. The primary end point was overall survival. RESULTS: The rates of surgery-related complications among patients assigned to D2 lymphadenectomy alone and those assigned to D2 lymphadenectomy plus PAND were 20.9% and 28.1%, respectively ($P = .07$). There were no significant differences between the two groups in the frequencies of anastomotic leakage, pancreatic fistula, abdominal abscess, pneumonia, or death from any cause within 30 days after surgery (the rate of death was 0.8% in each group). The median operation time was 63 minutes longer and the median blood loss was 230 mL greater in the group assigned to D2 lymphadenectomy plus PAND. The 5-yearoverall survival rate was 69.2% for the group assigned to D2 lymphadenectomy alone and 70.3% for the group assigned to D2 lymphadenectomy plus PAND; the hazard ratio for death was 1.03 (95% confidence interval [CI], 0.77 to 1.37; $P = $ .85). There were no significant differences in recurrence-free survival between the two groups; the hazard ratio for recurrence was 1.08 (95% CI, 0.83 to 1.42; $P = $ .56). CONCLUSIONS: As compared with D2 lymphadenectomy alone, treatment with D2 lymphadenectomy plus PAND does not improve the survival rate in curable gastric cancer. (Copyright [2008] Massachusetts Medical Society. All rights reserved. Reprinted with permission.)

Editor's Summary and Comments: This multi-institution trial randomized patients to the standard D2 LND with or without PAND and found no difference in survival. Patients who underwent PAND had a longer operative time, more intraoperative blood loss, and required more blood transfusions than patients in the control group. The authors noted that there was no difference between groups with regard to major complications (ie, anastomotic leak) but minor complications such as ileus were more common in patients undergoing PAND. There was no difference in perioperative mortality, which to the credit of the investigators, was 0.8% overall. Despite there being no administration of adjuvant therapy, the 5-year survival was approximately 70% for each group. This impressive result potentially reflects stage distribution in this study. The Japanese surgeons once again have demonstrated that gastrectomy with extended LND can be performed with minimal morbidity and mortality in experienced hands. However, because only 8.5% of patients in the PAND had lymph node metastases, the extended lymph node dissection may essentially be for staging and not therapeutic.

(4) Randomized clinical trial of splenectomy versus splenic preservation in patients with proximal gastric cancer. Yu W, Choi G, Chung H. Br J Surg 2006;93:559–63.[10]

Hypothesis: Splenic preservation does not compromise outcome in patients with gastric cancer undergoing D2 lymphadenectomy.

No. Patients Randomized	Study Groups	Stratification	Significance Demonstrated	% Change Identified in Trial
207	Total gastrectomy with splenectomy N = 104 Total gastrectomy without splenectomy N = 103	None	No Survival	50% (no splenectomy) versus 56% (splenectomy) 5-year survival

Published Abstract: BACKGROUND: Preservation or removal of the spleen during total gastrectomy for proximal gastric cancer is a matter of debate. METHODS: A randomized clinical trial included patients with gastric adenocarcinoma who underwent total gastrectomy either with (104 patients) or without (103) splenectomy. Postoperative outcome in the two groups was compared, including morbidity, mortality, and survival. RESULTS: Gastrectomy combined with splenectomy tended to be associated with slightly higher morbidity and mortality rates, a slightly greater incidence of lymph node metastasis at the splenic hilum and along the splenic artery, and marginally better survival, but there were no statistically significant differences between the groups. Splenectomy had no impact on survival in patients with meta-static lymph nodes at the hilum of the spleen or in those with metastatic lymph nodes along the splenic artery. CONCLUSION: These results do not support the use of prophylactic splenectomy to remove macroscopically negative lymph nodes near the spleen in patients undergoing total gastrectomy for proximal gastric cancer. (Copyright 2006 John Wiley & Sons Inc. Reprinted with permission.)

Editor's Summary and Comments: As demonstrated by the Dutch and other trials, splenectomy confers significant risk for morbidity and mortality during extended LND. Yu and colleagues set out to demonstrate that a proper D2 LND could be per-formed without splenectomy and have no impact on oncologic outcome. Interestingly, there was no difference between the groups with regard to operative complications. The number of lymph nodes harvested was not statistically different between groups indicating that splenic preservation does not necessarily compromise the D2 LND. There was a slight trend toward more positive nodes along the splenic artery and hilum, but these differences were not significant. The authors conclude that routine splenectomy is not justified during extended LND for gastric cancer.

(5) Perioperative chemotherapy versus surgery alone for resectable gastro-esophageal cancer. Cunningham D, Allum W, Stenning S, et al. N Engl J Med 2006;355:11–20.[26]

Hypothesis: The addition of perioperative ECF chemotherapy would improve the survival of patients with resectable gastroesophageal junction cancer.

No. Patients Randomized	Study Groups	Stratification	Significance Demonstrated	% Change Identified in Trial
503	Surgery N = 253 Surgery + ECF N = 250	Age Tumor site WHO performance status Surgeon	Yes Survival	23% (control) versus 36% (treated) 5-year survival

Abbreviation: WHO, World Health Organization.

Published Abstract: BACKGROUND: A regimen of epirubicin, cisplatin, and infused fluorouracil (ECF) improves survival among patients with incurable locally advanced or metastatic gastric adenocarcinoma. We assessed whether the addition of a perio-perative regimen of ECF to surgery improves outcomes among patients with poten-tially curable gastric cancer. METHODS: We randomly assigned patients with resectable adenocarcinoma of the stomach, esophagogastric junction, or lower esophagus to either perioperative chemotherapy and surgery (250 patients) or surgery alone (253 patients). Chemotherapy consisted of three preoperative and three postoperative cycles of intravenous epirubicin (50 mg per m^2 of body surface area) and cisplatin (60 mg per m^2) on day one, and a continuous intravenous infusion of fluorouracil (200 mg per m^2 per day) for 21 days. The primary end point was overall survival. RESULTS: ECF-related adverse effects were similar to those previously re-ported among patients with advanced gastric cancer. Rates of postoperative compli-cations were similar in the perioperative-chemotherapy group and the surgery group (46% and 45%, respectively), as were the numbers of deaths within 30 days after surgery. The resected tumors were significantly smaller and less advanced in the perioperative-chemotherapy group. With a median follow-up of 4 years, 149 patients in the perioperative-chemotherapy group and 170 in the surgery group had died. As compared with the surgery group, the perioperative-chemotherapy group had a higher likelihood of overall survival (hazard ratio for death, 0.75; 95% confidence interval, 0.60 to 0.93; P = .009; 5-year survival rate, 36% versus 23%) and of progression-free survival (hazard ratio for progression, 0.66; 95% confidence interval, 0.53 to 0.81; P < .001). CONCLUSIONS: In patients with operable gastric or lower esophageal adenocarcinomas, a perioperative regimen of ECF decreased tumor size and stage and significantly improved progression-free and overall survival. (Copyright [2006] Massachusetts Medical Society. All rights reserved. Reprinted with permission.)

Editors' Comments: This important, multicenter trial successfully demonstrated the benefit of perioperative epirubicin, cisplatin, and fluorouracil (ECF) chemotherapy for treatment of localized gastroesophageal adenocarcinoma. The staging protocol and extent of LND performed were not standardized, although these presumably did not differ between study groups. Of the 250 patients assigned to receive perioperative chemotherapy, a total of 215 (86%) completed preoperative therapy and 209 (84%) went on to resection. Of these 209, only 137 (55%) began postoperative chemotherapy and 104 (42%) eventually completed all three cycles. Of the 219 patients in the perioperative chemotherapy group who went on to surgery, 29 (13.2%) did not undergo resection. On pathologic analysis, tumor size was significantly smaller in the chemotherapy group (3 cm versus 5 cm; P < .001), suggesting tumor downstaging. There was also a significantly higher percentage of patients with T1 and T2 tumors in the chemotherapy group (51.7% versus 36.8%; P = .002). Grade 3 or 4 gastrointestinal toxicity (nausea and vomiting) occurred less frequently during the preoperative than the postoperative regimen of chemotherapy. Interestingly, despite the fact that only 42% of patients in the perioperative-chemotherapy group completed all protocol treatment, patients in this group still had a significant survival advantage (36% versus 23% 5-year overall survival) over patients receiving surgery alone. Two criticisms of this study include a lack of a standard preoperative staging protocol to include diagnostic laparoscopy and peritoneal cytology. Also, there was no assessment of histologic response in treated patients to help guide decisions about effective adjuvant therapy.

(6) Chemoradiotherapy after surgery compared with surgery alone for adenocarcinoma of the stomach or gastroesophageal junction. Macdonald J, Smalley S, Benedetti J, et al. N Engl J Med 2001;345:725–730.[30]

Hypothesis: Adjuvant chemoradiotherapy would improve the survival of patients with resectable gastric or gastroesophageal junction cancer.

No. Patients Randomized	Study Groups	Stratification	Significance Demonstrated	% Change Identified in Trial
556	Surgery N = 275 Surgery plus chemoradiotherapy N = 281	Tumor stage Nodal status	Yes Survival	27 months (control) versus 36 months (treatment) Median overall survival

Published Abstract: BACKGROUND: Surgical resection of adenocarcinoma of the stomach is curative in fewer than 40% of cases. We investigated the effect of surgery plus postoperative (adjuvant) chemoradiotherapy on the survival of patients with resectable adenocarcinoma of the stomach or gastroesophageal junction. METHODS: A total of 556 patients with resected adenocarcinoma of the stomach or gastroesophageal junction were randomly assigned to surgery plus postoperative chemoradiotherapy or surgery alone. The adjuvant treatment consisted of 425 mg of fluorouracil per m^2 of body-surface area per day, plus 20 mg of leucovorin per m^2 per day, for 5 days, followed by 4500 cGy of radiation at 180 cGy per day, given 5 days per week for 5 weeks, with modified doses of fluorouracil and leucovorin on the first 4 and the last 3 days of radiotherapy. One month after the completion of radiotherapy, two 5-day cycles of fluorouracil (425 mg/m^2 per day) plus leucovorin (20 mg/m^2 per day) were given 1 month apart. RESULTS: The median overall survival in the surgery-only group was 27 months, as compared with 36 months in the chemoradiotherapy group; the hazard ratio for death was 1.35 (95% confidence interval, 1.09 to 1.66; $P = .005$). The hazard ratio for relapse was 1.52 (95% confidence interval, 1.23 to 1.86; $P < .001$). Three patients (1%) died from toxic effects of the chemoradiotherapy; grade 3 toxic effects occurred in 41% of the patients in the chemoradiotherapy group, and grade 4 toxic effects occurred in 32%. CONCLUSIONS: Postoperative chemoradiotherapy should be considered for all patients at high risk for recurrence of adenocarcinoma of the stomach or gastroesophageal junction who have undergone curative resection. (Copyright [2001] Massachusetts Medical Society. All rights reserved. Reprinted with permission.)

Editors' Comments: This seminal trial demonstrated the benefit of adjuvant chemoradiotherapy (CRT) in patients with completely resected adenocarcinoma of the stomach or gastroesophageal junction. Three-year survival was also significantly improved by the addition of CRT to surgery (50% versus 41%). This improvement was seen although only 64% of patients assigned to the chemoradiotherapy group completed planned therapy. Patients were highly selected, with requirements for consumption of at least 1500 kcal per day and Southwest Oncology group performance status of 2 or less within 3 to 6 weeks after gastrectomy. One of the most concerning findings in this study was the lack of surgical quality control. The extent of lymphadenectomy in this trial was inadequate in most patients even for accurate staging if not treatment; 54% of patients in the study underwent D0 LND. Although the trial included patients with early-stage disease, most patients had T3 or T4 tumors and 85% had nodal metastases. CRT was not without toxicity and there were three deaths attributed to this therapy. The toxicity of the radiation therapy fields were all reviewed, and many were altered (35%) to avoid potential serious radiation-associated toxicity; although there was no long-term evaluation of toxicity. As most patients in the study received a D0 LND, some interpret these findings as adjuvant therapy compensating for inadequate surgery.

(7) Adjuvant chemotherapy for gastric cancer with S-1, an oral fluoropyrimidine. Sakuramoto S, Sasako M, Yamaguchi T, et al. N Engl J Med 2007;357: 1810–20.[32]

Hypothesis: Adjuvant S-1 chemotherapy improves survival of patients with resectable gastric cancer.

No. Patients Randomized	Study Groups	Stratification	Significance Demonstrated	% Change Identified in Trial
1059	Surgery N = 530 Surgery plus S-1 N = 529	Stage	Yes Survival	70.1% (control) versus 80.1% (treatment) 3-year overall survival

Published Abstract: BACKGROUND: Advanced gastric cancer can respond to S-1, an oral fluoropyrimidine. We tested S-1 as adjuvant chemotherapy in patients with curatively resected gastric cancer. METHODS: Patients in Japan with stage II or III gastric cancer who underwent gastrectomy with extended (D2) lymph-node dissection were randomly assigned to undergo surgery followed by adjuvant therapy with S-1 or to undergo surgery only. In the S-1 group, administration of S-1 was started within 6 weeks after surgery and continued for 1 year. The treatment regimen consisted of 6-week cycles in which, in principle, 80 mg of oral S-1 per square meter of body surface area per day was given for 4 weeks and no chemotherapy was given for the following 2 weeks. The primary end point was overall survival. RESULTS: We randomly assigned 529 patients to the S-1 group and 530 patients to the surgery-only group between October 2001 and December 2004. The trial was stopped on the recommendation of the independent data and safety monitoring committee, because the first interim analysis, performed 1 year after enrollment was completed, showed that the S-1 group had a higher rate of overall survival than the surgery-only group (P = .002). Analysis of follow-up data showed that the 3-year overall survival rate was 80.1% in the S-1 group and 70.1% in the surgery-only group. The hazard ratio for death in the S-1 group, as compared with the surgery-only group, was 0.68 (95% confidence interval, 0.52 to 0.87; P = .003). Adverse events of grade 3 or grade 4 (defined according to the Common Toxicity Criteria of the National Cancer Institute) that were relatively common in the S-1 group were anorexia (6.0%), nausea (3.7%), and diarrhea (3.1%). CONCLUSIONS: S-1 is an effective adjuvant treatment for East Asian patients who have undergone a D2 dissection for locally advanced gastric cancer. (Copyright [2007] Massachusetts Medical Society. All rights reserved. Reprinted with permission.)

Editors' Comments: This large randomized multicenter Japanese trial demonstrated the efficacy of S-1, an oral fluoropyrimidine, in the adjuvant treatment of Asian patients undergoing complete D2 resection of stage II or III gastric adenocarcinoma. The authors maintained high surgical quality control for D2 lymph node dissection in that centers included performed at least 100 operations for gastric cancer annually. All but one patient in this trial had a D2 or D3 operation, and nearly 90% had at least one positive node. Accrual to this trial was rapid and was discontinued at the first interim analysis, as it was predicted at that time that there would be a 99.3% chance that the S-1 group would fare significantly better than patients treated with surgery alone. S-1 improved survival and also significantly reduced disease recurrence despite remarkable local control with surgery alone. Interestingly, subgroup analysis revealed that stage II patients derived more of a survival benefit from S-1 therapy than stage III patients. In contrast to the trial by Macdonald et al, S-1 was extremely well tolerated in the adjuvant setting with minimal toxicity; 65.8% of patients completed the full 12 months of therapy.[30] This study was very well designed and conducted, however it is hard to know whether this treatment is generalizable to Western patient populations.

(8) Phase III study of docetaxel and cisplatin plus fluorouracil compared with cisplatin and fluorouracil as first-line therapy for advanced gastric cancer: a report of the V325 Study Group. Van Cutsem E, Moiseyenko V, Tjulandin S, et al. J Clin Oncol 2006;24:4991–97.[38]

Hypothesis: Addition of docetaxel to cisplatin and fluorouracil would reduce time to progression in patients with advanced gastric and gastroesophageal junction cancer.

No. Patients Randomized	Study Groups	Stratification	Significance Demonstrated	% Change Identified in Trial
445	DCF N = 221 CF N = 224	Center Liver metastases Prior gastrectomy Measurable versus assessable cancer Weight loss during prior 3 months (≤versus≥5%)	Yes Time to progression Overall survival	*Time to progression:* 32% risk reduction (DCF) *Overall survival:* 23% risk reduction (DCF)

Published Abstract: PURPOSE: In the randomized, multinational phase II/III trial (V325) of untreated advanced gastric cancer patients, the phase II part selected docetaxel, cisplatin, and fluorouracil (DCF) over docetaxel and cisplatin for comparison against cisplatin and fluorouracil (CF; reference regimen) in the phase III part. PATIENTS AND METHODS: Advanced gastric cancer patients were randomly assigned to docetaxel 75 mg/m^2 and cisplatin 75 mg/m^2 (day 1) plus fluorouracil 750 mg/m^2/d (days 1 to 5) every 3 weeks or cisplatin 100 mg/m^2 (day 1) plus fluorouracil 1000 mg/m^2/d (days 1 to 5) every 4 weeks. The primary end point was time-to-progression (TTP). **Results** In 445 randomly assigned and treated patients (DCF = 221; CF = 224), TTP was longer with DCF versus CF (32% risk reduction; log-rank $P < .001$). Overall survival was longer with DCF versus CF (23% risk reduction; log-rank $P = .02$). Two-year survival rate was 18% with DCF and 9% with CF. Overall response rate was higher with DCF ($\chi^2 P = .01$). Grade 3 to 4 treatment-related adverse events occurred in 69% (DCF) versus 59% (CF) of patients. Frequent grade 3 to 4 toxicities for DCF versus CF were: neutropenia (82% versus 57%), stomatitis (21% versus 27%), diarrhea (19% versus 8%), and lethargy (19% versus 14%). Complicated neutropenia was more frequent with DCF than CF (29% versus 12%). CONCLUSION: Adding docetaxel to CF significantly improved TTP, survival, and response rate in gastric cancer patients, but resulted in some increase in toxicity. Incorporation of docetaxel, as in DCF or with other active drug(s), is a new therapy option for patients with untreated advanced gastric cancer. (Copyright 2006 American Society of Clinical Oncology. Reprinted with permission.)

Editors' Comments: One of the common questions we have for our patients is whether or not small improvements in survival or time to progression matters. This is the first of three published reports from the V325 study group; the primary end point was time to progression. The significance noted was a 32% risk reduction for progression (which translates into an improvement in median TTP of 3.7 months to 5.6 months). Secondary end points such as clinical response to therapy and survival were also significantly, but minimally improved. The subsequent analyses from this study showed that DCF not only improved these objective parameters but also translated into a delay in decline of Karnofsky performance status and improved quality of life. Despite the reported benefits, the toxicity of DCF remains significant and as a result is given only to select, highly functioning patients.

(9) S-1 plus cisplatin versus S-1 alone for first-line treatment of advanced gastric cancer (SPIRITS trial): a phase III trial. Koizumi W, Narahara H, Hara T, et al. Lancet Oncol 2008;9:215–21.[43]

Hypothesis: The addition of cisplatin to S-1 chemotherapy would improve the survival of patients with advanced gastric cancer over treatment with S-1 alone.

No. Patients Randomized	Study Groups	Stratification	Significance Demonstrated	% Change Identified in Trial
305	S-1 N = 152 S-1 + cisplatin N = 153	ECOG performance status Unresectable or recurrent disease Clinical center Postoperative adjuvant therapy	Yes Survival	11 months S-1 versus 13 months S-1 + cisplatin Median survival

Published Abstract: BACKGROUND: Phase I/II clinical trials of S-1 plus cisplatin for advanced gastric cancer have yielded good responses and the treatment was well tolerated. In this S-1 Plus cisplatin versus S-1 In RCT In the Treatment for Stomach cancer (SPIRITS) trial, we aimed to verify that overall survival was better in patients with advanced gastric cancer treated with S-1 plus cisplatin than with S-1 alone. METHODS: In this phase III trial, chemotherapy-naive patients with advanced gastric cancer were enrolled between March 26, 2002, and November 30, 2004, at 38 centers in Japan, and randomly assigned to S-1 plus cisplatin or S-1 alone. In patients assigned to S-1 plus cisplatin, S-1 (40–60 mg depending on patient's body surface area) was given orally, twice daily for 3 consecutive weeks, and 60 mg/m^2 cisplatin was given intravenously on day 8, followed by a 2-week rest period, within a 5-week cycle. Those assigned to S-1 alone received the same dose of S-1 twice daily for 4 consecutive weeks, followed by a 2-week rest period, within a 6-week cycle. The primary end point was overall survival. Secondary end points were progression-free survival, proportions of responders, and safety. Analysis was by intention to treat. This trial is registered with http://ClinicalTrials.gov, number NCT00150670. FINDINGS: A total of 305 patients were enrolled; 7 patients were ineligible or withdrew consent. Therefore, 148 patients were assigned to S-1 plus cisplatin and 150 patients were assigned to S-1 alone. Median overall survival was significantly longer in patients assigned to S-1 plus cisplatin (13.0 months [IQR 7.6–21.9]) than in those assigned to S-1 alone (11.0 months [5.6–19.8]; hazard ratio for death, 0.77; 95% CI 0.61–0.98; P = .04). Progression-free survival was significantly longer in patients assigned to S-1 plus cisplatin than in those assigned to S-1 alone (median progression-free survival 6.0 months [3.3–12.9] versus 4.0 months [2.1–6.8]; P < .0001). Additionally, of 87 patients assigned S-1 plus cisplatin who had target tumors, 1 patient had a complete response and 46 patients had partial responses, ie, a total of 54% (range 43–65). Of 106 patients assigned S-1 alone who had target tumors, one patient had a complete response and 32 had partial responses, ie, a total of 31% (23–41). We recorded more grade 3 or 4 adverse events, including leucopenia, neutropenia, anemia, nausea, and anorexia, in the group assigned to S-1 plus cisplatin than in the group assigned to S-1 alone. There were no treatment-related deaths in either group. INTERPRETATION: S-1 plus cisplatin holds promise of becoming a standard first-line treatment for patients with advanced gastric cancer. (Copyright Elsevier 2008. Reprinted with permission.)

Editors' Comments: The oral chemotherapeutic agent S-1 is used as first-line treatment for advanced gastric cancer in Japan; however, a recent phase I/II trial demonstrated the efficacy of a combination of S-1 with cisplatin. This multicenter randomized phase III trial confirms improvements in overall and progression-free survival using the latter regimen. Subgroup analyses showed that the effect of adding cisplatin was most pronounced among patients with peritoneal metastases and in those patients without measurable tumors. Toxicity was more common in the S-1 plus cisplatin group than in the S-1 alone group, but less common than in comparable trials using other regimens. A multicenter, international trial comparing S-1 plus cisplatin to 5-FU plus cisplatin has been performed; preliminary results are negative however.

(10) Effect of eradication of *Helicobacter pylori* on incidence of metachronous gastric carcinoma after endoscopic resection of early gastric cancer: an open-label, randomized controlled trial. Fukase K, Kato M, Kikuchi S, et al. Lancet 2008;372:392–97.[37]

Hypothesis: Eradicating *Helicobacter pylori* infection decreases the incidence of metachronous gastric cancer after endoscopic mucosal resection of early gastric cancer.

No. Patients Randomized	Study Groups	Stratification	Significance Demonstrated	% Change Identified in Trial
544	Endoscopic resection N = 272 Endoscopic resection + H pylori eradication N = 272	Newly diagnosed versus post-resection	Yes	3.3% (control) versus 8.8% (treated) 3-year incidence of metachronous cancer

Published Abstract: BACKGROUND: The relation between *Helicobacter pylori* infection and gastric cancer has been proven in epidemiologic studies and animal experiments. Our aim was to investigate the prophylactic effect of *H pylori* eradication on the development of metachronous gastric carcinoma after endoscopic resection for early gastric cancer. METHODS: In this multicenter, open-label, randomized controlled trial, 544 patients with early gastric cancer, either newly diagnosed and planning to have endoscopic treatment or in post-resection follow-up after endoscopic treatment, were randomly assigned to receive an *H pylori* eradication regimen (n = 272) or control (n = 272). Randomization was done by a computer-generated randomization list and was stratified by whether the patient was newly diagnosed or post-resection. Patients in the eradication group received lansoprazole 30 mg twice daily, amoxicillin 750 mg twice daily, and clarithromycin 200 mg twice daily for a week; those in the control group received standard care, but no treatment for *H pylori*. Patients were examined endoscopically at 6, 12, 24, and 36 months after allocation. The primary end point was diagnosis of new carcinoma at another site in the stomach. Analyses were by intention to treat. This trial is registered with the University hospitals Medical Information Network (UMIN) Clinical Trials Registry, number UMIN000001169. FINDINGS: At 3-year follow-up, metachronous gastric carcinoma had developed in nine patients in the eradication group and 24 in the control group. In the full intention-to-treat population, including all patients irrespective of length of follow-up (272 patients in each group), the odds ratio for metachronous gastric carcinoma was 0.353 (95% CI 0.161–0.775; $P = .009$); in the modified intention-to-treat population, including patients with at least one post-randomization assessment of tumor status and adjusting for loss to follow-up (255 patients in the eradication group, 250 in the control group), the hazard ratio for metachronous gastric carcinoma was 0.339 (95% CI 0.157–0.729; $P = .003$). In the eradication group, 19 (7%) patients had diarrhea and 32 (12%) had soft stools. INTERPRETATION: Prophylactic eradication of *H pylori* after endoscopic resection of early gastric cancer should be used to prevent the development of metachronous gastric carcinoma. (Copyright Elsevier 2008. Reprinted with permission.)

Editors' Comments: This trial included patients with early gastric cancer and active *H pylori* infection who had undergone or were about to undergo endoscopic treatment. To determine if *H pylori* eradication could reduce the rate of metachronous gastric cancer development, patients were randomized to receive an *H pylori* eradication regimen consisting of a proton pump inhibitor and two antibiotics or no treatment. *H pylori* infection was successfully eradicated in 75% of the treated group and spontaneously resolved in 5% of patients in the control group. A significant odds ratio for metachronous cancer of 0.353 in favor of *H pylori* eradication was found.

DISCLOSURE

Authors have nothing to disclose.

REFERENCES

1. Weber SM, Karpeh MS. Randomized clinical trials in gastric cancer. Surg Oncol Clin N Am 2002;11(1):111–31, ix.
2. Bonenkamp JJ, Hermans J, Sasako M, et al. Extended lymph-node dissection for gastric cancer. N Engl J Med 1999;340(12):908–14.
3. Cuschieri A, Weeden S, Fielding J, et al. Patient survival after D1 and D2 resections for gastric cancer: long-term results of the MRC randomized surgical trial. Surgical Co-operative Group. Br J Cancer 1999;79(9–10):1522–30.
4. Hartgrink HH, van de Velde CJ, Putter H, et al. Extended lymph node dissection for gastric cancer: who may benefit? Final results of the randomized Dutch gastric cancer group trial. J Clin Oncol 2004;22(11):2069–77.
5. Wu CW, Hsiung CA, Lo SS, et al. Nodal dissection for patients with gastric cancer: a randomised controlled trial. Lancet Oncol 2006;7(4):309–15.
6. Sasako M, Sano T, Yamamoto S, et al. D2 lymphadenectomy alone or with para-aortic nodal dissection for gastric cancer. N Engl J Med 2008;359(5):453–62.
7. Yonemura Y, Wu CC, Fukushima N, et al. Randomized clinical trial of D2 and extended paraaortic lymphadenectomy in patients with gastric cancer. Int J Clin Oncol 2008;13(2):132–7.
8. Sasako M, Sano T, Yamamoto S, et al. Left thoracoabdominal approach versus abdominal-transhiatal approach for gastric cancer of the cardia or subcardia: a randomised controlled trial. Lancet Oncol 2006;7(8):644–51.
9. Csendes A, Burdiles P, Rojas J, et al. A prospective randomized study comparing D2 total gastrectomy versus D2 total gastrectomy plus splenectomy in 187 patients with gastric carcinoma. Surgery 2002;131(4):401–7.
10. Yu W, Choi GS, Chung HY. Randomized clinical trial of splenectomy versus splenic preservation in patients with proximal gastric cancer. Br J Surg 2006; 93(5):559–63.
11. Huscher CG, Mingoli A, Sgarzini G, et al. Laparoscopic versus open subtotal gastrectomy for distal gastric cancer: five-year results of a randomized prospective trial. Ann Surg 2005;241(2):232–7.
12. Kitano S, Shiraishi N, Fujii K, et al. A randomized controlled trial comparing open vs laparoscopy-assisted distal gastrectomy for the treatment of early gastric cancer: an interim report. Surgery 2002;131(Suppl 1):S306–11.

13. Hayashi H, Ochiai T, Shimada H, et al. Prospective randomized study of open versus laparoscopy-assisted distal gastrectomy with extraperigastric lymph node dissection for early gastric cancer. Surg Endosc 2005;19(9):1172–6.
14. Kim YW, Baik YH, Yun YH, et al. Improved quality of life outcomes after laparoscopy-assisted distal gastrectomy for early gastric cancer: results of a prospective randomized clinical trial. Ann Surg 2008;248(5):721–7.
15. Lee JH, Han HS, Lee JH. A prospective randomized study comparing open vs laparoscopy-assisted distal gastrectomy in early gastric cancer: early results. Surg Endosc 2005;19(2):168–73.
16. Mohri Y, Tonouchi H, Kobayashi M, et al. Randomized clinical trial of single-versus multiple-dose antimicrobial prophylaxis in gastric cancer surgery. Br J Surg 2007;94(6):683–8.
17. Ishikawa M, Kitayama J, Kaizaki S, et al. Prospective randomized trial comparing Billroth I and Roux-en-Y procedures after distal gastrectomy for gastric carcinoma. World J Surg 2005;29(11):1415–20 [discussion: 1421].
18. Iivonen MK, Koskinen MO, Ikonen TJ, et al. Emptying of the jejunal pouch and Roux-en-Y limb after total gastrectomy—a randomised, prospective study. Eur J Surg 1999;165(8):742–7.
19. Fein M, Fuchs KH, Thalheimer A, et al. Long-term benefits of Roux-en-Y pouch reconstruction after total gastrectomy: a randomized trial. Ann Surg 2008;247(5):759–65.
20. Kim J, Lee J, Hyung WJ, et al. Gastric cancer surgery without drains: a prospective randomized trial. J Gastrointest Surg 2004;8(6):727–32.
21. Alvarez Uslar R, Molina H, Torres O, et al. Total gastrectomy with or without abdominal drains. A prospective randomized trial. Rev Esp Enferm Dig 2005;97(8):562–9.
22. Doglietto GB, Papa V, Tortorelli AP, et al. Nasojejunal tube placement after total gastrectomy: a multicenter prospective randomized trial. Arch Surg 2004; 139(12):1309–13 [discussion: 1313].
23. Yoo CH, Son BH, Han WK, et al. Nasogastric decompression is not necessary in operations for gastric cancer: prospective randomised trial. Eur J Surg 2002; 168(7):379–83.
24. Lee JH, Hyung WJ, Noh SH. Comparison of gastric cancer surgery with versus without nasogastric decompression. Yonsei Med J 2002;43(4):451–6.
25. Yang Z, Zheng Q, Wang Z. Meta-analysis of the need for nasogastric or nasojejunal decompression after gastrectomy for gastric cancer. Br J Surg 2008;95(7):809–16.
26. Cunningham D, Allum WH, Stenning SP, et al. Perioperative chemotherapy versus surgery alone for resectable gastroesophageal cancer. N Engl J Med 2006; 355(1):11–20.
27. Wang XL, Wu GX, Zhang MD, et al. A favorable impact of preoperative FPLC chemotherapy on patients with gastric cardia cancer. Oncol Rep 2000;7(2):241–4.
28. Hartgrink HH, van de Velde CJ, Putter H, et al. Neo-adjuvant chemotherapy for operable gastric cancer: long term results of the Dutch randomised FAMTX trial. Eur J Surg Oncol 2004;30(6):643–9.
29. Stahl M, Walz MK, Stuschke M, et al. Phase III comparison of preoperative chemotherapy compared with chemoradiotherapy in patients with locally advanced adenocarcinoma of the esophagogastric junction. J Clin Oncol 2009;27(6):851–6.
30. Macdonald JS, Smalley SR, Benedetti J, et al. Chemoradiotherapy after surgery compared with surgery alone for adenocarcinoma of the stomach or gastroesophageal junction. N Engl J Med 2001;345(10):725–30.
31. Coit D. Adjuvant therapy for gastric cancer. J Am Coll Surg 2007;205(Suppl 4):S54–8.
32. Sakuramoto S, Sasako M, Yamaguchi T, et al. Adjuvant chemotherapy for gastric cancer with S-1, an oral fluoropyrimidine. N Engl J Med 2007;357(18):1810–20.

33. Di Costanzo F, Gasperoni S, Manzione L, et al. Adjuvant chemotherapy in completely resected gastric cancer: a randomized phase III trial conducted by GOIRC. J Natl Cancer Inst 2008;100(6):388–98.
34. De Vita F, Giuliani F, Orditura M, et al. Adjuvant chemotherapy with epirubicin, leucovorin, 5-fluorouracil and etoposide regimen in resected gastric cancer patients: a randomized phase III trial by the Gruppo Oncologico Italia Meridionale (GOIM 9602 Study). Ann Oncol 2007;18(8):1354–8.
35. Cascinu S, Labianca R, Barone C, et al. Adjuvant treatment of high-risk, radically resected gastric cancer patients with 5-fluorouracil, leucovorin, cisplatin, and epidoxorubicin in a randomized controlled trial. J Natl Cancer Inst 2007;99(8):601–7.
36. Yu W, Whang I, Chung HY, et al. Indications for early postoperative intraperitoneal chemotherapy of advanced gastric cancer: results of a prospective randomized trial. World J Surg 2001;25(8):985–90.
37. Fukase K, Kato M, Kikuchi S, et al. Effect of eradication of *Helicobacter pylori* on incidence of metachronous gastric carcinoma after endoscopic resection of early gastric cancer: an open-label, randomised controlled trial. Lancet 2008; 372(9636):392–7.
38. Van Cutsem E, Moiseyenko VM, Tjulandin S, et al. Phase III study of docetaxel and cisplatin plus fluorouracil compared with cisplatin and fluorouracil as first-line therapy for advanced gastric cancer: a report of the V325 Study Group. J Clin Oncol 2006;24(31):4991–7.
39. Ajani JA, Moiseyenko VM, Tjulandin S, et al. Clinical benefit with docetaxel plus fluorouracil and cisplatin compared with cisplatin and fluorouracil in a phase III trial of advanced gastric or gastroesophageal cancer adenocarcinoma: the V-325 Study Group. J Clin Oncol 2007;25(22):3205–9.
40. Ajani JA, Moiseyenko VM, Tjulandin S, et al. Quality of life with docetaxel plus cisplatin and fluorouracil compared with cisplatin and fluorouracil from a phase III trial for advanced gastric or gastroesophageal adenocarcinoma: the V-325 Study Group. J Clin Oncol 2007;25(22):3210–6.
41. Cunningham D, Starling N, Rao S, et al. Capecitabine and oxaliplatin for advanced esophagogastric cancer. N Engl J Med 2008;358(1):36–46.
42. Ross P, Nicolson M, Cunningham D, et al. Prospective randomized trial comparing mitomycin, cisplatin, and protracted venous-infusion fluorouracil (PVI 5-FU) with epirubicin, cisplatin, and PVI 5-FU in advanced esophagogastric cancer. J Clin Oncol 2002;20(8):1996–2004.
43. Koizumi W, Narahara H, Hara T, et al. S-1 plus cisplatin versus S-1 alone for first-line treatment of advanced gastric cancer (SPIRITS trial): a phase III trial. Lancet Oncol 2008;9(3):215–21.
44. Cocconi G, Carlini P, Gamboni A, et al. Cisplatin, epirubicin, leucovorin and 5-fluorouracil (PELF) is more active than 5-fluorouracil, doxorubicin and methotrexate (FAMTX) in advanced gastric carcinoma. Ann Oncol 2003;14(8):1258–63.
45. Al-Batran SE, Hartmann JT, Probst S, et al. Phase III trial in metastatic gastroesophageal adenocarcinoma with fluorouracil, leucovorin plus either oxaliplatin or cisplatin: a study of the Arbeitsgemeinschaft Internistische Onkologie. J Clin Oncol 2008;26(9):1435–42.
46. Dank M, Zaluski J, Barone C, et al. Randomized phase III study comparing irinotecan combined with 5-fluorouracil and folinic acid to cisplatin combined with 5-fluorouracil in chemotherapy naive patients with advanced adenocarcinoma of the stomach or esophagogastric junction. Ann Oncol 2008;19(8):1450–7.

Randomized Clinical Trials in Gastrointestinal Stromal Tumors

Peter A. Learn, MD, Jason K. Sicklick, MD,
Ronald P. DeMatteo, MD*

KEYWORDS

- Gastrointestinal stromal tumor • Disease-free survival
- Recurrence-free survival

Gastrointestinal (GI) stromal tumor (GIST) is recognized as the most common mesen-chymal tumor of the GI tract. It constitutes 80% of all GI mesenchymal tumors and approximately 20% of all small bowel malignancies, excluding lymphomas. It is believed that there are up to 5000 new cases of GIST diagnosed each year in the United States.[1] GIST first gained recognition as a distinct tumor type in the 1980s, before which it was considered a type of leiomyomatous tumor. Further research has demonstrated that approximately 90% of GISTs contain an activating KIT (CD117) mutation, while 5% carry a mutation in platelet-derived growth factor receptor alpha (PDGFRα). Accordingly, the treatment of GIST has changed radically with the evolution of targeted therapies in oncology. Six prospective, randomized controlled trials have been published on the treatment of this disease during the brief period since its molecular and pathologic characterization.

SURGERY AND RADIATION

There are no data from randomized controlled trials regarding the surgical manage-ment of GIST. By consensus, surgical resection with negative microscopic margins remains the primary treatment and is the only modality that appears to offer a signifi-cant chance of cure. Aggressive surgical therapy to debulk progressive, nonlocalized disease or to resect metastatic disease is advocated in select circumstances, but these approaches have not been evaluated in prospective, controlled studies.

Disclosure: See last page of article.
Department of Surgery, Memorial Sloan-Kettering Cancer Center, 1275 York Avenue, Box 203, New York, NY 10065, USA
* Corresponding author.
E-mail address: dematter@mskcc.org (R.P. DeMatteo).

Similarly, no randomized controlled trials have been published on the use of radiation therapy for GIST. In fact, retrospective data are sparse. Current applications for this treatment modality remain limited.

CHEMOTHERAPY AND METASTATIC DISEASE

In general, traditional chemotherapeutic agents, including doxorubicin, alone or with gemcitabine, or ifosfamide with etoposide or temozolomide, have not been efficacious in treating patients with GIST.[2–7] The application of imatinib mesylate in the treatment of GIST reflects a major advance in the treatment of solid tumors with specific, therapeutic, molecular targeting. Imatinib, a product of rational drug development, demonstrates inhibitory activity against BCR-ABL, PDGFRα, and KIT kinases. By binding to the adenosine triphosphate (ATP)-binding pocket of these proteins, imatinib blocks the transfer of a phosphate group to the substrate molecule and leads to inhibition of KIT or PDGFRα signal transduction.[8] Given these effects, and regardless of the KIT or PDGFRα mutation status, imatinib has become the first-line medical treatment for metastatic, unresectable, or recurrent GIST. Surgery alone for metastatic disease often has limited value. The initial starting dose of imatinib is 400 mg/d administered orally, although some studies have compared this starting dose with an 800 mg/d dose. The data from these randomized trials will be discussed later, but 400 mg/d remain the standard initial therapy in most patients. The task of characterizing tumor mutation status (KIT/PDGFRα), assessing disease progression, and integrating surgery and targeted therapy has led to the necessity for a multidisciplinary approach to treating patients with GIST. A team including radiologists, pathologists, medical oncologists, and surgeons is required for successful care of these patients.[9]

All of the currently available randomized controlled trials in the treatment of GIST address the use of targeted biologic agents, primarily in advanced (surgically unresectable or metastatic) disease but more recently in the adjuvant setting as well. Although initially advanced for use in chronic myelogenous leukemia, the dramatic benefits of imatinib mesylate for treating GIST were demonstrated by Demetri and colleagues with an initial case report in 2001[10] followed by report of their phase 2 trial in 2002.[11] This latter study demonstrated unprecedented early improvements in progression-free survival (PFS) and overall survival in patients treated with either 400 mg/d or 600 mg/d of imatinib. A subsequent long-term follow-up study[12] demonstrated a median survival of 57 months in patients for whom a 20-month median survival traditionally would have been estimated.

Subsequent studies of imatinib in GIST have addressed some of the questions regarding dosing and duration of therapy. Verweij and colleagues,[7] reporting in 2004 for the European Organization for Research and Treatment of Cancer (EORTC) Soft Tissue and Bone Sarcoma Group, the Italian Sarcoma Group (ISG), and the Australasian Gastrointestinal Trials Group (AGITG), demonstrated a small but statistically significant improvement in progression-free survival among patients receiving 800 mg/d of imatinib over those receiving 400 mg/d. A concurrent study of similar design published by Blanke and colleagues[13] (SWOG S0033), however, failed to demonstrate significant improvements in the higher-dose group. Nevertheless, some clinical benefit, in the form of delayed progression of disease, was identified in both trials among patients who crossed over to high-dose therapy after progressing on conventional-dose imatinib.[13,14] In 2007, Van Glabbeke and colleagues[15] presented results of the MetaGIST analysis, which combined 1640 patients from the SWOG S0033 and the EORTC-ISG-AGITG phase 3 trials. This meta-analysis affirmed a small but statistically significant improvement in PFS in the higher-dose arm (800 mg/d), although no difference in overall survival was demonstrated. In particular, patients with exon 9 KIT mutations demonstrated worse PFS, which may have been improved somewhat by higher-dose imatinib. Because the original trials were not stratified for mutation location, however, the results of this post-hoc subgroup analysis require further validation.

As for the question of therapy duration, Blay and colleagues,[16] reporting for the French Sarcoma Group in 2007, clearly demonstrated the risks of interrupting imatinib therapy after 1 year. Eighty-one percent of patients with stable or responsive disease who interrupted imatinib therapy demonstrated prompt disease progression. In summary, these results suggest that initiating therapy with conventional-dose imatinib is appropriate for most patients with surgically unresectable disease, and interruption in therapy should be avoided in patients with responsive or stable disease.

For patients whose disease progresses on imatinib or who are unable to tolerate the drug, Demetri and colleagues[17] demonstrated the viability of sunitinib as a second-line treatment. Although the response rates in this group are not nearly as dramatic as with first-line imatinib, sunitinib clearly offers improvement in PFS over no treatment.

Finally, DeMatteo and colleagues,[18] reporting for the American College of Surgeons Oncology Group, published in 2009 the results of the first randomized controlled trial addressing the role of imatinib in the adjuvant setting. Early results from this trial demonstrated that imatinib 400 mg/d, administered for 1 year after complete resection of localized, primary GIST, provided a 15% absolute reduction in recurrence events compared with placebo at 1 year. Reductions in risk of recurrence were observed among all subgroups as stratified by tumor size. The impact on overall survival will require longer follow-up to establish but is not different at this time.

At the time of this writing, no randomized trials evaluating the neoadjuvant use of imatinib have been reported, although phase 2 data support its safety.[19] In the absence of randomized data, retrospective data would suggest that patients can be treated in a neoadjuvant setting to improve resectability or reduce the extent of the operation.

ONGOING TRIALS

Several active and recently closed trials should help answer important questions regarding the optimal use of imatinib in adjuvant or neoadjuvant settings. The Scandinavian Sarcoma Group has completed enrollment and is currently in the data collection phase on a randomized, controlled trial evaluating adjuvant therapy with imatinib (400 mg/d) administered as a short (12 months) versus long (36 months) course of treatment, following complete gross resection of GIST at high risk for recurrence. Recurrence-free survival is the primary endpoint. The EORTC recently closed their trial (protocol 62024) comparing 2 years of adjuvant therapy with imatinib versus observation alone in patients undergoing complete resection of localized primary GIST. Because overall survival is the primary endpoint, results are not expected for about 9 years. Additionally, the EORTC is accruing subjects for a phase 3 randomized study (protocol 62063) evaluating resection of residual disease in patients with metastatic GIST responding to imatinib.

LEVEL IA EVIDENCE: RANDOMIZED CLINICAL TRIALS IN GIST

1. Efficacy and safety of imatinib mesylate in advanced gastrointestinal stromal tumors.

Demetri GD, von Mehren M, Blanke CD, et al. N Engl J Med 2002 Aug 15; 347(7):472–80.[11]

Hypothesis: Imatinib, evaluated at two different dose regimens, improves PFS in patients with unresectable or metastatic GIST beyond historical expectations.

# Patients Randomized	Study Groups	Stratification	Significance Demonstrated	% Change Identified in Trial
147	400 mg imatinib daily n = 73 600 mg imatinib daily n = 74	None	No difference in PFS	*P* = not significant

Published abstract: BACKGROUND: Constitutive activation of KIT receptor tyrosine kinase is critical in the pathogenesis of GISTs. Imatinib mesylate, a selective tyrosine kinase inhibitor, has been shown in preclinical models and preliminary clinical studies to have activity against such tumors. METHODS: The authors conducted an open-label, randomized, multicenter trial to evaluate the activity of imatinib in patients with advanced gastrointestinal stromal tumor. They assessed antitumor response and the safety and tolerability of the drug. Pharmacokinetics were assessed in a subgroup of patients. RESULTS: One-hundred forty-seven patients were randomly assigned to receive 400 mg or 600 mg of imatinib daily. Overall, 79 patients (53.7%) had a partial response; 41 patients (27.9%) had stable disease, and for technical reasons, response could not be evaluated in 7 patients (4.8%). No patient had a complete response to the treatment. The median duration of response had not been reached after a median follow-up of 24 weeks after the onset of response. Early resistance to imatinib was noted in 20 patients (13.6%). Therapy was tolerated well, although mild-to-moderate edema, diarrhea, and fatigue were common. GI or intra-abdominal hemorrhage occurred in approximately 5% of patients. There were no significant differences in toxic effects or response between the two doses. Imatinib was absorbed well, with pharmacokinetics similar to those reported in patients with chronic myeloid leukemia. CONCLUSIONS: Imatinib induced a sustained objective response in more than half of patients with an advanced unresectable or metastatic GIST. Inhibition of the KIT signal transduction pathway is a promising treatment for advanced GISTS that resist conventional chemotherapy. (Copyright [2002] Massachusetts Medical Society. All rights reserved.)

Editor's summary and comments: In this seminal, multicenter, phase 2 study, Demetri and colleagues demonstrated the unprecedented efficacy of imatinib in unresectable or metastatic KIT-positive GIST. Beginning as a proof-of-concept study, promising early results prompted expanded enrollment. Following a 6-month follow-up of the first 100 patients, interim analysis demonstrated no difference in PFS but illustrated a dramatic response over historical expectations. The study was closed as enrollment into a phase 3trial was initiated. Of the 147 patients enrolled, 120 patients (81.6%) demonstrated either disease regression or stabilization. Although differences in efficacy were not observed between the two administered doses, the vast improvements in overall survival and PFS seen in both arms over historical controls established the benefits of imatinib in advanced GIST. In a subsequent follow-up study,[12] the investigators demonstrated the sustained benefit of imatinib administered at either dose. With longer follow-up, objective radiological responses, as determined by Response Evaluation Criteria In Solid Tumors (RECIST) criteria, increased from 54% to 68%. More importantly, survival was shown to be independent of the extent of response, such that patients with partial responses or with stable disease experienced similar survival benefits. This may reflect the inadequacy of RE-CIST criteria in categorizing responses to molecular therapy. More specifically, changes in tumor density do not always correlate with alterations in tumor size (**Fig. 1**).[20]

2. Phase III randomized, intergroup trial assessing imatinib mesylate at two dose levels in patients with unresectable or metastatic gastrointestinal stromal tumors expressing the kit receptor tyrosine kinase: S0033.
  Blanke CD, Rankin C, Demetri GD, et al. J Clin Oncol 2008 Feb 1;26(4):626–32.[13]
  Hypothesis: High-dose imatinib (400 mg twice daily) achieves better PFS and overall survival than conventional-dose imatinib (400 mg once daily).
  Published abstract: PURPOSE: To assess potential differences in PFS or overall survival when imatinib mesylate is administered to patients with incurable GIST at

# Patients Randomized	Study Groups	Stratification	Significance Demonstrated	% Change Identified in Trial
746	Imatinib 400 mg daily n = 345 Imatinib 400 mg twice daily n = 349	By Zubrod performance status (0–2 versus 3) and by disease status (measurable versus unmeasurable)	No significant differences in PFS or overall survival	P = not significant

a standard dose (400 mg daily) versus a high dose (400 mg twice daily). PATIENTS AND METHODS: Patients with metastatic or surgically unresectable GIST were eligible for this phase 3 open-label clinical trial. At registration, patients were assigned randomly to either standard or high-dose imatinib, with close-interval follow-up. If objective progression occurred by RECIST, patients on the standard-dose arm could reregister to the trial and receive the high-dose imatinib regimen. RESULTS: Seven hundred forty-six patients with advanced GIST from 148 centers across the United States and Canada were enrolled onto this trial in 9 months. With a median follow-up of 4.5 years, median PFS was 18 months for patients on the standard-dose arm and 20 months for those receiving high-dose imatinib. Median overall survival was 55 and 51 months, respectively. There were no statistically significant differences in objective response rates, PFS, or overall survival. After progression on standard-dose imatinib, 33% of patients who crossed over to the high-dose imatinib regimen achieved either an objective response or stable disease. There were more grade 3, 4, and 5 toxicities noted on the high-dose imatinib arm. CONCLUSION: This trial confirms the effectiveness of imatinib as primary systemic therapy for patients with incurable GIST but did not show any advantage to higher dose treatment. It appears reasonable to initiate therapy with 400 mg daily and to consider dose escalation on progression of disease. (Copyright [2008] American Society of Clinical Oncology, reprinted with permission.)
  Editor's summary and comments: This multicenter, phase 3 trial was designed to investigate the appropriate dose of imatinib in patients with surgically incurable GIST, following on results of the earlier phase 2 trial. Imatinib was tolerated fairly well at both doses, although dose reductions and grade 3 to 5 toxicities were more common

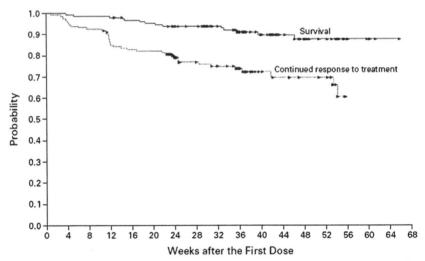

Fig. 1. Kaplain-Meier estimates of overall survival and time to treatment failure for all patients. Each arrowhead represents the point at which a patient's data were censored. (*Reprinted from* Demetri GD, von Mehren M, Blanke CD, et al. N Engl J Med 2002;15;347(7):472–80; with permission.)

in the high-dose arm. No significant differences were identified in PFS or overall survival on intention-to-treat analyses. Of the 133 patients who crossed over, however, 118 could be assessed for response, and among these, median PFS was 5 months. These results suggest a possible benefit to increasing treatment dose consequent to conventional dose failure. Based on the results of this study, it is reasonable to presume that conventional-dose imatinib is appropriate for most patients, with high-dose therapy reserved for patients progressing on a conventional dose.

3. Progression-free survival in gastrointestinal stromal tumors with high-dose imatinib: randomized trial.

Verweij J, Casali PG, Zalcberg J, et al. Lancet 2004 Sep 25-Oct 1;364(9440):1127–34.[7]

Hypothesis: High-dose imatinib (400 mg twice daily) achieves better PFS than low-dose imatinib (400 mg once daily).

# Patients Randomized	Study Groups	Stratification	Significance Demonstrated	% Change Identified in Trial
946	400 mg imatinib once daily n = 473 400 mg imatinib twice daily n = 473	None	400 mg imatinib daily results in partial response of disease while a dose of 400 mg imatinib twice daily improves PFS	PFS: hazard ratio (HR) 0.82 (95% confidence interval (CI) 0.69–0.98, $P = .026$)

Published abstract: BACKGROUND: Imatinib is approved worldwide for use in GISTs. The authors aimed to assess dose dependency of response and PFS with imatinib for metastatic GIST. METHODS: Nine-hundred forty-six patients were allocated randomly imatinib 400 mg either once or twice a day. Those assigned the once-a-day regimen who had progression were offered the option of crossover. The primary endpoint was PFS. Analysis was by intention to treat. FINDINGS: At median follow-up of 760 days (interquartile range [IQR] 644-859), 263 (56%) of 473 patients allocated imatinib once daily had progressed compared with 235 (50%) of 473 patients who were assigned treatment twice daily (estimated hazard ratio [HR] 0.82 [95% CI 0.69 to 0.98]; $P = .026$). Side effects arose in 465 of 470 (99%) patients allocated the once-daily regimen compared with 468 of 472 (99%) assigned treatment twice daily. By comparison with the group treated once daily, more dose reductions (77 [16%] versus 282 [60%]) and treatment interruptions (189 [40%] versus 302 [64%]) were recorded in patients allocated the twice-daily regimen, but treatment in both arms was tolerated fairly well. Fifty-two (5%) patients achieved a complete response, 442 (47%) a partial response, and 300 (32%) stable disease, with no difference between groups. Median time to best response was 107 days (IQR 58-172). INTERPRETATION: If response induction is the only aim of treatment, a daily dose of 400 mg of imatinib is sufficient; however, a dose of 400 mg twice a day achieves significantly longer PFS. (Copyright [2004] Elsevier.)

Editor's summary and comments: The European Organization for Research and Treatment of Cancer (EORTC) Soft Tissue and Bone Sarcoma Group, the Italian Sarcoma Group (ISG), and the Australasian Gastrointestinal Trials Group (AGITG) performed a worldwide, prospective, randomized trial to investigate once- versus twice-daily imatinib for metastatic GIST. At a median follow-up of just over 2 years, only 6% fewer patients had disease progression with the twice-daily dosing. While this did translate into a statistically significant increase in PFS, the effect was modest. Patients in the higher-dose arm had slightly more dose reductions and treatment interruptions because of toxicities. Moreover, in the intention-to-treat analysis, treatment responses were remarkably similar between the two treatment groups. This trial both suggests that a lower dose of imatinib is adequate for treatment if a response is seen and establishes 400 mg daily as the standard dose of imatinib for treating advanced GIST.

A subsequent follow-up study[14] evaluated the feasibility, safety, and efficacy of crossing-over from low-dose to high-dose imatinib upon progression of disease. Of the patients possible for crossover, 55% (133 of 241 patients) crossed over. Although toxicities were often not high grade, slightly more than half of patients did not tolerate the dose escalation. Crossover resulted in a 33% increase in time to progression. Based on this post-hoc analysis, crossover to high-dose imatinib is feasible and safe in GIST patients who progress on low-dose therapy, and it also appears to delay disease progression, suggesting that there is therapeutic utility to an imatinib dose increase in patients with progression of disease.

4. Prospective multicentric randomized phase III study of imatinib in patients with advanced gastrointestinal stromal tumors comparing interruption versus continuation of treatment beyond 1 year: the French Sarcoma Group.
    Blay JY, Le Cesne A, Ray-Coquard I, et al. J Clin Oncol 2007 Mar 20;25(9): 1107–13.[16]
    Hypothesis: Continuous imatinib improves PFS in patients with advanced GIST as compared with interrupted imatinib beyond 1 year of treatment.

# Patients Randomized	Study Groups	Stratification	Significance Demonstrated	% Change Identified in Trial
58	Interrupted imatinib n = 32 Continuous imatinib n = 26	None	Improvement in PFS with continuous imatinib therapy versus interrupted imatinib therapy	Median PFS 18 months (95% CI 15.0–23.6) versus 6.1 months (95% CI 3.5–9.7), $P<.0001$)

Published abstract: PURPOSE: Imatinib is the standard treatment of advanced GISTs. It is not known whether imatinib may be stopped in patients in whom disease is controlled. METHODS: This prospective, randomized, multicentric phase 3 study was designed to compare continuous with interrupted imatinib beyond 1 year of treatment in patients with advanced GIST. The primary end point was PFS. Secondary end points included overall survival, response rate after reinitiation of imatinib, and quality of life. Early stopping rules in cases of rapid progression of disease were defined, with preplanned interim analyses. RESULTS: Between May 2002 and April 2004, 182 patients with advanced GIST were enrolled. Between May 2003 and April 2004, 98 patients in response or stable disease under imatinib reached more than 1 year of follow-up. Forty patients were not eligible for randomization, and 58 patients were randomly assigned, 32 and 26 patients in the interrupted and continuous arms, respectively. As of Oct. 15, 2005, 8 of 26 patients in the continuous group and 26 of 32 patients in the interrupted group had documented disease progression ($P<.0001$). Twenty-four of 26 patients with documented progression in the interrupted arm responded to imatinib reintroduction. No differences in overall survival or imatinib resistance were observed between the two arms. Quality of life evaluated 6 months after random assignment using the 30-item quality of life questionnaire was not significantly different between the two groups of randomly assigned patients. CONCLUSION: Imatinib interruption results in rapid progression in most patients with advanced GIST, and cannot be recommended in routine practice unless patients experience significant toxicity. (Copyright [2007] American Society of Clinical Oncology, reprinted with permission.)

Editor's summary and comments: This prospective, randomized, multicenter phase 3 trial was designed to determine whether imatinib therapy may be discontinued in patients whose disease is controlled following 1 year of treatment. The data suggested that therapy should be administered without interruption. During a 2-year period, 182 patients were enrolled. Following 1 year of treatment with imatinib, patients with metastatic or unresectable GIST who had either stable or partially responsive disease randomly were assigned either to continue or to discontinue imatinib therapy. Patients who were randomized to interrupted therapy were able to cross over to the treatment arm if they had progression of disease. Of this arm, 81% (26 of 32 patients) crossed over. Of these patients, 92% (24 of 26) responded to reintroduction of therapy. This suggested that even if there is no disease seen on a computed tomography (CT) scan, viable microscopic disease remains after imatinib therapy. Lending further validity to this concept, no patients in the continuous treatment arm had progression of disease at undetectable disease sites. Although there was no difference in overall survival, Imatinib resistance, or quality of life, continuous treatment resulted in a significantly longer PFS. This trial affirmed that imatinib therapy should not be sporadic and demonstrated that for patients wherein imatinib is discontinued, early progression is expected.

5. Efficacy and safety of sunitinib in patients with advanced gastrointestinal stromal tumor after failure of imatinib: a randomized controlled trial.

Demetri GD, van Oosterom AT, Garrett CR, et al. Lancet 2006 Oct 14; 368(9544):1329–38.[17]

Hypothesis: Sunitinib improves PFS in patients with unresectable GIST who have failed imatinib therapy compared with placebo.

# Patients Randomized	Study Groups	Stratification	Significance Demonstrated	% Change Identified in Trial
312	Sunitinib n = 207 Placebo n = 105	Based on prior outcome on imatinib treatment: progression within 6 months versus progression beyond 6 months or intolerance to imatinib	Improvement in PFS	Hazard ratio 0.33 (95% CI 0.23– 0.47, *P*<.0001)

Published abstract: BACKGROUND: No effective therapeutic options for patients with unresectable imatinib-resistant GIST are available. The authors did a randomized, double-blind, placebo-controlled, multicenter, international trial to assess tolerability and anticancer efficacy of sunitinib, a multitargeted tyrosine kinase inhibitor, in patients with advanced GIST who were resistant to or intolerant of previous treatment with imatinib. METHODS: Blinded sunitinib or placebo was given orally once daily at a 50-mg starting dose in 6-week cycles, with 4 weeks on and 2 weeks off treatment. The primary endpoint was time to tumor progression. Intention-to-treat, modified intention-to-treat, and per-protocol analyses were done. This study is registered at http://www.ClinicalTrials.gov, number NCT00075218. FINDINGS: Three hundred-twelve patients were randomized in a 2:1 ratio to receive sunitinib (n = 207) or placebo (n = 105); the trial was unblinded early when a planned interim analysis showed significantly longer time to tumor progression with sunitinib. Median time to tumor progression was 27.3 weeks (95% CI 16.0 to 32.1) in patients receiving sunitinib and 6.4 weeks (95% CI 4.4 to 10.0) in those on placebo (HR 0.33; *P*<.0001). Therapy was tolerated reasonably well; the most common treatment-related adverse events were fatigue, diarrhea, skin discoloration, and nausea. INTERPRETATION: The authors noted significant clinical benefit, including disease control and superior survival, with sunitinib compared with placebo in patients with advanced GIST after failure and discontinuation of imatinib. Tolerability was acceptable. (Copyright [2006] Elsevier.)

Editor's summary and comments: In this international trial involving 56 centers, Demetri and colleagues validated the efficacy of sunitinib as a second-line therapy in advanced GIST. Patients who had failed imatinib therapy, either by disease progression or drug intolerance, were enrolled. Initially powered to detect a 50% improvement in median PFS, the study was unblinded early after a planned interim analysis. Using intention-to-treat analysis, PFS was superior in the sunitinib arm, extending the median time to progression by over 4 months. The threshold for difference in outcome was low, because sunitinib was being compared with placebo. Although not designed to evaluate overall survival, early data suggested an overall survival advantage in the sunitinib arm (HR of death 0.49, 95% CI 0.29 to 0.83). Given the limited options for patients who fail imatinib therapy, this study affirmed the viability of sunitinib as a second-line therapy.

6. Adjuvant imatinib mesylate after resection of localized, primary gastrointestinal stromal tumor: a randomized, double-blind, placebo-controlled trial.
Dematteo RP, Ballman KV, Antonescu CR, et al. Lancet 2009 Mar 28;373(9669):1097–104.[18]

Hypothesis: Imatinib 400 mg daily administered for 1 year after complete resection of localized, primary GIST improves recurrence-free survival over placebo.

# Patients Randomized	Study Groups	Stratification	Significance Demonstrated	% Change Identified in Trial
713	Imatinib 400 mg daily n = 359 Placebo n = 354	By tumor size: ≥3–<6 cm, ≥6–<10 cm, or ≥10 cm	Improvement in recurrence-free survival	HR 0.35 (95% CI 0.22–0.53, P<.0001)

Published abstract: BACKGROUND: GIST is the most common sarcoma of the intestinal tract. Imatinib mesylate is a small molecule that inhibits activation of the KIT and PDGFRα proteins, and is effective in first-line treatment of metastatic GIST. The authors postulated that adjuvant treatment with imatinib would improve recurrence-free survival compared with placebo after resection of localized, primary GIST. METHODS: The authors undertook a randomized phase 3, double-blind, placebo-controlled, multicenter trial. Eligible patients had complete gross resection of a primary GIST at least 3 cm in size and positive for the KIT protein by immunohistochemistry. Patients were randomly assigned, by a stratified biased coin design, to imatinib 400 mg (n = 359) or to placebo (n = 354) daily for 1 year after surgical resection. Patients and investigators were blinded to the treatment group. Patients assigned to placebo were eligible to cross over to imatinib treatment in the event of tumor recurrence. The primary endpoint was recurrence-free survival, and analysis was by intention to treat. Accrual was stopped early, because the trial results crossed the interim analysis efficacy boundary for recurrence-free survival. This study is registered with http://www.ClinicalTrials.gov, number NCT00041197. FINDINGS: All randomized patients were included in the analysis. At median follow-up of 19.7 months (range 0 to 56.4 months), 30 (8%) patients in the imatinib group and 70 (20%) in the placebo group had tumor recurrence or died. Imatinib significantly improved recurrence-free survival compared with placebo (98% [95% CI 96 to 100] versus 83% [95% CI 78 to 88] at 1 year; HR 0.35 [0.22 to 0.53]; one-sided P<.0001). Adjuvant imatinib was tolerated well, with the most common serious events being dermatitis (11 [3%] versus 0), abdominal pain (12 [3%] versus 6 [1%]), and diarrhea (10 [2%] versus 5 [1%]) in the imatinib group and hyperglycemia (two [<1%] versus seven [2%]) in the placebo group. INTERPRETATION: Adjuvant imatinib therapy is safe and seems to improve recurrence-free survival compared with placebo after the resection of primary GIST.

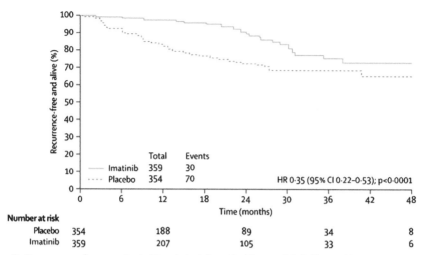

Fig. 2. Recurrence-free survival. (*Reprinted from* DeMatteo RP, Ballman KV, Antonescu CR, et al. Adjuvant imatinib mesylate after resection of localized, primary gastrointestinal stromal tumor: a randomized, double-blind, placebo-controlled trial. Lancet 2009;373(9669):1097–104; with permission.)

FUNDING: Funding was provided by the US National Institutes of Health and Novartis Pharmaceuticals. (Copyright [2009] Elsevier.)

Editor's summary and comments: While all other randomized controlled trials to date have explored the use of therapies in surgically incurable GIST, DeMatteo and colleagues evaluated the use of imatinib in an adjuvant setting, recognizing the significant risk of tumor recurrence following complete surgical resection. This trial originally was designed with overall survival as the primary end point, at a time when the efficacy of imatinib in advanced GIST had not yet been recognized fully. As the efficacy of imatinib became apparent, the study was redesigned to detect a 40% improvement in recurrence-free survival with a 90% power. The trial was closed early after interim analysis demonstrated efficacy in the therapy arm. With a median follow-up of nearly 20 months, a clear improvement in recurrence-free survival in the treatment arm was demonstrated. This effect was observed across all groups of the trial stratification. Differences in overall survival have not been demonstrated so far. In addition, the recurrence rate in the imatinib group was noted to increase appreciably around 18 months after surgery, raising the concern that 1 year of therapy may be inadequate for patients at high risk for recurrence. Although this study clearly demonstrates that empiric adjuvant imatinib reduces the rates of early recurrence, it is not yet clear whether this strategy improves overall survival over a strategy of watchful waiting. Furthermore, optimal patient selection criteria remain to be determined (**Fig. 2**).

DISCLOSURE

Dr. DeMatteo has received honoraria and served as a consultant for Novartis.

REFERENCES

1. Katz SC, DeMatteo RP. Gastrointestinal stromal tumors and leiomyosarcomas. J Surg Oncol 2008;97:350.

2. Dematteo RP, Heinrich MC, El-Rifai WM, et al. Clinical management of gastrointestinal stromal tumors: before and after STI-571. Hum Pathol 2002; 33:466.
3. Edmonson JH, Marks RS, Buckner JC, et al. Contrast of response to dacarbazine, mitomycin, doxorubicin, and cisplatin (DMAP) plus GM-CSF between patients with advanced malignant gastrointestinal stromal tumors and patients with other advanced leiomyosarcomas. Cancer Invest 2002;20:605.
4. Trent JC, Beach J, Burgess MA, et al. A two-arm phase II study of temozolomide in patients with advanced gastrointestinal stromal tumors and other soft tissue sarcomas. Cancer 2003;98:2693.
5. Von Burton G, Rankin C, Zalupski MM, et al. Phase II trial of gemcitabine as first-line chemotherapy in patients with metastatic or unresectable soft tissue sarcoma. Am J Clin Oncol 2006;29:59.
6. Blair SC, Zalupski MM, Baker LH. Ifosfamide and etoposide in the treatment of advanced soft tissue sarcomas. Am J Clin Oncol 1994;17:480.
7. Verweij J, Casali PG, Zalcberg J, et al. Progression-free survival in gastrointestinal stromal tumours with high-dose imatinib: randomised trial. Lancet 2004; 364:1127.
8. Nilsson B, Nilsson O, Ahlman H. Treatment of gastrointestinal stromal tumours: imatinib, sunitinib—and then? Expert Opin Investig Drugs 2009;18:457.
9. Kingham TP, DeMatteo RP. Multidisciplinary treatment of gastrointestinal stromal tumors. Surg Clin North Am 2009;89:217.
10. Joensuu H, Roberts PJ, Sarlomo-Rikala M, et al. Effect of the tyrosine kinase inhibitor STI571 in a patient with a metastatic gastrointestinal stromal tumor. N Engl J Med 2001;344:1052.
11. Demetri GD, von Mehren M, Blanke CD, et al. Efficacy and safety of imatinib mesylate in advanced gastrointestinal stromal tumors. N Engl J Med 2002;347:472.
12. Blanke CD, Demetri GD, von Mehren M, et al. Long-term results from a randomized phase II trial of standard- versus higher-dose imatinib mesylate for patients with unresectable or metastatic gastrointestinal stromal tumors expressing KIT. J Clin Oncol 2008;26:620.
13. Blanke CD, Rankin C, Demetri GD, et al. Phase III randomized, intergroup trial assessing imatinib mesylate at two dose levels in patients with unresectable or metastatic gastrointestinal stromal tumors expressing the kit receptor tyrosine kinase: S0033. J Clin Oncol 2008;26:626.
14. Zalcberg JR, Verweij J, Casali PG, et al. Outcome of patients with advanced gastro-intestinal stromal tumours crossing over to a daily imatinib dose of 800 mg after progression on 400 mg. Eur J Cancer 2005;41:1751.
15. Van Glabbeke M, Owzar K, Rankin C, et al. Comparisonof two doses of imatinib for the treatment of gastrointestinal stromal tumors (GIST): a meta-analysis based on 1,640 patients [supplement]. J Clin Oncol 2007;25:S546.
16. Blay JY, Le Cesne A, Ray-Coquard I, et al. Prospective multicentric randomized phase III study of imatinib in patients with advanced gastrointestinal stromal tumors comparing interruption versus continuation of treatment beyond 1 year: the French Sarcoma Group. J Clin Oncol 2007;25:1107.
17. Demetri GD, van Oosterom AT, Garrett CR, et al. Efficacy and safety of sunitinib in patients with advanced gastrointestinal stromal tumour after failure of imatinib: a randomised controlled trial [see comment]. Lancet 2006;368:1329.
18. Dematteo RP, Ballman KV, Antonescu CR, et al. Adjuvant imatinib mesylate after resection of localised, primary gastrointestinal stromal tumour: a randomised, double-blind, placebo-controlled trial. Lancet 2009;373:1097.

19. Eisenberg BL, Harris J, Blanke CD, et al. Phase II trial of neoadjuvant/adjuvant imatinib mesylate (IM) for advanced primary and metastatic/recurrent operable gastrointestinal stromal tumor (GIST): early results of RTOG 0132/ACRIN 6665. J Surg Oncol 2009;99:42.
20. Benjamin RS, Choi H, Macapinlac HA, et al. We should desist using RECIST, at least in GIST. J Clin Oncol 2007;25:1760.

Randomized Clinical Trials in Pancreatic Adenocarcinoma

Udo Rudloff, MD, PhD, Ajay V. Maker, MD,
Murray F. Brennan, MD, Peter J. Allen, MD*

KEYWORDS

- Pancreas cancer • Randomized controlled trials
- Literature review • Level Ia evidence

The authors of this article have identified 107 prospective, randomized controlled trials (RCT) for pancreatic adenocarcinoma through a standard MEDLINE literature search strategy that were published between 2000 and 2008. The articles are critically reviewed and ranked according to a standardized, previously published 3-tiered system (Ia, Ib, and Ic).[1] All trials included in this article are Ia or Ib.

Overall, there was a near 2-fold increase in RCT published per year on pancreas cancer compared with the previous study period (1977–2000). This surge was due mostly to an increase for advanced disease trials, the increased reporting of endoscopic stent trials, and advances in targeted molecular therapies.

RANDOMIZED CONTROLLED TRIALS IN PANCREAS CANCER BETWEEN 1977 AND 2000

The authors previously reported surgical trials conducted within this time period with the largest impact on clinical practice.[2] These trials included studies of the role of extended retroperitoneal lymphadenectomy for periampullary cancers, the type of pancreaticoenteric reconstruction after pancreaticoduodenectomy, and the use of prophylactic gastrojejunostomy for unresectable pancreatic cancer.[3–5] There was no evidence that a distal gastrectomy with perigastric and extensive retroperitoneal lymphadenectomy improved outcome,[3] and there was no advantage for pancreaticogastrostomy versus pancreaticojejunostomy following pancreaticoduodenectomy.[4] Although the randomized trial on prophylactic gastrojejunostomy for unresectable periampullary cancer indicated a decrease in the incidence of late gastric outlet obstruction and related complications in the prophylactic bypass group, the authors alluded to the emerging role of duodenal stents that would diminish the role of this procedure in the palliation of unresectable pancreas cancer in the near future.[5]

Disclosure: See last page of article.
Department of Surgery, Memorial Sloan-Kettering Cancer Center, Hepatopancreaticobiliary Service, C-896, 1275 York Avenue, NY 10021, USA
* Corresponding author.
E-mail address: allenp@mskcc.org (P. J. Allen).

Surg Oncol Clin N Am 19 (2010) 115–150
doi:10.1016/j.soc.2009.09.009
1055-3207/09/$ – see front matter © 2010 Elsevier Inc. All rights reserved.

There were 2 landmark chemotherapy/chemoradiation trials during this period, including a small randomized trial of gemcitabine use in advanced pancreas cancer.[6] Quality of life was improved in the gemcitabine arm compared with the 5-fluorouracil (5-FU) arm (24% vs 5%; $P = .002$), and there were also improvements in median survival (5.7 vs 4.4 months; $P = .003$), time to disease progression (9 vs 4 weeks; $P = .002$), and 12-month survival (18% vs 2% for the gemcitabine arm; $P = .0025$). Although the results were limited because of the single-blinded design of the study, they represent the first implications of superior clinical efficacy of gemcitabine-based systemic chemotherapy.[6] The EORTC GTCCG trial was a small study that observed a trend toward improved survival ($P = .09$) in patients who were randomized to adjuvant radiation therapy and 5-FU after surgery.[7] Randomized trials investigating nutritional interventions and the prophylactic use of octreotide to prevent pancreatic fistulas did not demonstrate any advantage in outcome in the intervention groups.[8–11]

SURGERY

There were 14 surgical trials reported, of which three compared pylorus preserving pancreaticoduodenectomy (PPPD) to a standard Whipple procedure (**Table 1**).[12–16] Both procedures were shown to be equally effective for the treatment of pancreatic and periampullary cancers, with similar overall long-term and disease-free survival rates. Both procedures were associated with comparable operating time, blood loss, hospital stay, mortality (5.3%), morbidity, positive resection margins, and quality of life (QOL). The two largest trials reported similar rates of delayed gastric emptying between groups, and only a minor postoperative increase in capacity to work at 6 months in the PPPD group (56 vs 77%; $P = .019$).[12,13] Previous findings of reduced blood loss and operating time in the PPPD group were not confirmed by these larger trials. These studies demonstrate the long-term oncologic equivalency of the two procedures and suggest only minor short-term advantages associated with PPPD.

Two trials evaluated the extent of lymphadenectomy at the time of pancreatectomy.[17,18] In both studies extended pancreaticoduodenectomy (PD) was performed with similar perioperative mortality but increased morbidity compared with standard pancreaticoduodenal resection. The overall complication rates were 29% for the standard group versus 43% for the extended group ($P = .01$).[17,19] Extended retroperitoneal lymphadenectomy was associated with longer hospital stay (11.3 vs 14.3 days; $P = .003$), increased rates of pancreatic fistula (13% vs 6%; $P = .05$), delayed gastric emptying (16% vs 6%; $P = .006$), and decreased early QOL.[18,19] There were no long-term differences in quality of life or overall survival (75% and 13% vs 73% and 29%; $P = .13$ for 1- and 5-year survival).[19,20] A consequent feasibility study to address this question concluded that more than 200,000 patients would be required to adequately power a trial that would detect any overall survival benefit, and will not be completed.[21,22]

Four trials examined various types of pancreaticoenteric reconstruction. Two studies examined the effect of pancreatic duct occlusion with fibrin glue versus standard pancreaticoenteric anastomosis after PD.[23,24] Duct occlusion without pancreaticojejunostomy was associated with significantly higher fistula rates (17% vs 5%) and a marked increase in the occurrence of diabetes mellitus. Of note, there were similar rates of exocrine insufficiency, as measured by the use of pancreatic enzyme substitution, between the study groups at 1-year follow-up (58 vs 59%).[23] Temporary duct occlusion with a pancreaticoenteric anastomosis did not decrease the rate or severity of intra-abdominal complications, including pancreatic fistula rates, after resection.[24] Pancreaticoenteric anastomosis remains the standard after PD.

One surgical trial compared pancreaticogastrostomy (PG) with pancreaticojejunostomy (PJ) following PD.[25] When compared with PJ, PG did not show any significant differences in overall postoperative complication rate or incidence of pancreatic fistula (13% in PG and 16% in PJ; P = not significant [NS]), confirming results of prior RCTs.[4,26] However, the trial identified minor perioperative advantages of PG over PJ such as a lower frequency of postoperative collections, delayed gastric emptying (P = NS), multiple surgical complications (P = .002), and pancreatic fistulae (13% in PG and 16% in PJ; P = NS).[25,26] PG or PJ can both be performed with similar perioperative morbidity and mortality.

Another trial compared an end-to-end telescoping invaginating ("binding") PJ to conventional PJ reconstruction.[27] In this trial, patients undergoing a "binding" PJ experienced decreased postoperative complications and a shortened hospital stay compared with conventional PJ. Pancreatic leaks occurred in 0 of 106 versus 8 of 111 patients (P = .014).[27]

One study examined the value of routine intraperitoneal drainage after pancreatic resection (n = 139, PD; n = 40, distal pancreatectomy).[28] The study failed to show a significant reduction in overall complications with peritoneal drainage (63% vs 57%). There was a trend toward an increased proportion of patients with drains that developed intraperitoneal sepsis, fluid collections, or a fistula (8/27 patients vs 19/27 patients; $P<.02$), suggesting that routine drain placement might have detrimental effects. Drains failed to reduce either the need for interventional radiologic drainage or surgical exploration for abdominal sepsis, and should not be considered mandatory or standard after pancreatic resection.

Two surgical trials studied the role of in locally advanced pancreatic head cancer. In a Japanese study, patients were randomized to resection versus no resection but chemoradiation. One-year survival (62% vs 32%, P = .05) and mean survival (>17 months vs 11 months, $P<.03$) were better in the surgical group.[29] In another study, patients were randomized to resection plus chemotherapy or to a palliative gastrobiliary bypass plus chemotherapy.[30] At 2 years, 82% of patients with resection were alive versus no patients in the palliative surgery group.

One trial investigated two different bypass operations for unresectable cancer of the pancreatic head.[31] Patients were randomized to isoperistaltic or antiperistaltic gastrojejunostomy. Both procedures yielded satisfactory results for palliation of unresectable carcinoma of the head of the pancreas without significant differences in gastric emptying time. Another group evaluated open versus laparoscopic isoperistaltic gastrojejunostomy as palliation in patients with gastric outlet obstruction. In 24 randomized patients, there was decreased blood loss, quicker return to solid oral intake, and less delayed gastric emptying in the laparoscopic group.[32]

There were two RCTs identified that are currently ongoing: the DROP trial (DRainage vs (direct) OPeration), a randomized multicenter trial addressing whether biliary drainage should be performed in patients with obstructive jaundice due to periampullary cancer, and the DISPACT trial (DIStal PAnCreaTectomy), evaluating stapled ligation versus hand-sewn closure of the pancreatic remnant.

CHEMOTHERAPY

Five of 38 chemotherapy trials reviewed examined the role of adjuvant chemotherapy or chemoradiation following potentially curative resection for pancreatic adenocarcinoma. The remainder compared different types and combinations of chemotherapeutic agents for patients with locally advanced or metastatic disease.

Table 1
Randomized surgical trials in pancreas cancer

Trial	Randomization	N	Significance Demonstrated	Classification
Tran[12]	PPPD vs standard PD	170	No difference in operation time, blood loss, hospital stay, delayed gastric emptying, morbidity, mortality, or oncologic outcome	Ia
Seiler[13]	PPPD vs standard	214	Both procedures are equally effective, PPPD offers minor advantages in early postop period	Ia
Lin[14]	PPPD vs standard	36	No significant difference in terms of operation time and blood loss. Delayed gastric emptying more common in PPPD group	Ib
Yeo[17]	standard PD (PPPD) vs extended PD	294	Similar mortality, increased morbidity; no difference in survival	Ib
Farnell[18]	standard PD vs PD with ELND	132	No difference in survival or complications but decrement in QOL at 4 months with ELND	Ib
Tran[23]	Duct occlusion vs pancreaticojejunostomy	169	Duct occlusion does not reduce postop complications but increases endocrine insufficiency	Ib
Suc[24]	PD vs PD with temporary duct occlusion	182	Ductal occlusion by intracanal injection of fibrin glue has no impact on severity of intra-abdominal complications	Ib
Bassi[25]	PD with PJ vs PD with PG	151	PG did not show any significant advantage in overall postop complications but had lower rate of collections and DGE	Ib
Peng[27]	conventional PJ after PD vs binding PJ	217	Binding pancreaticojejunostomy after PD significantly decreases postop complications and leak rates	Ib
Conlon[28]	Surgery + intraperitoneal drain vs Surgery + no drain	179	No reduction in deaths or complications (need for interventional radiology or surgical intervention)	Ia

(continued on next page)

| | | | Significance | |
Trial	Randomization	N	Demonstrated	Classification
Imamura[29]	Resection vs no resection + chemoradiation	42	Locally invasive, but resectable pancreas cancer is best treated with resection	Ib
Lygidakis[30]	Radical pancreatectomy vs palliative gastro-biliary bypass	56	Radical pancreatectomy, splenectomy, and vascular reconstruction is superior to bypass in patients with pancreas cancer and vascular invasion	Ib
Yilmaz[31]	Isoperistaltic gastrojejunostomy vs antiperistaltic gastrojejunostomy	44	Both operations suitable for patients Ib with unresectable PC	Ib
Navarra[32]	Open palliative gastrojejunostomy vs laparoscopic gastrojejunostomy	24	Laparoscopic gastrojejunostomy is a safe and feasible alternative to open gastrojejunostomy	Ib

Table 1
(continued)

Abbreviations: DGE, delayed gastric emptying; ELND, elective lymph node dissection; PD, pancreaticoduodenectomy; PG, pancreaticogastrostomy; PJ, pancreaticojejunostomy; PPPD, pyloruspreserving pancreaticoduodenectomy; QOL, quality of life.

Adjuvant Chemotherapy and Chemoradiation After Surgical Resection

The CONKO-001 trial randomized 368 patients after surgical resection to six cycles of standard-dose gemcitabine or observation (**Table 2**).[33] Intention-to-treat analysis was designed to determine if addition of gemcitabine would prolong disease-free survival by at least 6 months. Patients randomized to receive gemcitabine had a median disease-free survival of 13.9 months (confidence interval [CI] 11.4–15.3), and those who underwent surgery alone had a median disease-free survival of 6.9 months (CI 6.1–7.8; $P<.01$). There was no statistically significant difference in overall survival (22.1 vs 20.2 months, respectively; $P = .06$), but there were differences in estimated 3-year and 5-year survival. The study was criticized for its high local failure rate (92% in observation arm). However, this study further confirmed the efficacy of gemcitabine-based chemotherapy for patients who have undergone resection.

There were three RCTs investigating the role of adjuvant chemoradiation in resected pancreas cancer. The EORTC trial 40891 was performed to investigate the 1985 results of the 43-patient GITSG trial, and has reported their 5- and 10-year follow-up.[7,34,35] Two hundred and eighteen patients with resected cancers of the pancreatic head or periampullary region were randomized to surgery alone or surgery and chemoradiation (40 Gy and 5-FU). Subgroup analysis of 114 patients with pancreatic head cancers revealed a trend toward improved overall survival for those who received adjuvant therapy compared with the surgery-only arm (median 17.1 months vs 12.6 months), but this difference was not statistically significant ($P = .099$). Long-term ($\geq$ 10 years) follow-up results reported median survivals of 1.3 and 1.0 years

Table 2
Overall survival data from prospective, randomized trials of adjuvant therapy in resected pancreas cancer

Trial	N	Randomization	Overall Survival (Months)	P	Classification
CONKO-001[33]	368	Chemotherapy (gemcitabine) vs observation	22.1 vs 20.1 Disease-free survival 13.4 vs 6.9	0.06 <.001	Ia
ESPAC-1[36,37]	541	Chemoradiation (5-FU, 20 Gy) vs no chemoradiation Chemotherapy vs observation	15.9 vs 17.9 20.6 vs 15.5	0.05 0.009	Ia
Kosuge[39]	88	Chemotherapy (5-FU + cisplatin) vs observation	15.8 vs 12.5	0.94	Ib
EORTC 40,891[35]	218	Chemoradiation (5-FU + 40 Gy EBRT) vs observation	15.6 vs 12.0	0.165	Ib
RTOG 9704[40]	451	Gemcitabine and 5-FU + 50.4 Gy EBRT vs 5-FU + 50.4 Gy EBRT	20.5 vs 16.9	0.05	Ia

(P = NS), respectively, for pancreatic head cancers.[35] In contrast to the previous, much smaller GITSG trial, EORTC-40891 did not support the benefit of 5-FU based chemoradiation.[7,34]

A multicenter trial organized by the European Study Group for Pancreatic Cancer (ESPAC) investigated the impact of chemotherapy and chemoradiation on patient survival after surgery for pancreatic cancer.[36,37] ESPAC-1 enrolled 541 patients. Patients were randomized to one of four arms: observation, chemotherapy with bolus 5-FU and leucovorin, radiation (20 Gy) plus bolus 5-FU during the first 3 days of split-course external beam radiation therapy (EBRT), or radiation followed by 6 months of chemotherapy with bolus 5-FU and leucovorin. The study analyzed the survival outcomes using a 2 × 2 factorial design, pooling survival data based on randomization to chemotherapy (yes or no), or chemoradiation (yes or no). There were no differences in overall survival among the four original groups, but the combined patients who received chemoradiation did worse (median survival 15.9 months vs 17.9 months; P = .05) than those not receiving chemoradiation. Patients who received chemotherapy but no radiation gained a survival advantage (median survival 20.6 months vs 15.5 months; P = .009).[36] There was no survival benefit associated with chemoradiation even in the margin-positive group.[38] The investigators concluded that adjuvant chemotherapy improves survival, and that adjuvant chemoradiation failed to benefit patients, potentially reducing survival when provided before chemotherapy. The trial has been criticized for its lack of standardized trial methodology, the large number of patients who did not receive the intended therapy (31% to receive chemotherapy and 19% to receive chemoradiation did not receive it), lack of standardized pathology review, and its high local recurrence rate (>60%). ESPAC-1 remains the first RCT demonstrating a statistically significant benefit of adjuvant systemic therapy alone in resected pancreas cancer. A much smaller study from Japan randomizing patients after radical resection to adjuvant chemotherapy containing 5-FU and cisplatin or observation did not observe any survival benefit.[39]

The Radiation Therapy Oncology Group (RTOG) performed a prospective randomized trial (RTOG 9704) evaluating infusional 5-FU and radiation with and without gemcitabine.[40] Five hundred and thirty-eight patients were enrolled into the study, with most patients having tumors of the pancreatic head. There was no difference in overall survival between the two groups. For patients with pancreatic head tumors, the addition of gemcitabine to adjuvant 5-FU based chemoradiation was associated with a survival benefit that approached statistical significance (20.5 months vs 16.9 months; $P = .05$). Major criticisms of the trial include the lack of a radiation-only arm, and that at least 50% of patients had an unknown or positive margin.

Despite shortcomings of the aforementioned trials that include absent standardized margin evaluation (therapy for incompletely resected disease), lack of pretreatment/postoperative imaging, and heterogeneous patient populations; adjuvant chemotherapy appears to improve survival following resection, with a −001 supporting gemcitabine-based regimen being the preferred option. Ongoing adjuvant trials in pancreatic cancer include ESPAC-3, whereby patients are randomized to gemcitabine or bolus 5-FU and leucovorin; EORTC 40013, investigating gemcitabine-based chemoradiation versus systemic gemcitabine alone; and ACOSOG Z05031, a phase two trial evaluating a regimen of infusional 5-FU, cisplatin, subcutaneous interferon-α, and EBRT.[41]

Chemotherapy and Chemoradiation for Locally Unresectable or Advanced Disease

Gemcitabine plus platinum analogue versus gemcitabine alone
Five randomized trials compared the combination of gemcitabine plus a platinum analogue with gemcitabine alone (**Table 3**).[42–46] Overall, combination chemotherapy of gemcitabine and platinum analogues offers modest survival advantages in advanced pancreas cancer.

Table 3
Survival outcomes in advanced pancreatic adenocarcinoma of gemcitabine plus platinum analogue vs gemcitabine alone

Trial	N	Randomization	ORR (%)	P	Median PFS/ TTP (Mo)	P	Median Survival (Mo)	P	Class
Colucci[42]	107	Gem	9.2		2.0		5.0		Ib
		Gem + cisplatin	26.4	0.02	5.0	0.048	7.5	0.48	
Viret[43]	83	Gem	5		2.5		6.7		Ib
		Gem + cisplatin	7	—	2.2	ns	8.0	0.73	
Louvet[44]	313	Gem	17.3		3.7		7.1		Ib
		Gem + oxaliplatin	26.8	0.04	5.8	0.04	9.0	0.13	
Poplin[45]	832	Gem (standard)	5		—		4.9		Ib
		Gem (fixed dose rate)	10		—		6.0		
		Gem + oxaliplatin	9	—	—	—	5.9	ns	Ib
Heinemann[46]	195	Gem	8.2		3.1		6.0		Ib
		Gem + cisplatin	10.2	—	5.3	0.053	7.5	0.15	

Abbreviations: Gem, gemcitabine; ORR, overall response rate; PFS, progression-free survival; TTP, time-to-progression.

Gemcitabine plus fluoropyrimidine versus gemcitabine alone

The combination of gemcitabine with a fluoropyrimidine was tested in 6 randomized trials (**Table 4**).[47–52] A modest survival benefit may be expected from the combination gemcitabine with a fluoropyrimidine.

Gemcitabine plus other cytotoxic agent(s) versus gemcitabine alone

Four randomized trials evaluated the combination of gemcitabine with the multitarget antifolate pemetrexed or the topoisomerase inhibitors irinotecan and exatecan (**Table 5**).[53–56] Survival analysis failed to provide any benefit from chemotherapy including these agents. Compared with the results of gemcitabine with a platinum analogue or fluoropyrimidine, neither pemetrexed nor topoisomerase I inhibitors revealed any effect on survival. One trial examining the effect of gemcitabine plus epirubicin, 5-FU, and cisplatin (PEFG) versus gemcitabine alone showed higher toxicity, but improved progression-free survival.[57] Clinically relevant improvement in QOL was observed more often after PEFG than after gemcitabine, and deserves further evaluation (see **Table 5**).[58]

Gemcitabine plus other cytotoxic agent(s) versus other combination chemotherapy

One 3-armed trial compared gemcitabine plus oxaliplatin to gemcitabine plus capeci-tabine to oxaliplatin plus capecitabine.[59] All three regimens had similar clinical efficacy and a distinct but manageable side effect profile. EORTC 40984 examined taxane-based cytotoxic regimens that showed no clinically significant superiority of docetaxel in combination with gemcitabine or cisplatin (**Table 6**).[60]

5-Fluorouracil plus other cytotoxic agent versus single-agent 5-fluorouracil

There were four RCTs investigating 5-FU based chemotherapy regimens (**Table 7**).[61–64] One small trial compared 5-FU, leucovorin, and cisplatin to observation alone.[64] No advantage of the evaluated chemotherapy regimens was observed. In general, response rates of 5-FU based regimens were lower compared with other single-agent

Table 4
Gemcitabine plus fluoropyrimidine vs single-agent gemcitabine

Trial	N	Randomization	ORR (%)	P	Median PFS/ TTP (Mo)	P	Median Survival (Mo)	P	Classification
ECOG 2297[47]	322	Gem	5.6		2.2		5.4		Ib
		Gem + 5-FU	6.9	—	3.4	0.022	6.7	0.09	
Scheithauer[48]	83	Gem	14		4.0		8.2		Ib
		Gem + capecitabine	—		5.1	—	9.5	—	
Riess[49]	473	Gem	7.2		3.5		6.2		Ib
		Gem + 5-FU	4.8	—	3.5	0.44	5.9	0.68	
GOIRC[50]	91	Gem	8		3.5		7.8		Ib
		Gem + 5-FU	11	—	4.5	—	7.5	—	
Herrmann[51]	319	Gem	7.9		4.0		7.3		Ib
		Gem + capecitabine	10.1	—	4.8	0.21	8.4	0.31	
Cunningham[52]	533	Gem	7.1		—		6.0		Ib
		Gem + capecitabine	14.2	0.008	—	—	7.4	0.026	

Table 5
Gemcitabine plus other cytotoxic agent(s) vs single agent gemcitabine

Trial	N	Randomization	ORR (%)	P	Median PFS/ TTP (Mo)	P	Median Survival (Mo)	P	Classification
Rocha Lima[53]	360	Gem	4.4		3.0		6.6		Ib
		Gem + irinotecan	16.1	<0.001	3.5	0.352	6.3	0.79	
Oettle[54]	565	Gem	7.1		3.3		6.3		Ib
		Gem + pemetrexed	14.8	0.004	3.9	0.11	6.2	0.85	
Stathopoulos[55]	130	Gem	10		2.9		6.5		Ib
		Gem + irinotecan	15	0.387	2.8	0.795	6.4	0.97	
Abou-Alfa[56]	349	Gem	7.1		3.8		6.2		Ib
		Gem + exatecan	8.2	—	4.1	0.22	6.7	0.52	
Reni[57]	99	Gem	8.5		3.3				Ib
		Gem + PEFG (epirubicin, 5-FU, cisplatin)	38.5	0.0008	5.4	0.003			

cytotoxic agents. Although there was a trend of multiagent 5-FU based chemotherapy regimens toward improved outcome, the limited number of cycles of chemotherapy received hinders application of those findings into clinical decision making (see **Table 7**).[62,63]

Chemoradiation for locally advanced pancreatic cancer

Four RCTs examined the role of adjuvant chemoradiation for unresected locally advanced pancreas cancer. One trial compared EBRT (50.4) and infusional 5-FU to observation alone.[65] EBRT plus concurrent continuous 5-FU increased the length

Table 6
Gemcitabine plus other cytotoxic agent(s) vs other combination chemotherapy

Trial	N	Randomization	ORR (%)	P	Median PFS/ TTP (Mo)	P	Median Survival (Mo)	P	Classification
Boeck[59]	190	Gem + capecitabine	25		5.7		9.0		Ib
		Gem + oxaliplatin	13		3.9		6.9		
		Capecitabine + oxaliplatin	13	0.13	4.2	0.67	8.1	0.56	
EORTC 40,984[60]	96	Gem + docetaxel	19.4		3.9		7.4		Ib
		Docetaxel + cisplatin	23.5	—	2.8		7.1	—	

Table 7
5-FU plus other cytotoxic agent vs single-agent 5-FU

Trial	N	Randomization	ORR (%)	P	Median PFS/TTP (Mo)	P	Median Survival (Mo)	P	Classification
Maisey[61]	208	5-FU	8.4		2.8		5.1		Ib
		5-FU + mitomycin	17.6	0.04	3.8	0.14	6.5	0.34	
Ducreux[62]	207	5-FU	0		2.0				Ib
		5-FU + cisplatin	12	<0.01	2.4	0.08			
Ducreux[63]	63	5-FU	0		1.5		2.4		Ib
		5-FU + oxaliplatin	4.2		9.0				
		Oxaliplatin	0	—	2.0	—	3.4		
Huguier[64]	55	5-FU + oxaliplatin + leucovorin	—	—	8.6	0.33	—	—	Ib
		Observation	—		7.0		—		

(median survival 13.2 vs 6.4 months; $P = .0009$) and quality of survival compared with no chemoradiotherapy.[65] However, when chemoradiation was compared with chemotherapy alone in another study, overall survival was shorter with induction chemoradiotherapy (60 Gy, infusional 5-FU, and intermittent cisplatin) followed by gemcitabine compared with gemcitabine alone (8.6 months vs 13 months; $P = .03$), despite a small advantage for chemoradiation in median survival (14.5 vs 7.1 months, $P = .07$) and median time to progression (7.7 vs 2.7 months, $P = .019$).[66] EORTC E8282 randomized 114 patients to 59.4 Gy EBRT alone or in combination with 5-FU and mitomycin.[67] The addition of 5-FU and mitomycin-C to radiotherapy increased toxicity without improving disease-free or overall survival. A smaller study that compared gemcitabine-concurrent chemoradiation to 5-FU concurrent chemoradiation revealed improved response rates, median survival, and median time to progression in the gemcitabine based group.[68] The exact role of chemoradiation in advanced pancreas cancer remains to be elucidated.

Others

There was one randomized controlled trial examining resection rates of potentially resectable pancreas cancer after neoadjuvant gemcitabine or gemcitabine plus cisplatin. Nine of 27 patients in the gemcitabine arm were resectable versus 18 of 27 in the gemcitabine plus cisplatin arm.[69]

Ongoing Trials

Important ongoing studies include investigating the effect of neoadjuvant chemoradiation in locally resectable cancer of the pancreatic head compared with primary surgery by the Interdisciplinary Study Group of Gastrointestinal Tumors of the German Cancer Aid.[70] Adjuvant chemotherapy is integrated into both arms. The CapRI study is comparing adjuvant 5-FU to postoperative 5-FU, cisplatin, and interferon-α2b.[71] JASPAC-01 is randomizing patients after resection to gemcitabine or S-1, an oral fluoropyrimidine analogue, which showed efficacy in gastric cancer.[72]

Table 8
Outcomes of advanced pancreatic adenocarcinoma treated with molecular therapy

Trial	N	Randomization	Significance Demonstrated	Classification
Bramhall[93]	414	MMP inhibitor Marimastat vs gemcitabine	No difference in survival but dose response in Marimastat group	Ib
Bramhall[94]	239	Marimastat + gemcitabine vs gemcitabine alone	No difference in overall survival (OS), response rate, PFS or time to treatment failure	Ib
Moore[95]	277	MMP inhibitor BAY 12-9566 vs gemcitabine	Gemcitabine significantly superior in survival compared with BAY 12-9566 alone	Ib
Moore[73]	569	Gemcitabine alone vs gemcitabine + erlotinib	Improved overall and PFS with erlotinib	Ia
Cascinu[74]	84	Gemcitabine + cisplatin vs gemcitabine + cisplatin + cetuximab	ADDITION of cetuximab does not increase response rates or survival	Ib
Chen[76]	26	Imatinib vs gemcitabine	treatment with imatinib was not associated with clinical benefit	Ib
Friess[96]	89	Gemcitabine alone vs gemcitabine + EMD121974	Angiogenesis inhibitor EMD121974 did not show any clinically important efficacy on OS or other secondary end points	Ib
Spano[97]	103	Gemcitabine alone vs gemcitabine + axitinib	Addition of Axitinib has no impact on survival in patients with advanced pancreas cancer	Ib
Richards[77]	174	Gemcitabine alone vs gemcitabine and CI-994	Oral histone deacetylase inhibitor CI-994 inferior to gemcitabine alone	Ib
Alberts[78]	81	PS-341 alone vs PS-341 + gemcitabine	Use of proteasome inhibitor PS-341 alone or in combination with gemcitabine showed no clinical benefit	Ib
Van Cutsem[79]	688	Gemcitabine vs gemcitabine + tipifarnib (farnesyltransferase inhibitor)	Addition of tipifarnib does not improve survival and does not add clinical benefit to gem alone	Ib
Chau[80]	116	Observation vs gastrazole (JB05008) vs 5-FU	Gastrazole (JB95008) improves survival compared with placebo but offers no advantage in comparison to 5-FU	Ib

Table 9
Randomized gastroenterology trials in pancreas cancer

Trial	N	Randomization	Significance Demonstrated	Classification
Van Berkel[98]	60	Tannenbaum stent vs standard PE stent	No improved patency of Tannenbaum- type Teflon coated stent	Ib
Catalano[99]	106	Tannenbaum (Teflon) stent vs standard polyethylene stent	No difference in ease of placement or patency	Ib
Terruzi[100]	57	Teflon stent (Tannenbaum) vs standard polyethylene stent	No advantage in length of patency	Ib
Costamagna[101]	83	Hydromer-coated polyurethane stents (HCPS) vs standard polyethylene stent	No advantage in terms of stent longevity	Ib
Tringali[102]	120	DoubleLayer stent vs standard PE stent	DoubleLayer stent have a longer patency period than PE stents ($P = .005$)	Ib
Katsinelos[81]	47	Tannenbaum (Teflon) stent vs self-expanding metal stent (SEMS)	Stent patency of SEMS superior	Ib
Soderlund[82]	100	Standard PE stent vs SEMS	Median patency times are higher in SEMS; failure rates are higher in PE stents	Ia
Isayama[83]	112	Covered EMS vs uncovered metal stent	Covered metal stents are superior to uncovered stents in preventing tumor ingrowth and occlusion	Ib
Katsinelos[103]	92	Uncovered Hanaro metal stent vs uncovered Luminex metal stent	The 2 uncovered metal stents are comparable in terms of placement, occlusion rate, stent patency	Ib
Giorgio[104]	172	PE stent placement vs PE stent + sphincterotomy	Sphincterotomy does not seem to be necessary for successful PE stent placement	Ib
Artifon[105]	74	Covered SEMS with ES vs covered SEMS without prior ES	Deployment of covered SEMS without prior sphincterotomy is feasible and preferable in view of risk of stent migration	Ib

(continued on next page)

Table 9 (continued)				
Trial	N	Randomization	Significance Demonstrated	Classification
Pinol[106]	54	Percutaneous metal stent vs endoscopic PE stent	Placement of percutaneous metal stent is alternative to endoscopic PE stent	Ib
Halm[107]	52	Ursodeoxycholic acid (URSO) vs URSO + ofloxacin	Ofloxacin in combination with URSO not superior to URSO alone to prevent stent occlusion	Ib
Fogel[108]	102	Cytolong brush vs standard Geenen brush	No improved cancer detection rate with Cytolong brush	Ib

MOLECULAR THERAPY

Trials investigating molecular targeted therapy were limited to locally advanced or metastatic pancreatic cancer. To date, with the exception of the epidermal growth factor receptor (EGFR) tyrosine kinase inhibitor erlotinib, statistically significant differences in outcome have been reported (**Table 8**).

A randomized multinational trial of the EGFR receptor tyrosine kinase inhibitor erlotinib in combination with first-line gemcitabine-based chemotherapy has led to Food and Drug Administration approval of this agent for locally advanced, unresectable pancreas cancer.[73] The addition of erlotinib to gemcitabine led to improved overall survival versus gemcitabine alone (6.24 months vs 5.91 months; hazard ratio [HR] = 0.82; CI 0.69–0.99; P = .038). One-year survival (23% vs 17%; P = .023) and progression-free survival (HR = 0.77; CI 0.64–0.92; P = .004) was significantly longer in the erlotinib group. However, the EGFR receptor tyrosine kinase inhibitor cetuximab, a monoclonal antibody against the extracellular component of the human EGFR receptor, did not show any efficacy in two randomized trials.[74,75] Cetuximab added to gemcitabine plus cisplatin or gemcitabine (SWOG S0205 Phase III) did not show any superiority to gemcitabine plus cisplatin or gemcitabine alone. Because it is conceivable that unknown downstream targets of erlotinib explain its efficacy compared with cetuximab, further consideration of this agent seems to be justified.[75] In a small randomized trial, the tyrosine kinase inhibitor imatinib did not inhibit pancreatic cancer progression.[76]

Trials investigating the role of antiangiogenesis agents in pancreas cancer are inconclusive at this point. Results are awaited of the ongoing AViTA trial, which examines the addition of bevacizumab to gemcitabine and erlotinib in advanced pancreatic cancer.

Other compounds that were compared in combination with gemcitabine to gemcitabine alone in randomized trials in advanced pancreas cancer were: CI-994, an oral histone deacetylase inhibitor; PS-341, a proteasomes inhibitor; and tipifarnib, a farnesyltransferase inhibitor.[77–79] None of these agents increased overall survival or response rates, and can currently not be recommended outside clinical trials. Gastrazole (JB95008), a novel CCK2/gastrin receptor antagonist, similarly did not exhibit any significant survival difference in comparison with 5-FU or placebo.[80]

Table 10				
Outcomes of nutritional intervention and modulation in pancreas cancer				
Trial	**N**	**Randomization**	**Significance Demonstrated**	**Classification**
Braga[109]	257	Postop total parenteral nutrition (TPN) vs Early enteral nutrition (EEN)	No difference in postop morbidity or mortality; no difference in nutritional, immunologic, and inflammatory variables	Ib
Hyltander[110]	126	Supportive parenteral or enteral postop vs oral nutrition only	After major surgery, specialized supportive enteral or parenteral nutrition are not superior to oral nutrition only	Ib
Lobo[111]	120	Jejunostomy feeding vs jejunostomy feeding with immune modulating diet	Early postop feeding with immune modulating diet no advantage when compared with standard feed	Ib
Fearon[112]	200	Protein + energy dense supplement vs isocaloric supplement enriched with n-3 fatty acids	Enrichment with n-3 fatty acids did not provide therapeutic advantage	Ib
Moses[113]	24	Protein + energy dense supplement vs isocaloric supplement enriched with n-3 fatty acids	Enrichment with n-3 fatty acids might increase total energy expenditure through increase in physical activity	Ib
Johnson[114]	278	Low-dose intravenous lithium gamolenate (LiGLA) vs high-dose LiGLA	High-dose IV treatment appeared to have an adverse effect; no difference in survival	Ib
Gordon[115]	50	Thalidomide vs placebo	Thalidomide is effective in attenuating weight loss in patients with cachexia	Ib
Heller[116]	44	Postop TPN vs postop TPN and omega-3 polyunsaturated fatty acids	Improved liver function and tendency to shorter intensive care unit stay in fatty acid receiving group	Ib
Giger[117]	46	Preoperative immunonutrition vs regular formula (enriched with glycine)	Improved inflammatory markers and reduced length of stay	Ib

GASTROENTEROLOGY

The majority of randomized prospective trials in gastroenterology addressed endo-scopically placed stents as treatment for malignant biliary obstruction (**Table 9**). Patients with biliary obstruction randomized to self-expanding metal stents (SEMS) had higher median patency times and lower failure rates than patients who underwent standard polyethylene (PE) or Teflon (Tannenbaum) stent placement.[81,82] The more effective SEMS are recommended in unresectable patients with malignant common bile duct strictures who are expected to survive 4.5 months or longer.[82] Less costly plastic stents are a reasonable alternative in patients with a very limited life expec-tancy. Covered metal stents were shown in one randomized trial to be superior to uncovered SEMS in preventing tumor in growth and occlusion, and are particularly advantageous for long-term palliation.[83]

NUTRITION

A summary of nutrition trials is given in **Table 10**.

RADIATION THERAPY

Two trials investigated new radiation sensitizers for intraoperative radiation therapy (IORT) for locally advanced pancreas cancer.[84,85] The addition of the radiosensitizer

Table 11 Randomized radiotherapy trials in pancreas cancer				
Trial	N	Randomization	Significance Demonstrated	Classification
Karasawa[85]	46	Intraoperative radiation therapy (IORT) vs IORT + doranidazol	Sensitizer might be effective in improving long-term survival for pancreas cancer	Ib
Sunamura[84]	48	IORT alone vs IORT + PR-350	Improved response rates with addition of radiosensitizer PR-350 but no effect on OS	Ib
Rosemurgy[86]	30	5-FU + gemcitabine vs 5-FU + gemcitabine + (32)P	(32)P promotes tumor liquefaction but does not decrease tumor size and but does not impact on survival	Ib
Hishinuma[87]	65	Curative resection vs Resection + prophylactic hepatic radiation	Prophylactic hepatic irradiation was associated with decreased risk of liver metastases and increased OS	Ib
Chung[88]	48	Gemcitabine-based concurrent chemoradiation (CCRT) + doxifluridine vs Paclitaxel-based CCRT + doxifluridine	Both regimens equally effective	Ib

Table 12
Randomized immunotherapy trials

Trial	N	Randomization	Significance Demonstrated	Classification
Kobari[89]	29	Tumor resection + IORT vs tumor resection + IORT + intraportal infusion of lymphokine-activated killer cells and recombinant interleukin (IL)-2	Reduced incidence of recurrence in treatment group ($P<.05$)	Ib
Wagener[90]	36	5-FU + cisplatin vs 5-FU + cisplatin + interferon-2b	No benefit; significant toxicity	Ib
Caprotti[91]	30	Surgery vs preop IL-2 and surgery	Short period of preop immunotherapy with IL-2 may improve time to progression and OS	Ib

PR-350 to IORT showed improved response rates at 6 months, though no effect on overall survival was observed,[84] and the radiation sensitizer doranidazole improved 3-year survival (23% vs 0% in control group; $P = .0102$).[85] In another small trial, the addition of intratumoral (32)P to 5-FU, gemcitabine, and radiation therapy promoted tumor liquefaction but no clinical response or effect on survival.[86] Another small trial investigating the role of prophylactic hepatic radiation (PHI) after curative resection found that the incidence of liver metastases was significantly lower in the PHI group ($P = .0455$).[87] Because patients also had an improved survival in the PHI group, a larger trial on this intervention seems to be justified (**Table 11**). A small trial comparing gemcitabine-based concurrent chemoradiation (CCRT) and paclitaxel-based CCRT plus doxifluridine revealed that both regimens had comparable efficacy (see **Table 11**).[88]

Table 13
Palliative interventions in pancreas cancer

Trial	N	Randomization	Significance Demonstrated	Classification
Wong[118]	100	Systemic analgesic therapy vs systemic analgesic therapy + neurolytic celiac plexus blockade (NCPB)	Celiac plexus blockade improves pain relief but not opioid consumption, QOL, or survival	Ib
Suleyman[119]	39	Celiac plexus block vs splanchnic nerve block	Splanchnic nerve block may be an alternative to celiac plexus block for tumors of the pancreatic body/tail	Ib

Table 14 RCT in pancreatic cancer—other				
Trial	N	Randomization	Significance Demonstrated	Classification
Gouillat[120]	75	PD vs PD + 7 days continuous octreotide infusion	Reduced incidence of pancreatic fistula and pancreatic stump-related complications	Ib
Shan[121]	54	PD vs PD + 7 day continuous IV somatostatin infusion	Incidence of overall morbidity and stump-related complications reduced by 50%	Ib
Hesse[122]	105	PD vs PD + low-dose octreotide for 7 days	Perioperative use of low-dose somatostatin for 7 d does not reduce complications or fistula formation	Ib
Burch[123]	84	Octreotide vs 5-FU or 5-FU + leucovorin	Octreotide only inferior; trial prematurely stopped	Ib
Jang[124]	56	PD vs PD + lansoprazole	Increased mean volume of distal pancreatic remnant and higher postoperative insulin levels	Ib
Wiedenmann[125]	89	Gemcitabine alone vs gemcitabine + infliximab	Addition of infliximab to gemcitabine in patients with cachexia and pancreas does not increase lean-body mass	Ib
Kuchler[92]	271	Standard care vs program of psychotherapeutic support	Increased overall survival with formal psychotherapeutic intervention post surgery	Ib
Horwha[126]	84	Endoscopic ultrasound-guided fine-needle aspiration (EUS-FNA) vs CT/US-FNA	EUS-FNA is superior to CT/US-FNA for the diagnosis of pancreatic malignancy	Ib
Imbriaco[127]	60	Dual phase vs single phase helical CT	Single phase as effective as dual phase; less radiation	Ib
Yanaga[128]	78	Fixed contrast material dose vs weight-tailored contrast injection	Dose protocol tailored to patient's body weight yielded satisfactory pancreatic imaging	Ib

IMMUNOTHERAPY

There were three trials investigating different forms of immunotherapy. One study evaluated the effect of adoptive immunotherapy using intraportal infusion of lymphokine-activated killer cells plus IORT after resection in advanced pancreas cancer.[89] Based on the observed trend toward improved overall survival as well as a significantly decreased incidence of liver metastasis, this approach justifies further study (**Table 12**). A randomized study of 5-FU plus cisplatin with or without interferon-α2b in patients with advanced pancreas cancer showed considerable toxicity and little activity in both arms.[90] A 3-day course of preoperative interleukin-2 (IL-2) was associated with improved progression-free and overall survival at 36 months (see **Table 12**).[91]

PALLIATIVE THERAPY

A summary of palliative therapy trials is given in **Table 13**.

OTHERS

Patients randomized to receive formal psychotherapeutic support started preoperatively plus routine care on the surgical wards were found have superior long-term survival compared with patients that received routine care alone (**Table 14**).[92] The authors attribute these findings, which are superior to other psychotherapeutic intervention trials, to initiating psychotherapeutic support in the preoperative period as well as focusing on all aspects of surgical and oncological treatments.[92]

LEVEL IA EVIDENCE: RANDOMIZED CLINICAL TRIALS IN PANCREAS CANCER

1. Pancreaticoduodenectomy with or without distal gastrectomy and extended retroperitoneal lymphadenectomy for periampullary adenocarcinoma, part 2: randomized controlled trial evaluating survival, morbidity, and mortality. Yeo CJ, Cameron JL, Lillemoe KD, et al. Ann Surg 2002;236:355–68.[17]

Hypothesis: Pancreaticoduodenectomy with extended lymphadenectomy and distal gastrectomy improves survival for periampullary cancers, and can be performed with similar morbidity and mortality as in standard pancreaticoduodenectomy.

No. of Patients Randomized	Study Groups	Stratification	Significance	Actual Change (%) P value
294	Standard PD N = 146 Radical PD N = 148	Age, gender	No difference in 1-, 3-, and 5-year survival No difference in mortality; Increase in −pancreatic fistula −delayed gastric emptying−overall complication	80%, 44%, 23% vs 77%, 44%, 29%; P = .79 6% vs 13%; P = .05 6% vs 16%; P = .006 29% vs 43%; P = .01

Published abstract: OBJECTIVE: To evaluate, in a prospective, randomized single-institution trial, the end points of operative morbidity, operative mortality, and survival in patients undergoing standard versus radical (extended) pancreaticoduodenectomy. SUMMARY BACKGROUND DATA: Numerous retrospective reports and a few prospective randomized trials have suggested that the performance of an extended lymphadenectomy in association with a pancreaticoduodenal resection may improve survival for patients with pancreatic and other periampullary adenocarcinomas. METHODS: Between April 1996 and June 2001, 299 patients with periampullary adenocarcinoma were enrolled in a prospective, randomized single-institution trial. After intraoperative verification (by frozen section) of margin-negative resected peri-ampullary adenocarcinoma, patients were randomized to either a standard pancrea-ticoduodenectomy (removing only the peripancreatic lymph nodes en bloc with the specimen) or a radical (extended) pancreaticoduodenectomy (standard resection plus distal gastrectomy and retroperitoneal lymphadenectomy). All pathology speci-mens were reviewed, fully categorized, and staged. The postoperative morbidity, mortality, and survival data were analyzed. RESULTS: Of the 299 patients randomized, five (1.7%) were subsequently excluded because their final pathology failed to reveal periampullary adenocarcinoma, leaving 294 patients for analysis (146 standard vs 148 radical). The two groups were statistically similar with regard to age (median 67 years) and gender (54% male). All the patients in the radical group underwent distal gastric resection, while 86% of the patients in the standard group underwent pylorus preser-vation ($P<.0001$). The mean operative time in the radical group was 6.4 hours, compared with 5.9 hours in the standard group ($P = .002$). There were no significant differences between the two groups with respect to intraoperative blood loss, trans-fusion requirements (median zero units), location of primary tumor (57% pancreatic, 22% ampullary, 17% distal bile duct, 3% duodenal), mean tumor size (2.6 cm), posi-tive lymph node status (74%), or positive margin status on final permanent section (10%). The mean total number of lymph nodes resected was significantly higher in the radical group. Of the 148 patients in the radical group, only 15% (n = 22) had meta-static adenocarcinoma in the resected retroperitoneal lymph nodes, and none had retroperitoneal nodes as the only site of lymph node involvement. One patient in the radical group with negative pancreaticoduodenectomy specimen lymph nodes had a micrometastasis to one perigastric lymph node. There were six perioperative deaths (4%) in the standard group versus three perioperative deaths (2%) in the radical group ($P = $ NS). The overall complication rates were 29% for the standard group versus 43% for the radical group ($P = .01$), with patients in the radical group having significantly higher rates of early delayed gastric emptying and pancreatic fistula and a significantly longer mean postoperative stay. With a mean patient follow-up of 24 months, there were no significant differences in 1-, 3-, or 5-year and median survival when comparing the standard and radical groups. CONCLUSIONS: Radical (extended) pan-creaticoduodenectomy can be performed with similar mortality but some increased morbidity compared with standard pancreaticoduodenectomy. The data to date fail to indicate that a survival benefit is derived from the addition of a distal gastrectomy and retroperitoneal lymphadenectomy to a pylorus-preserving pancreaticoduodenec-tomy. (Copyright 2002, Lippincott Williams & Wilkins. Reprinted with permission.)

Editor's comments: This study is a prospective, randomized single-institution trial examining the end points of operative morbidity, operative mortality, and survival in patients undergoing standard versus radical (extended) PD. No significant differences in survival were observed when evaluating subgroups of patients with pancreas cancer stratified by number of resected lymph nodes comparing standard and radical PD. Extended PD was associated with a significantly higher operative morbidity but not mortality. Overall, patients can only benefit from extended PD when

- involved nodes are located around the pancreas
- more involved nodes are removed during extended resection
- increased number of involved nodes translates into improved survival

Assuming an 80% R0 resection rate, 10% second-order only nodal involvement, and a 5% node-positive M0 rate, a mathematical model showed that thousands of patients would be required to demonstrate a difference in survival. The associated perioperative morbidity of extended resection seems prohibitive without a survival benefit. The lack of a demonstrable survival advantage for surgical lymphadenectomy is not limited to pancreas cancer. Most data from prospective randomized trials in gastric adenocarcinoma have failed to reveal a survival advantage for extended lymphadenectomy. The study, however, supports the use of pylorus preservation with lower rates of early delayed gastric emptying, pancreatic fistula, and hospital stay. PD without extended resections should continue to be the standard operative approach to tumors of the pancreatic head.

2. Pylorus preserving pancreaticoduodenectomy versus standard Whipple procedure. A prospective, randomized, multicenter analysis of 170 patients with pancreatic and periampullary tumors.
Tran KTC, Smeenk HG, van Eijck CHJ, et al. Ann Surg 2004;240:738–45.[12]
Hypothesis: Results of PPPD are equal to those of standard pancreaticoduodenectomy in terms of survival, delayed gastric emptying (DGE), blood loss, and hospital stay.

No. of Patients Randomized	Study Groups	Stratification	Significance	Actual Median Survival (P value)
170	Standard PD N = 83 PPPD N = 87	Age, gender, preoperative weight	No difference in median disease-free survival. No difference in DGE, blood loss, operative time, postoperative weight loss	14 vs 15 months; P = .80

Published abstract: OBJECTIVE: A prospective randomized multicenter study was performed to assess whether the results of PPPD equal those of the standard Whipple (SW) operation, especially with respect to duration of surgery, blood loss, hospital stay, DGE, and survival. SUMMARY BACKGROUND DATA: PPPD has been associated with a higher incidence of DGE, resulting in a prolonged period of postoperative nasogastric suctioning. Another criticism of the PPPD for patients with a malignancy is the radicalness of the resection. On the other hand, PPPD might be associated with a shorter operation time and less blood loss. METHODS: A prospective, randomized multicenter study was performed in a nonselected series of 170 consecutive patients. All patients with suspicion of pancreatic or periampullary tumor were included and randomized for a SW or a PPPD resection. Data concerning patients' demographics, intraoperative and histologic findings, as well as postoperative mortality, morbidity, and follow-up up to 115 months after discharge, were analyzed. RESULTS: There were no significant differences noted in age, sex distribution, tumor localization, and staging. There were no differences in median blood loss and duration of operation between the two techniques. DGE was observed equally in the two groups. There was only a marginal difference in postoperative weight loss in favor of the standard Whipple procedure. Overall operative mortality was 5.3%. Tumor positive resection margins were found for 12 patients of the SW group and 19 patients of the PPPD group (P<.23). Long-term follow-up showed no significant statistical differences in survival between the two groups (P<.90). CONCLUSIONS: The SW and PPPD operations were associated with comparable operation time, blood loss, hospital stay, mortality, morbidity, and incidence of DGE. The overall long-term and disease-free survival was comparable in both groups. Both surgical procedures are equally effective for the treatment of pancreatic and periampullary carcinoma. (Copyright 2004, Lippincott Williams & Wilkins. Reprinted with permission.)

Editor's comments: Previous studies have shown that pyloric preservation may lead to long-term improvement in gastrointestinal function, increased postoperative weight gain, fewer peptic ulcers, less dumping, shorter operations, and less intraoperative blood loss. Initial studies reported a high incidence of complications, including delayed gastric emptying, ulcerative lesions at the anastomosis, and concern about resection margins and overall oncologic outcome. This study compared PPPD to standard Whipple procedure. No difference in complication rates, length of stay, incidence of delayed gastric emptying (22 vs 23%; $P = .80$), margin positivity (17 vs 26%; $P = .23$), or overall median disease-free survival (14 vs 15 months; $P = .80$) was found. The PPPD seems to have the same oncologic outcome as standard PD. Long-term survival and disease-free survival did not exhibit significant differences. Both procedures are equally effective for the treatment of pancreatic cancer.

3. Prospective randomized clinical trial of the value of intraperitoneal drainage after pancreatic resection
Conlon KC, Labow D, Leung D, et al. Ann Surg 2001;234:487–94.[28]

Hypothesis: The presence or absence of surgically placed drains has no impact on the rate of either death or complications after pancreatic resections.

No. of Patients Randomized	Study Groups	Stratification	Significance	Actual Change (%); P value
171	Drain N = 88 No drain N = 91	Age, gender, site of disease, prior therapy	No difference in operative mortality No difference in need for interventional radiologic drainage or surgical exploration Increased incidence of intra-abdominal sepsis (abscess and fistula) in drain group	2% vs 2%; P = NS 19% vs 8%; P<.02

Published abstract: OBJECTIVE: To test the hypothesis that routine intraperitoneal drainage is not required after pancreatic resection. SUMMARY BACKGROUND DATA: The use of surgically placed intraperitoneal drains has been considered routine after pancreatic resection. Recent studies have suggested that for other major upper abdominal resections, routine postoperative drainage is not required and may be associated with an increased complication rate. METHODS: After informed consent, eligible patients with peripancreatic tumors were randomized during surgery either to have no drains placed or to have closed suction drainage placed in a standardized fashion after pancreatic resection. Clinical, pathologic, and surgical details were recorded. RESULTS: One hundred seventy-nine patients were enrolled in the study, 90 women and 89 men. Mean age was 65.4 years (range 23–87). The pancreas was the tumor site in 142 (79%) patients, with the ampulla (n = 24), duodenum (n = 10), and distal common bile duct (n = 3) accounting for the remainder. A pancreaticoduodenectomy was performed in 139 patients and a distal pancreatectomy in 40 cases.

Eighty-eight patients were randomized to have drains placed. Demographic, surgical, and pathologic details were similar between both groups. The overall 30-day death rate was 2% (n = 4). A postoperative complication occurred during the initial admission in 107 patients (59%). There was no significant difference in the number or type of complications between groups. In the drained group, 11 patients (12.5%) developed a pancreatic fistula. Patients with a drain were more likely to develop a significant intra-abdominal abscess, collection, or fistula. CONCLUSIONS: This randomized prospective clinical trial failed to show a reduction in the number of deaths or complications with the addition of surgical intraperitoneal closed suction drainage after pancreatic resection. The data suggest that the presence of drains failed to reduce either the need for interventional radiologic drainage or surgical exploration for intra-abdominal sepsis. Based on these results, closed suction drainage should not be considered mandatory or standard after pancreatic resection. (Copyright 2001, Lippincott Williams & Wilkins. Reprinted with permission.)

Editor's comments: This study is a prospective, single-institution trial on the value of routine intraperitoneal drainage after pancreatic resections. The investigators find in their well-conducted study that the use of peritoneal drains does not decrease perioperative morbidity or mortality, and they suggest in their secondary end-point analysis that certain intra-abdominal complications may actually be increased with the use of drains. The incidence of CT-guided drainage for intra-abdominal abscesses was similar in the drain group and "no drain" group. Surgically placed intraperitoneal drains did not reduce the rate of either death or complications associated with pancreatic resections. These results are consistent with those of other prospective trials that have examined the role of drainage after a variety of other abdominal procedures, including colorectal resections, hepatic and gastric resection, closure of perforated duodenal ulcers, and cholecystectomy, suggesting that the routine placement of drains after pancreatic resection is unnecessary and may be harmful to the patient.

4. Adjuvant chemotherapy with gemcitabine versus observation in patients undergoing curative-intent resection of pancreatic cancer. A randomized controlled trial.
Oettle H, Post S, Neuhaus P, et al. JAMA 2007;297(3):267–77.[33]

Hypothesis: Adjuvant chemotherapy with gemcitabine administered after complete resection of pancreas cancer improves disease-free survival by at least 6 months.

No. of Patients Randomized	Study Groups	Stratification	Significance	Actual Median Disease-free Survival; P value
355	Gemcitabine N = 179 Observation alone N = 175	Age, gender, surgery, primary tumor size, nodal status, grading, histology	Improvement in median disease-free survival No improvement in overall survival	13.4 vs 6.9 months; P<.001 22.1 vs 20.2 months; P = .06

Published abstract: CONTEXT: The role of adjuvant therapy in resectable pancreatic cancer is still uncertain, and no recommended standard exists. OBJECTIVE: To test the hypothesis that adjuvant chemotherapy with gemcitabine administered after complete resection of pancreatic cancer improves disease-free survival by 6 months or more. DESIGN, SETTING, and PATIENTS: Open, multicenter, randomized controlled phase

III trial with stratification for resection, tumor, and node status. Conducted from July 1998 to December 2004 in the outpatient setting at 88 academic and community-based oncology centers in Germany and Austria. A total of 368 patients with gross complete (R0 or R1) resection of pancreatic cancer and no prior radiation or chemotherapy were enrolled into two groups. Intervention: Patients received adjuvant chemotherapy with six cycles of gemcitabine on days 1, 8, and 15 every 4 weeks (n = 179), or observation ([control] n = 175). MAIN OUTCOME MEASURE: Primary end point was disease-free survival, and secondary end points were overall survival, toxicity, and quality of life. Survival analysis was based on all eligible patients (intention-to-treat). RESULTS: More than 80% of patients had R0 resection. The median number of chemotherapy cycles in the gemcitabine group was 6 (range, 0–6). Grade three or four toxicities rarely occurred, with no difference in quality of life (by Spitzer index) between groups. During median follow-up of 53 months, 133 patients (74%) in the gemcitabine group and 161 patients (92%) in the control group developed recurrent disease. Median disease-free survival was 13.4 months in the gemcitabine group (95% confidence interval, 11.4–15.3) and 6.9 months in the control group (95% confidence interval, 6.1–7.8; $P<.001$, log-rank). Estimated disease-free survival at 3 and 5 years was 23.5% and 16.5% in the gemcitabine group, and 7.5% and 5.5% in the control group, respectively. Subgroup analyses showed that the effect of gemcitabine on disease-free survival was significant in patients with either R0 or R1 resection. There was no difference in overall survival between the gemcitabine group (median, 22.1 months; 95% confidence interval, 18.4–25.8; estimated survival, 34% at 3 years and 22.5% at 5 years) and the control group (median, 20.2 months; 95% confidence interval, 17–23.4; estimated survival, 20.5% at 3 years and 11.5% at 5 years; $P = .06$, log-rank). CONCLUSIONS: Postoperative gemcitabine significantly delayed the development of recurrent disease after complete resection of pancreatic cancer compared with observation alone. These results support the use of gemcitabine as adjuvant chemotherapy in resectable carcinoma of the pancreas. (Copyright 2007, American Medical Association. All rights reserved. Reprinted with permission.)

Editor's comments: The objective of the trial was to determine whether gemcitabine prolonged disease-free survival after pancreatectomy with curative intent compared with observation alone. Inclusion criteria included carcinoembryonic antigen and carbohydrate antigen 19-9 less than 2.5 times the upper limit of normal post-resection. Three hundred and sixty-eight patients who underwent a complete resection for pancreatic adenocarcinoma were randomly assigned to undergo observation, or to receive six cycles of standard-dose gemcitabine (1000 mg/m^2 over 30 minutes) on days 1, 8, and 15, every 28 days. Patients randomized to receive gemcitabine had a median disease-free survival of 13.9 months (95% CI, 11.4–15.3), and those who underwent surgery alone had a median disease-free survival of 6.9 months (95% CI, 6.1–7.8; $P<.001$). There was no statistically significant difference in overall survival between those assigned to receive adjuvant gemcitabine and those assigned to observation (median 22.1 months vs 20.2 months; $P = .06$), but there were differences in estimated 3-year and 5-year survival rates.

The trial was consequently criticized for its lack of standardized pretreatment imaging, high local recurrence rate (35% of patients in gemcitabine arm; 41% of patients in observation arm), and lack of standardized histopathological evaluation. Furthermore, most follow-up was performed with ultrasonography, raising a concern for underreporting of local recurrence or R1 resection states. However, the finding of a similar survival benefit in patients with R1 resections as well as the fact that nearly all patients in the control arm received gemcitabine on relapse at a later stage (which is a delayed cross-over and reduces the survival difference between the two study groups) reaffirm the investigators' conclusions. Adjuvant treatment with gemcitabine has minimal toxicity and prolongs disease-free survival in patients undergoing R0 and R1 resection for pancreatic cancer.

5. A randomized trial of chemoradiotherapy and chemotherapy after resection of pancreatic cancer.
Neoptolemos JP, Stocken DD, Friess H, et al. N Engl J Med 2004;350:1200–10.[36]

Hypothesis: There is a survival difference between patients with resectable pancreas cancer treated with curative resection alone versus those treated with resection and adjuvant chemoradiation or chemotherapy.

No. of Patients Randomized	Study Groups	Stratification	Significance	% Change P value
289	Two-by-two factorial analysis: No chemoradio-therapy N = 144 versus Chemoradio-therapy N = 145 No chemotherapy N = 142 vs Chemotherapy N = 147	Age, gender, surgery including resection margins, maximal tumor size, nodal status, grading, histology, medical comorbidities, postoperative complications	Adjuvant 5-FU based chemoradio-therapy had deleterious effect on survival (chemoradio-therapy vs no chemoradio-therapy) Adjuvant 5-FU based chemotherapy prolongs overall median survival (chemothera-py vs no chem-otherapy)	15.9 months vs 17.9 months; $P = .05$ 20.1 months vs 15.5 months; $P = .009$

Published abstract: BACKGROUND: The effect of adjuvant treatment on survival in pancreatic cancer is unclear. We report the final results of the European Study Group for Pancreatic Cancer 1 Trial and update the interim results. METHODS: In a multicenter trial using a 2-by-2 factorial design, we randomly assigned 73 patients with resected pancreatic ductal adenocarcinoma to treatment with chemoradiotherapy alone (20 Gy over a 2-week period plus fluorouracil), 75 patients to chemotherapy alone (fluorouracil), 72 patients to both chemoradiotherapy and chemotherapy, and 69 patients to observation. RESULTS: The analysis was based on 237 deaths among the 289 patients (82%) and a median follow-up of 47 months (interquartile range, 33–62). The estimated 5-year survival rate was 10% among patients assigned to receive chemoradiotherapy and 20% among patients who did not receive chemoradiotherapy ($P = .05$). The 5-year survival rate was 21% among patients who received chemotherapy and 8% among patients who did not receive chemotherapy ($P = .009$). The benefit of chemotherapy persisted after adjustment for major prognostic factors. CONCLUSIONS: Adjuvant chemotherapy has a significant survival benefit in patients with resected pancreatic cancer, whereas adjuvant chemoradiotherapy has a deleterious effect on survival. (Copyright 2004, Massachusetts Medical Society. All rights reserved.)

Editor's comments: This study enrolled 289 patients. After pancreatic resection, patients were randomized to one of four arms: observation; chemotherapy with bolus

5-FU (425 mg/m^2) and leucovorin (20 mg/m^2) daily for 5 days every 28 days for 6 months, chemoradiation with bolus 5-FU (500 mg/m^2) provided during the first 3 days of split-course EBRT, or chemoradiation followed by 6 months of chemotherapy with bolus 5-FU and leucovorin. The study analyzed the survival outcomes based on randomization to chemotherapy or chemoradiation. There were no survival differences between the four original arms. When the results were pooled by the 2 × 2 factorial design analysis, patients who received chemoradiation had a decreased survival versus no chemoradiation (median survival 15.9 vs 17.9 months; HR 1.28; CI 0.99–1.66; P = .05), whereas patients who received chemotherapy derived a survival benefit (20.6 vs 15.5 months; HR 0.71; CI 0.55–0.92; P = .009). The ESPAC-1 trial sparked a lot of criticism because of its complicated, nonstandard design and analysis. The current study attempted to address some of the concerns of the earlier study by analyzing only randomized patients and extending the median follow-up to 47 months. However, the high rate of nonadherence to the assigned treatment arm and the potential for bias into the randomization by a sequential-therapy design (2 × 2 factorial design) continue to weaken the validity of the analysis and its conclusions. Other points of criticism include the accrual of patients with positive margins and the high local recurrence rate. The absence of standardized pretreatment imaging and histopathological evaluation make it unclear what the pretreatment disease burdens were. The finding that chemoradiation has a negative effect on survival is biologically unexpected, and the finding that the original, nonpooled chemotherapy group (N = 75) did not experience any difference in survival questions the conclusions. Based on this trial, it is premature to state that standard of care for patients with resectable pancreatic cancer should consist of curative surgery followed by adjuvant fluorouracil-based systemic chemotherapy.

6. Long-term survival and metastatic pattern of pancreatic and periampullary cancer after adjuvant chemoradiation or observation: long-term results of EORTC trial 40,891.

Smeenk HG, van Eijck CHJ, Hop WC, et al. Ann Surg 2007;246:734–40.[35]

Hypothesis: Adjuvant chemoradiation in resected pancreatic cancer influences long-term survival.

No. of Patients Randomized	Study Groups	Stratification	Significance	% Change P value
218	Observation N = 179 Chemoradiation N = 175	Age, gender, surgery, grade, pathologic type, T stage, nodal status, time from surgery	Overall and progression-free survival was not influenced by treatment	1.6 years vs 1.8 years; P = .54 1.2 years vs 1.5 years; P = .663

Published abstract: BACKGROUND: The role of adjuvant chemoradiation in pancreatic cancer remains unclear. This report presents the long-term follow-up results of EORTC trial 40891, which assessed the role of chemoradiation in resectable pancreatic cancer. METHODS: Two hundred eighteen patients were randomized after resection of the primary tumor. Eligible patients had T1-2 N0-N1a M0 pancreatic cancer or T1-3 N0-N1a M0 periampullary cancers, all histologic proven. Patients in the treatment group (n = 110) underwent postoperative chemoradiation (40 Gy plus 5-FU). Patients in the control group (n = 108) had no further adjuvant treatment. FINDINGS: After a median follow-up of 11.7 years, 173 deaths (79%) have been reported. The overall survival did not differ between the 2 treatment groups (Chemoradiation treatment vs Controls: death rate ratio 0.91, 95% CI: 0.68–1.23, P value 0.54). The 10-year overall survival was 18% in the whole population of patients (8% in the pancreatic head cancer group and 29% in the periampullary cancer group). INTERPRETATION: These results confirm the previous short-term analysis, indicating no benefit of adjuvant chemoradiation over observation in patients with resected pancreatic cancer or periampullary cancer. Patients with pancreatic cancer may survive more than 10 years. Only 1 of 31 cases recurred after year 7. (Copyright 2007, Lippincott Williams & Wilkins. Reprinted with permission.)

Editor's comments: The EORTC 40891 trial evaluated the effect of adjuvant treatment with radiotherapy and fluorouracil after potentially curative resection in patients with cancer of the pancreatic head and periampullary region. This study reported its long-term findings (11.7 years median follow-up). 5-FU was given concomitantly as a continuous infusion with radiation therapy. Radiotherapy was started 2 to 8 weeks after surgery and was delivered over a period of 6 weeks with a 2-week break. A total of 40 Gy was delivered in two courses of 20 Gy (2 Gy/d, 5 days per week at weeks 1–2 and 5–6). During each course, 5-FU (25 mg/kg/d) was administered with a maximal daily dose of 1500 mg. At 11.7 years of follow-up there was no evidence that survival was influenced by treatment (HR = 0.91; CI 0.68–1.23; P = .54). Median survival was 1.6 and 1.8 years in the two groups, respectively. Also, no advantage of adjuvant treatment on progression-free survival was shown (for all patients HR = 0.94; CI 0.70–1.26; P = .663 with median progression-free survival of 1.2 vs 1.5 years). EORTC 40891 has been criticized for its long accrual period and its limited sample size. Both control and study groups were reduced by about 20% over time, contributing to the lack of statistical power in their final conclusions. Furthermore, 21% of patients had positive margins, and resection status was not controlled for in the study, potentially confounding the ability to discriminate small differences, Despite these limitations, with the adequate long-term follow-up, fluorouracil-based adjuvant chemoradiation is unlikely to provide a survival benefit to patients who undergo resection for pancreatic and periampullary tumors.

7. Erlotinib plus gemcitabine compared with gemcitabine alone in patients with advanced pancreatic cancer: a phase III trial of the National Cancer Institute of Canada Clinical Trials Group.
Moore MJ, Goldstein D, Hamm J, et al. JCO 2007;25:1960–66.[73]

Hypothesis: The addition of erlotinib to first-line gemcitabine based chemotherapy in the treatment of chemotherapy-naïve locally advanced and metastatic pancreas cancer improves outcome.

No. of Patients Randomized	Study Groups	Stratification	Significance	Overall Survival; P value
569	Erlotinib and gemcitabine N = 285 Gemcitabine alone N = 284	Age, sex, performance status, extent of disease (locally advanced vs metastatic), prior therapy	Improved overall median survival with the addition of erlotinib Improved progression-free survival by the addition of erlotinib	6.24 vs 5.91 months; P = .038 3.75 vs 3.55 months; P = .004

Published abstract: PURPOSE: Patients with advanced pancreatic cancer have a poor prognosis and there have been no improvements in survival since the introduction of gemcitabine in 1996. Pancreatic tumors often overexpress human epidermal growth factor receptor type 1 (HER1/EGFR) and this is associated with a worse prognosis. We studied the effects of adding the HER1/EGFR-targeted agent erlotinib to gemcitabine in patients with unresectable, locally advanced, or metastatic pancreatic cancer. PATIENTS and METHODS: Patients were randomly assigned 1:1 to receive standard gemcitabine plus erlotinib (100 or 150 mg/d orally) or gemcitabine plus placebo in a double-blind, international phase III trial. The primary end point was overall survival. RESULTS: A total of 569 patients were randomly assigned. Overall survival based on an intent-to-treat analysis was significantly prolonged on the erlotinib/gemcitabine arm with a hazard ratio (HR) of 0.82 (95% CI, 0.69–0.99; $P = .038$, adjusted for stratification factors; median 6.24 months vs 5.91 months). One-year survival was also greater with erlotinib plus gemcitabine (23% vs 17%; $P = .023$). Progression-free survival was significantly longer with erlotinib plus gemcitabine with an estimated HR of 0.77 (95% CI, 0.64–0.92; $P = .004$). Objective response rates were not significantly different between the arms, although more patients on erlotinib had disease stabilization. There was a higher incidence of some adverse events with erlotinib plus gemcitabine, but most were grade 1 or 2. CONCLUSION: To our knowledge, this randomized phase III trial is the first to demonstrate statistically significantly improved survival in advanced pancreatic cancer by adding any agent to gemcitabine. The recommended dose of erlotinib with gemcitabine for this indication is 100 mg/d. (Copyright 2007, American Society of Clinical Oncology. Reprinted with permission.)

Editor's comments: This trial organized by the National Cancer Institute of Canada Clinical Trials Group investigated the role of erlotinib plus gemcitabine in advanced pancreatic cancer. Human epidermal growth factor receptor type 1 (HER1/ERRB1) is overexpressed in many pancreatic cancers, and is associated with poor prognosis and disease progression, thus the addition of an EGFR inhibitor is a useful and interesting strategy in pancreas cancer. Median overall survival was significantly improved with erlotinib and gemcitabine compared with placebo plus gemcitabine (6.24 vs 5.91 months; $P = .038$), resulting in an overall 22% improvement in survival, and the 1-year survival rate with erlotinib and gemcitabine was 23% vs 17% with gemcitabine alone ($P = .03$). A median change of 10 to 14 days would however seem to be clinically irrelevant despite statistical significance. There are 3 major caveats with this trial:

1. There was no difference in response rate (8.6% vs 8.0%; $P = .29$).
2. There was no association of erlotinib benefit to EGFR mutational status (as examined by immunohistochemistry).
3. Another large, randomized prospective study, SWOG S0205, which randomized patients with advanced pancreatic cancer to gemcitabine alone or gemcitabine plus cetuximab, an antibody directed against the EGFR receptor, showed no difference in survival between the two groups.

Although there was a statistically significant difference between the 2 groups, it is questionable if this represents a clinically meaningful difference. When calculating the mean average gain associated with the addition of erlotinib, the mean actuarial benefit was 12 to 14 days. Although this trial represents the first "positive" trial of targeted therapy in pancreas cancer, the results are so clinically irrelevant that a more positive trial should be provided to accept clinical efficacy of erlotinib. As the cost of 150 mg/d of erlotinib from Canada is $1650.00 per month, this 10-day survival improvement, if it exists, will cost 6 × $1,650 = $9,900 or approximately $1000 per day of gained survival.

DISCLOSURE

Authors have nothing to disclose.

REFERENCES

1. Stojadinovic A, Brooks A, Hoos A, et al. An evidence-based approach to the surgical management of resectable pancreatic adenocarcinoma. J Am Coll Surg 2003;196(6):954–64.
2. Stojadinovic A, Hoos A, Brennan MF, et al. Randomized clinical trials in pancreatic cancer. Surg Oncol Clin N Am 2002;11(1):207–29, x.
3. Yeo CJ, Cameron JL, Sohn TA, et al. Pancreaticoduodenectomy with or without extended retroperitoneal lymphadenectomy for periampullary adenocarcinoma: comparison of morbidity and mortality and short-term outcome. Ann Surg 1999; 229(5):613–22 [discussion: 622–4].
4. Yeo CJ, Cameron JL, Maher MM, et al. A prospective randomized trial of pancreaticogastrostomy versus pancreaticojejunostomy after pancreaticoduodenectomy. Ann Surg 1995;222(4):580–8 [discussion: 588–92].
5. Lillemoe KD, Cameron JL, Hardacre JM, et al. Is prophylactic gastrojejunostomy indicated for unresectable periampullary cancer? A prospective randomized trial. Ann Surg 1999;230(3):322–8 [discussion: 328–30].
6. Burris HA 3rd, Moore MJ, Andersen J, et al. Improvements in survival and clinical benefit with gemcitabine as first-line therapy for patients with advanced pancreas cancer: a randomized trial. J Clin Oncol 1997;15(6):2403–13.
7. Kalser MH, Ellenberg SS. Pancreatic cancer. Adjuvant combined radiation and chemotherapy following curative resection. Arch Surg 1985;120(8):899–903.
8. Brennan MF, Pisters PW, Posner M, et al. A prospective randomized trial of total parenteral nutrition after major pancreatic resection for malignancy. Ann Surg 1994;220(4):436–41 [discussion: 441–44].
9. Heslin MJ, Latkany L, Leung D, et al. A prospective, randomized trial of early enteral feeding after resection of upper gastrointestinal malignancy. Ann Surg 1997;226(4):567–77 [discussion: 577–80].
10. Lowy AM, Lee JE, Pisters PW, et al. Prospective, randomized trial of octreotide to prevent pancreatic fistula after pancreaticoduodenectomy for malignant disease. Ann Surg 1997;226(5):632–41.
11. Yeo CJ, Cameron JL, Lillemoe KD, et al. Does prophylactic octreotide decrease the rates of pancreatic fistula and other complications after pancreaticoduodenectomy? Results of a prospective randomized placebo-controlled trial. Ann Surg 2000;232(3):419–29.
12. Tran KT, Smeenk HG, van Eijck CH, et al. Pylorus preserving pancreaticoduodenectomy versus standard Whipple procedure: a prospective, randomized, multicenter analysis of 170 patients with pancreatic and periampullary tumors. Ann Surg 2004;240(5):738–45.
13. Seiler CA, Wagner M, Bachmann T, et al. Randomized clinical trial of pylorus-preserving duodenopancreatectomy versus classical Whipple resection-long term results. Br J Surg 2005;92(5):547–56.
14. Lin PW, Shan YS, Lin YJ, et al. Pancreaticoduodenectomy for pancreatic head cancer: PPPD versus Whipple procedure. Hepatogastroenterology 2005; 52(65):1601–4.
15. Seiler CA, Wagner M, Sadowski C, et al. Randomized prospective trial of pylorus-preserving vs. classic duodenopancreatectomy (Whipple procedure): initial clinical results. J Gastrointest Surg 2000;4(5):443–52.

16. Iqbal N, Lovegrove RE, Tilney HS, et al. A comparison of pancreaticoduodenec-tomy with pylorus preserving pancreaticoduodenectomy: a meta-analysis of 2822 patients. Eur J Surg Oncol 2008;34(11):1237–45.

17. Yeo CJ, Cameron JL, Lillemoe KD, et al. Pancreaticoduodenectomy with or without distal gastrectomy and extended retroperitoneal lymphadenectomy for periampullary adenocarcinoma, part 2: randomized controlled trial evaluating survival, morbidity, and mortality. Ann Surg 2002;236(3):355–66 [discussion: 366–68].

18. Farnell MB, Pearson RK, Sarr MG, et al. A prospective randomized trial comparing standard pancreatoduodenectomy with pancreatoduodenectomy with extended lymphadenectomy in resectable pancreatic head adenocarci-noma. Surgery 2005;138(4):618–28 [discussion: 628–30].

19. Riall TS, Cameron JL, Lillemoe KD, et al. Pancreaticoduodenectomy with or without distal gastrectomy and extended retroperitoneal lymphadenectomy for periampullary adenocarcinoma—part 3: update on 5-year survival. J Gastrointest Surg 2005;9(9):1191–204 [discussion: 1204–06].

20. Nguyen TC, Sohn TA, Cameron JL, et al. Standard vs. radical pancreaticoduo-denectomy for periampullary adenocarcinoma: a prospective, randomized trial evaluating quality of life in pancreaticoduodenectomy survivors. J Gastrointest Surg 2003;7(1):1–9 [discussion: 9–11].

21. Pawlik TM, Abdalla EK, Barnett CC, et al. Feasibility of a randomized trial of extended lymphadenectomy for pancreatic cancer. Arch Surg 2005;140(6): 584–9 [discussion: 589–91].

22. Farnell MB, Aranha GV, Nimura Y, et al. The role of extended lymphadenectomy for adenocarcinoma of the head of the pancreas: strength of the evidence. J Gastrointest Surg 2008;12(4):651–6.

23. Tran K, Van Eijck C, Di Carlo V, et al. Occlusion of the pancreatic duct versus pancreaticojejunostomy: a prospective randomized trial. Ann Surg 2002; 236(4):422–8 [discussion: 428].

24. Suc B, Msika S, Fingerhut A, et al. Temporary fibrin glue occlusion of the main pancreatic duct in the prevention of intra-abdominal complications after pancre-atic resection: prospective randomized trial. Ann Surg 2003;237(1):57–65.

25. Bassi C, Falconi M, Molinari E, et al. Reconstruction by pancreaticojejunostomy versus pancreaticogastrostomy following pancreatectomy: results of a compara-tive study. Ann Surg 2005;242(6):767–71 [discussion: 771–3].

26. Wente MN, Shrikhande SV, Muller MW, et al. Pancreaticojejunostomy versus pancreaticogastrostomy: systematic review and meta-analysis. Am J Surg 2007;193(2):171–83.

27. Peng SY, Wang JW, Lau WY, et al. Conventional versus binding pancreaticoje-nostomy after pancreaticoduodenectomy: a prospective randomized trial. Ann Surg 2007;245(5):692–8.

28. Conlon KC, Labow D, Leung D, et al. Prospective randomized clinical trial of the value of intraperitoneal drainage after pancreatic resection. Ann Surg 2001; 234(4):487–93 [discussion: 493–4].

29. Imamura M, Doi R, Imaizumi T, et al. A randomized multicenter trial comparing resection and radiochemotherapy for resectable locally invasive pancreatic cancer. Surgery 2004;136(5):1003–11.

30. Lygidakis NJ, Singh G, Bardaxoglou E, et al. Mono-bloc total spleno-pancreati-coduodenectomy for pancreatic head carcinoma with portal-mesenteric venous invasion. A prospective randomized study. Hepatogastroenterology 2004; 51(56):427–33.

31. Yilmaz S, Kirimlioglu V, Katz DA, et al. Randomised clinical trial of two bypass operations for unresectable cancer of the pancreatic head. Eur J Surg 2001;167(10):770–6.
32. Navarra G, Musolino C, Venneri A, et al. Palliative antecolic isoperistaltic gastro-jejunostomy: a randomized controlled trial comparing open and laparoscopic approaches. Surg Endosc 2006;20(12):1831–4.
33. Oettle H, Post S, Neuhaus P, et al. Adjuvant chemotherapy with gemcitabine vs observation in patients undergoing curative-intent resection of pancreatic cancer: a randomized controlled trial. JAMA 2007;297(3):267–77.
34. Klinkenbijl JH, Jeekel J, Sahmoud T, et al. Adjuvant radiotherapy and 5-fluorouracil after curative resection of cancer of the pancreas and periampullary region: phase III trial of the EORTC gastrointestinal tract cancer cooperative group. Ann Surg 1999;230(6):776–82 [discussion: 782–4].
35. Smeenk HG, van Eijck CH, Hop WC, et al. Long-term survival and metastatic pattern of pancreatic and periampullary cancer after adjuvant chemoradiation or observation: long-term results of EORTC trial 40891. Ann Surg 2007;246(5):734–40.
36. Neoptolemos JP, Stocken DD, Friess H, et al. A randomized trial of chemoradio-therapy and chemotherapy after resection of pancreatic cancer. N Engl J Med 2004;350(12):1200–10.
37. Neoptolemos JP, Dunn JA, Stocken DD, et al. Adjuvant chemoradiotherapy and chemotherapy in resectable pancreatic cancer: a randomised controlled trial. Lancet 2001;358(9293):1576–85.
38. Neoptolemos JP, Stocken DD, Dunn JA, et al. Influence of resection margins on survival for patients with pancreatic cancer treated by adjuvant chemoradiation and/or chemotherapy in the ESPAC-1 randomized controlled trial. Ann Surg 2001;234(6):758–68.
39. Kosuge T, Kiuchi T, Mukai K, et al. A multicenter randomized controlled trial to evaluate the effect of adjuvant cisplatin and 5-fluorouracil therapy after curative resection in cases of pancreatic cancer. Jpn J Clin Oncol 2006;36(3):159–65.
40. Regine WF, Winter KA, Abrams RA, et al. Fluorouracil vs gemcitabine chemo-therapy before and after fluorouracil-based chemoradiation following resection of pancreatic adenocarcinoma: a randomized controlled trial. JAMA 2008;299(9):1019–26.
41. Wolff RA, Varadhachary GR, Evans DB. Adjuvant therapy for adenocarcinoma of the pancreas: analysis of reported trials and recommendations for future prog-ress. Ann Surg Oncol 2008;15(10):2773–86.
42. Colucci G, Giuliani F, Gebbia V, et al. Gemcitabine alone or with cisplatin for the treatment of patients with locally advanced and/or metastatic pancreatic carci-noma: a prospective, randomized phase III study of the Gruppo Oncologia dell'Italia Meridionale. Cancer 2002;94(4):902–10.
43. Viret F, Ychou M, Lepille D, et al. Gemcitabine in combination with cisplatin (GP) versus gemcitabine (G) alone in the treatment of locally advanced or metastatic pancreatic cancer: final results of a multicenter randomized phase II. J Clin Oncol 2004;22(14S) [abstract 4118].
44. Louvet C, Labianca R, Hammel P, et al. Gemcitabine in combination with oxali-platin compared with gemcitabine alone in locally advanced or metastatic pancreatic cancer: results of a GERCOR and GISCAD phase III trial. J Clin Oncol 2005;23(15):3509–16.
45. Poplin E, Levy DE, Berlin J, et al. Phase III trial of gemcitabine (30-mintue infu-sion) versus gemcitabine (fixed-dose rate-infusion [FDR]) versus gemcitabine +

oxaliplatine (GEMOX) in patients with advanced pancreas cancer (E6201). J Clin Oncol 2006;24(18S) [abstract LBA4004].

46. Heinemann V, Quietzsch D, Gieseler F, et al. Randomized phase III trial of gemcitabine plus cisplatin compared with gemcitabine alone in advanced pancreatic cancer. J Clin Oncol 2006;24(24):3946–52.

47. Berlin JD, Catalano P, Thomas JP, et al. Phase III study of gemcitabine in combination with fluorouracil versus gemcitabine alone in patients with advanced pancreatic carcinoma: Eastern Cooperative Oncology Group Trial E2297. J Clin Oncol 2002;20(15):3270–5.

48. Scheithauer W, Schull B, Ulrich-Pur H, et al. Biweekly high-dose gemcitabine alone or in combination with capecitabine in patients with metastatic pancreatic adenocarcinoma: a randomized phase II trial. Ann Oncol 2003;14(1):97–104.

49. Riess H, Helm A, Niedergethmann M, et al. A randomised, prospective, multicenter phase III trial of gemcitabine, 5-fluorouracil (5-FU), folinic-acid vs. gemcitabine alone in patients with advanced pancreatic cancer. J Clin Oncol 2005;23(16S) [abstract 4009].

50. Di Costanzo F, Carlini P, Doni L, et al. Gemcitabine with or without continuous infusion 5-FU in advanced pancreatic cancer: a randomised phase II trial of the Italian oncology group for clinical research (GOIRC). Br J Cancer 2005; 93(2):185–9.

51. Herrmann R, Bodoky G, Ruhstaller T, et al. Gemcitabine plus capecitabine compared with gemcitabine alone in advanced pancreatic cancer: a randomized, multicenter, phase III trial of the Swiss Group for Clinical Cancer Research and the Central European Cooperative Oncology Group. J Clin Oncol 2007; 25(16):2212–7.

52. Cunningham D, Chau I, Stocken DD, et al. Phase III randomised comparison of gemcitabine (GEM) versus gemcitabine plus capecitabine (GEM-CAP) in patients with advanced pancreatic cancer. Eur J Cancer 2005;18(Suppl 7) [abstract PS11].

53. Rocha Lima CM, Green MR, Rotche R, et al. Irinotecan plus gemcitabine results in no survival advantage compared with gemcitabine monotherapy in patients with locally advanced or metastatic pancreatic cancer despite increased tumor response rate. J Clin Oncol 2004;22(18):3776–83.

54. Oettle H, Richards D, Ramanathan RK, et al. A phase III trial of pemetrexed plus gemcitabine versus gemcitabine in patients with unresectable or metastatic pancreatic cancer. Ann Oncol 2005;16(10):1639–45.

55. Stathopoulos GP, Syrigos K, Aravantinos G, et al. A multicenter phase III trial comparing irinotecan-gemcitabine (IG) with gemcitabine (G) monotherapy as first-line treatment in patients with locally advanced or metastatic pancreatic cancer. Br J Cancer 2006;95(5):587–92.

56. Abou-Alfa GK, Letourneau R, Harker G, et al. Randomized phase III study of exatecan and gemcitabine compared with gemcitabine alone in untreated advanced pancreatic cancer. J Clin Oncol 2006;24(27):4441–7.

57. Reni M, Cordio S, Milandri C, et al. Gemcitabine versus cisplatin, epirubicin, fluorouracil, and gemcitabine in advanced pancreatic cancer: a randomised controlled multicentre phase III trial. Lancet Oncol 2005;6(6):369–76.

58. Reni M, Bonetto E, Cordio S, et al. Quality of life assessment in advanced pancreatic adenocarcinoma: results from a phase III randomized trial. Pancreatology 2006;6(5):454–63.

59. Boeck S, Hoehler T, Seipelt G, et al. Capecitabine plus oxaliplatin (CapOx) versus capecitabine plus gemcitabine (CapGem) versus gemcitabine plus

oxaliplatin (mGemOx): final results of a multicenter randomized phase II trial in advanced pancreatic cancer. Ann Oncol 2008;19(2):340–7.

60. Lutz MP, Van Cutsem E, Wagener T, et al. Docetaxel plus gemcitabine or docetaxel plus cisplatin in advanced pancreatic carcinoma: randomized phase II study 40984 of the European Organisation for Research and Treatment of Cancer Gastrointestinal Group. J Clin Oncol 2005;23(36):9250–6.

61. Maisey N, Chau I, Cunningham D, et al. Multicenter randomized phase III trial comparing protracted venous infusion (PVI) fluorouracil (5-FU) with PVI 5-FU plus mitomycin in inoperable pancreatic cancer. J Clin Oncol 2002;20(14): 3130–6.

62. Ducreux M, Rougier P, Pignon JP, et al. A randomised trial comparing 5-FU with 5-FU plus cisplatin in advanced pancreatic carcinoma. Ann Oncol 2002;13(8): 1185–91.

63. Ducreux M, Mitry E, Ould-Kaci M, et al. Randomized phase II study evaluating oxaliplatin alone, oxaliplatin combined with infusional 5-FU, and infusional 5-FU alone in advanced pancreatic carcinoma patients. Ann Oncol 2004;15(3):467–73.

64. Huguier M, Barrier A, Valinas R, et al. Randomized trial of 5-fluorouracil, leucovorin and cisplatin in advanced pancreatic cancer. Hepatogastroenterology 2001;48(39):875–8.

65. Shinchi H, Takao S, Noma H, et al. Length and quality of survival after external-beam radiotherapy with concurrent continuous 5-fluorouracil infusion for locally unresectable pancreatic cancer. Int J Radiat Oncol Biol Phys 2002;53(1):146–50.

66. Chauffert B, Mornex F, Bonnetain F, et al. Phase III trial comparing intensive induction chemoradiotherapy (60 Gy, infusional 5-FU and intermittent cisplatin) followed by maintenance gemcitabine with gemcitabine alone for locally advanced unresectable pancreatic cancer. Definitive results of the 2000–01 FFCD/SFRO study. Ann Oncol 2008;19(9):1592–9.

67. Cohen SJ, Dobelbower R Jr, Lipsitz S, et al. A randomized phase III study of radiotherapy alone or with 5-fluorouracil and mitomycin-C in patients with locally advanced adenocarcinoma of the pancreas: Eastern Cooperative Oncology Group study E8282. Int J Radiat Oncol Biol Phys 2005;62(5):1345–50.

68. Li CP, Chao Y, Chi KH, et al. Concurrent chemoradiotherapy treatment of locally advanced pancreatic cancer: gemcitabine versus 5-fluorouracil, a randomized controlled study. Int J Radiat Oncol Biol Phys 2003;57(1):98–104.

69. Palmer DH, Stocken DD, Hewitt H, et al. A randomized phase 2 trial of neoadjuvant chemotherapy in resectable pancreatic cancer: gemcitabine alone versus gemcitabine combined with cisplatin. Ann Surg Oncol 2007;14(7): 2088–96.

70. Brunner TB, Grabenbauer GG, Meyer T, et al. Primary resection versus neoadjuvant chemoradiation followed by resection for locally resectable or potentially resectable pancreatic carcinoma without distant metastasis. A multi-centre prospectively randomised phase II-study of the Interdisciplinary Working Group Gastrointestinal Tumours (AIO, ARO, and CAO). BMC Cancer 2007;7:41.

71. Knaebel HP, Marten A, Schmidt J, et al. Phase III trial of postoperative cisplatin, interferon alpha-2b, and 5-FU combined with external radiation treatment versus 5-FU alone for patients with resected pancreatic adenocarcinoma—CapRI: study protocol [ISRCTN62866759]. BMC Cancer 2005;5:37.

72. Maeda A, Boku N, Fukutomi A, et al. Randomized phase III trial of adjuvant chemotherapy with gemcitabine versus S-1 in patients with resected pancreatic cancer: Japan Adjuvant Study Group of Pancreatic Cancer (JASPAC-01). Jpn J Clin Oncol 2008;38(3):227–9.

73. Moore MJ, Goldstein D, Hamm J, et al. Erlotinib plus gemcitabine compared with gemcitabine alone in patients with advanced pancreatic cancer: a phase III trial of the National Cancer Institute of Canada Clinical Trials Group. J Clin Oncol 2007;25(15):1960–6.

74. Cascinu S, Berardi R, Labianca R, et al. Cetuximab plus gemcitabine and cisplatin compared with gemcitabine and cisplatin alone in patients with advanced pancreatic cancer: a randomised, multicentre, phase II trial. Lancet Oncol 2008;9(1):39–44.

75. Philip PA. Improving treatment of pancreatic cancer. Lancet Oncol 2008;9(1):7–8.

76. Chen J, Rocken C, Nitsche B, et al. The tyrosine kinase inhibitor imatinib fails to inhibit pancreatic cancer progression. Cancer Lett 2006;233(2):328–37.

77. Richards DA, Boehm KA, Waterhouse DM, et al. Gemcitabine plus CI-994 offers no advantage over gemcitabine alone in the treatment of patients with advanced pancreatic cancer: results of a phase II randomized, double-blind, placebo-controlled, multicenter study. Ann Oncol 2006;17(7):1096–102.

78. Alberts SR, Foster NR, Morton RF, et al. PS-341 and gemcitabine in patients with metastatic pancreatic adenocarcinoma: a North Central Cancer Treatment Group (NCCTG) randomized phase II study. Ann Oncol 2005;16(10): 1654–61.

79. Van Cutsem E, van de Velde H, Karasek P, et al. Phase III trial of gemcitabine plus tipifarnib compared with gemcitabine plus placebo in advanced pancreatic cancer. J Clin Oncol 2004;22(8):1430–8.

80. Chau I, Cunningham D, Russell C, et al. Gastrazole (JB95008), a novel CCK2/gastrin receptor antagonist, in the treatment of advanced pancreatic cancer: results from two randomised controlled trials. Br J Cancer 2006;94(8): 1107–15.

81. Katsinelos P, Paikos D, Kountouras J, et al. Tannenbaum and metal stents in the palliative treatment of malignant distal bile duct obstruction: a comparative study of patency and cost effectiveness. Surg Endosc 2006;20(10): 1587–93.

82. Soderlund C, Linder S. Covered metal versus plastic stents for malignant common bile duct stenosis: a prospective, randomized, controlled trial. Gastrointest Endosc 2006;63(7):986–95.

83. Isayama H, Komatsu Y, Tsujino T, et al. A prospective randomised study of "covered" versus "uncovered" diamond stents for the management of distal malignant biliary obstruction. Gut 2004;53(5):729–34.

84. Sunamura M, Karasawa K, Okamoto A, et al. Phase III trial of radiosensitizer PR-350 combined with intraoperative radiotherapy for the treatment of locally advanced pancreatic cancer. Pancreas 2004;28(3):330–4.

85. Karasawa K, Sunamura M, Okamoto A, et al. Efficacy of novel hypoxic cell sensitiser doranidazole in the treatment of locally advanced pancreatic cancer: long-term results of a placebo-controlled randomised study. Radiother Oncol 2008;87(3):326–30.

86. Rosemurgy A, Luzardo G, Cooper J, et al. ^{32}P as an adjunct to standard therapy for locally advanced unresectable pancreatic cancer: a randomized trial. J Gastrointest Surg 2008;12(4):682–8.

87. Hishinuma S, Ogata Y, Tomikawa M, et al. Prophylactic hepatic irradiation following curative resection of pancreatic cancer. J Hepatobiliary Pancreat Surg 2005;12(3):235–42.

88. Chung HW, Bang SM, Park SW, et al. A prospective randomized study of gemcitabine with doxifluridine versus paclitaxel with doxifluridine in concurrent

chemoradiotherapy for locally advanced pancreatic cancer. Int J Radiat Oncol Biol Phys 2004;60(5):1494–501.

89. Kobari M, Egawa S, Shibuya K, et al. Effect of intraportal adoptive immunotherapy on liver metastases after resection of pancreatic cancer. Br J Surg 2000;87(1):43–8.

90. Wagener DJ, Wils JA, Kok TC, et al. Results of a randomised phase II study of cisplatin plus 5-fluorouracil versus cisplatin plus 5-fluorouracil with alpha-interferon in metastatic pancreatic cancer: an EORTC gastrointestinal tract cancer group trial. Eur J Cancer 2002;38(5):648–53.

91. Caprotti R, Brivio F, Fumagalli L, et al. Free-from-progression period and overall short preoperative immunotherapy with IL-2 increases the survival of pancreatic cancer patients treated with macroscopically radical surgery. Anticancer Res 2008;28(3B):1951–4.

92. Kuchler T, Bestmann B, Rappat S, et al. Impact of psychotherapeutic support for patients with gastrointestinal cancer undergoing surgery: 10-year survival results of a randomized trial. J Clin Oncol 2007;25(19):2702–8.

93. Bramhall SR, Rosemurgy A, Brown PD, et al. Marimastat as first-line therapy for patients with unresectable pancreatic cancer: a randomized trial. J Clin Oncol 2001;19(15):3447–55.

94. Bramhall SR, Schulz J, Nemunaitis J, et al. A double-blind placebo-controlled, randomised study comparing gemcitabine and marimastat with gemcitabine and placebo as first line therapy in patients with advanced pancreatic cancer. Br J Cancer 2002;87(2):161–7.

95. Moore MJ, Hamm J, Dancey J, et al. Comparison of gemcitabine versus the matrix metalloproteinase inhibitor BAY 12-9566 in patients with advanced or metastatic adenocarcinoma of the pancreas: a phase III trial of the National Cancer Institute of Canada Clinical Trials Group. J Clin Oncol 2003;21(17):3296–302.

96. Friess H, Langrehr JM, Oettle H, et al. A randomized multi-center phase II trial of the angiogenesis inhibitor Cilengitide (EMD 121974) and gemcitabine compared with gemcitabine alone in advanced unresectable pancreatic cancer. BMC Cancer 2006;6:285.

97. Spano JP, Chodkiewicz C, Maurel J, et al. Efficacy of gemcitabine plus axitinib compared with gemcitabine alone in patients with advanced pancreatic cancer: an open-label randomised phase II study. Lancet 2008;371(9630):2101–8.

98. van Berkel AM, Huibregtse IL, Bergman JJ, et al. A prospective randomized trial of Tannenbaum-type Teflon-coated stents versus polyethylene stents for distal malignant biliary obstruction. Eur J Gastroenterol Hepatol 2004;16(2):213–7.

99. Catalano MF, Geenen JE, Lehman GA, et al. "Tannenbaum" Teflon stents versus traditional polyethylene stents for treatment of malignant biliary stricture. Gastrointest Endosc 2002;55(3):354–8.

100. Terruzzi V, Comin U, De Grazia F, et al. Prospective randomized trial comparing Tannenbaum Teflon and standard polyethylene stents in distal malignant biliary stenosis. Gastrointest Endosc 2000;51(1):23–7.

101. Costamagna G, Mutignani M, Rotondano G, et al. Hydrophilic hydromer-coated polyurethane stents versus uncoated stents in malignant biliary obstruction: a randomized trial. Gastrointest Endosc 2000;51(1):8–11.

102. Tringali A, Mutignani M, Perri V, et al. A prospective, randomized multicenter trial comparing DoubleLayer and polyethylene stents for malignant distal common bile duct strictures. Endoscopy 2003;35(12):992–7.

103. Katsinelos P, Kountouras J, Paroutoglou G, et al. Uncovered Hanaro Versus Luminex metal stents for palliation of malignant biliary strictures. J Clin Gastroenterol 2008;42(5):539–45.

104. Giorgio PD, Luca LD. Comparison of treatment outcomes between biliary plastic stent placements with and without endoscopic sphincterotomy for inoperable malignant common bile duct obstruction. World J Gastroenterol 2004;10(8): 1212–4.

105. Artifon EL, Sakai P, Ishioka S, et al. Endoscopic sphincterotomy before deployment of covered metal stent is associated with greater complication rate: a prospective randomized control trial. J Clin Gastroenterol 2008;42(7): 815–9.

106. Pinol V, Castells A, Bordas JM, et al. Percutaneous self-expanding metal stents versus endoscopic polyethylene endoprostheses for treating malignant biliary obstruction: randomized clinical trial. Radiology 2002;225(1):27–34.

107. Halm U, Schiefke, Fleig WE, et al. Ofloxacin and ursodeoxycholic acid versus ursodeoxycholic acid alone to prevent occlusion of biliary stents: a prospective, randomized trial. Endoscopy 2001;33(6):491–4.

108. Fogel EL, deBellis M, McHenry L, et al. Effectiveness of a new long cytology brush in the evaluation of malignant biliary obstruction: a prospective study. Gastrointest Endosc 2006;63(1):71–7.

109. Braga M, Gianotti L, Gentilini O, et al. Early postoperative enteral nutrition improves gut oxygenation and reduces costs compared with total parenteral nutrition. Crit Care Med 2001;29(2):242–8.

110. Hyltander A, Bosaeus I, Svedlund J, et al. Supportive nutrition on recovery of metabolism, nutritional state, health-related quality of life, and exercise capacity after major surgery: a randomized study. Clin Gastroenterol Hepatol 2005;3(5): 466–74.

111. Lobo DN, Williams RN, Welch NT, et al. Early postoperative jejunostomy feeding with an immune modulating diet in patients undergoing resectional surgery for upper gastrointestinal cancer: a prospective, randomized, controlled, double-blind study. Clin Nutr 2006;25(5):716–26.

112. Fearon KC, Von Meyenfeldt MF, Moses AG, et al. Effect of a protein and energy dense n-3 fatty acid enriched oral supplement on loss of weight and lean tissue in cancer cachexia: a randomised double blind trial. Gut 2003;52(10):1479–86.

113. Moses AW, Slater C, Preston T, et al. Reduced total energy expenditure and physical activity in cachectic patients with pancreatic cancer can be modulated by an energy and protein dense oral supplement enriched with n-3 fatty acids. Br J Cancer 2004;90(5):996–1002.

114. Johnson CD, Puntis M, Davidson N, et al. Randomized, dose-finding phase III study of lithium gamolenate in patients with advanced pancreatic adenocarcinoma. Br J Surg 2001;88(5):662–8.

115. Gordon JN, Trebble TM, Ellis RD, et al. Thalidomide in the treatment of cancer cachexia: a randomised placebo controlled trial. Gut 2005;54(4):540–5.

116. Heller AR, Rossel T, Gottschlich B, et al. Omega-3 fatty acids improve liver and pancreas function in postoperative cancer patients. Int J Cancer 2004;111(4): 611–6.

117. Giger U, Buchler M, Farhadi J, et al. Preoperative immunonutrition suppresses perioperative inflammatory response in patients with major abdominal surgery-a randomized controlled pilot study. Ann Surg Oncol 2007;14(10): 2798–806.

118. Wong GY, Schroeder DR, Carns PE, et al. Effect of neurolytic celiac plexus block on pain relief, quality of life, and survival in patients with unresectable pancreatic cancer: a randomized controlled trial. JAMA 2004;291(9):1092–9.

119. Suleyman Ozyalcin N, Talu GK, Camlica H, et al. Efficacy of coeliac plexus and splanchnic nerve blockades in body and tail located pancreatic cancer pain. Eur J Pain 2004;8(6):539–45.
120. Gouillat C, Chipponi J, Baulieux J, et al. Randomized controlled multicentre trial of somatostatin infusion after pancreaticoduodenectomy. Br J Surg 2001;88(11): 1456–62.
121. Shan YS, Sy ED, Lin PW. Role of somatostatin in the prevention of pancreatic stump-related morbidity following elective pancreaticoduodenectomy in high-risk patients and elimination of surgeon-related factors: prospective, randomized, controlled trial. World J Surg 2003;27(6):709–14.
122. Hesse UJ, DeDecker C, Houtmeyers P, et al. Prospectively randomized trial using perioperative low-dose octreotide to prevent organ-related and general complications after pancreatic surgery and pancreatico-jejunostomy. World J Surg 2005;29(10):1325–8.
123. Burch PA, Block M, Schroeder G, et al. Phase III evaluation of octreotide versus chemotherapy with 5-fluorouracil or 5-fluorouracil plus leucovorin in advanced exocrine pancreatic cancer: a North Central Cancer Treatment Group study. Clin Cancer Res 2000;6(9):3486–92.
124. Jang JY, Kim SW, Han JK, et al. Randomized prospective trial of the effect of induced hypergastrinemia on the prevention of pancreatic atrophy after pancreatoduodenectomy in humans. Ann Surg 2003;237(4):522–9.
125. Wiedenmann B, Malfertheiner P, Friess H, et al. A multicenter, phase II study of infliximab plus gemcitabine in pancreatic cancer cachexia. J Support Oncol 2008;6(1):18–25.
126. Horwhat JD, Paulson EK, McGrath K, et al. A randomized comparison of EUS-guided FNA versus CT or US-guided FNA for the evaluation of pancreatic mass lesions. Gastrointest Endosc 2006;63(7):966–75.
127. Imbriaco M, Megibow AJ, Camera L, et al. Dual-phase versus single-phase helical CT to detect and assess resectability of pancreatic carcinoma. AJR Am J Roentgenol 2002;178(6):1473–9.
128. Yanaga Y, Awai K, Nakayama Y, et al. Pancreas: patient body weight tailored contrast material injection protocol versus fixed dose protocol at dynamic CT. Radiology 2007;245(2):475–82.

Randomized Clinical Trials in Hepatocellular Carcinoma

Adam C. Yopp, MD, William R. Jarnagin, MD*

KEYWORDS

- Evidence-based medicine • Hepatocellular carcinoma
- Management • Randomized controlled trials

Hepatocellular carcinoma (HCC) is among the most common solid tumors, ranking behind only lung and gastric for cancer-related deaths worldwide.[1] Despite improved surveillance programs in many countries, most patients present with advanced-stage cancer and chronic hepatic dysfunction limiting the available treatment options. This article reviews the most pertinent randomized controlled trials (RCT) with respect to surgical and adjuvant interventions that shape the current treatment algorithm for HCC.

LOCOREGIONAL THERAPY: SURGERY AND ABLATION

Potential curative therapies include surgery, either resection or orthotopic liver transplantation (OLT), and possibly ablation in selected patients. Locoregional interventions remain the cornerstone of treatment of early stage, localized HCC. Underlying chronic liver dysfunction in the form of viral or nonviral cirrhosis determines the appropriate surgical or locoregional treatment. Despite the absence of a prospective, randomized controlled trial comparing partial hepatectomy and OLT, surgical resection of early stage HCC remains the standard of care in well-compensated cirrhotic livers. A trial comparing resection with transplantation is difficult to perform, given the critical shortage of donor organs and the relatively small proportion of patients who are candidates for both treatments.

Historically, in patients with advanced cirrhosis undergoing hepatic resection for HCC closed suction drainage was used to evacuate perihepatic collections adjacent to the cut surface of the liver. One RCT showed no difference in overall survival and

Disclosure: See last page of article.
Division of Hepatobiliary Surgery, Department of Surgery, Memorial Sloan-Kettering Cancer Center, 1275 York Avenue, New York, NY 10065, USA
* Corresponding author.
E-mail address: jarnigiw@mskcc.org (W.R. Jarnagin).

Surg Oncol Clin N Am 19 (2010) 151–162
doi:10.1016/j.soc.2009.09.012
1055-3207/09/$ – see front matter © 2010 Elsevier Inc. All rights reserved.

morbidity in patients who did not have a closed suction drain placed following partial hepatectomy.[2] Most patients in this study had well-preserved hepatic function and the hepatectomies were done for reasons other than HCC. In a report by Liu and colleagues,[3] 104 patients were randomized to either closed suction drainage or no drainage following hepatic resection. The two cohorts consisted predominantly of patients with HCC and underlying viral-induced cirrhosis. There was no difference in overall in-hospital mortality or subsequent need for additional postoperative drainage but there was a significantly higher overall perioperative morbidity and hospital length of stay in the closed suction drainage group. This difference was most likely the result of a significantly higher rate (62% versus 21%; $P<.001$) of wound complications in the drainage group. The data do not support the routine use of closed suction drains following partial hepatectomy in the absence of a biliary-enteric anastomosis.

The use of low central venous pressure during liver mobilization and parenchymal transection has been advocated to reduce intraoperative blood loss and perioperative morbidity.[4] Until recently, no RCTs examined this practice during partial hepatectomy for HCC. Although this recent trial demonstrated the use of low central venous pressure reduced both intraoperative blood loss and the length of the hospital stay, the paucity of patients in each arm of the trial precluded finding differences in perioperative morbidity or mortality.[5] Because low central venous pressure anesthetic technique has been adopted as the standard of care in most high-volume centers and has shown to reduce perioperative morbidity in retrospective studies, it is unlikely that further, larger RCTs are possible.

The goals of partial hepatectomy for HCC are to resect the tumor with an adequate margin to prevent tumor recurrence and to preserve enough functional hepatic parenchyma to prevent perioperative hepatic failure. A recent trial attempted to determine the optimal margin of resection by randomizing patients with a solitary HCC tumor to a partial hepatectomy with either 1- or 2-cm gross, intraoperative margins.[6] Patients with an intended 2-cm operative margin had a significant recurrence-free and overall survival benefit compared with the 1-cm margin group. This study failed to comment on the number of positive margins in the 1-cm group and median period of follow-up. Because most recurrences in the narrow margin group occurred at the site of resection and the pathologic mean margin was only 0.7 cm in this group, it is conceivable that positive intraoperative margins could be a confounding factor.

Other technical aspects of partial hepatectomy for HCC have been evaluated through RCTs. The use of the anterior approach to right hepatectomy in large (>5 cm), solitary tumors, where initial vascular inflow and venous outflow and parenchymal dissection occurs before the right liver mobilization was compared with the more conventional approach, where the right liver is mobilized before vascular control and parenchymal dissection.[7] The median disease-free survival was similar in both resection approaches but patients undergoing the anterior approach had a significantly increased overall survival. This difference seemed to be caused by more frequent recurrences that were either multifocal or extrahepatic, and not amenable to salvage resection or ablation techniques. The authors postulated that early and frequent tumor manipulation as seen in the conventional approach promoted hematogenous tumor spread outside the site of local resection. This study was well done and provocative, because it is one of the few to show an impact of surgical technique on oncologic outcome; however, its applicability to the field as a whole is limited because of the paucity of patients with solitary, large HCC tumors limited to the right liver that are candidates for surgical resection.

Two additional studies compared percutaneous local therapies with partial hepatectomy for small HCC in patients with preserved hepatic function. The first trial demonstrated that patients undergoing percutaneous ethanol injection (PEI) had similar recurrence-free and overall survival rates when compared with a cohort undergoing partial hepatectomy.[8] The second trial also demonstrated similar rates of recurrence and overall survival when comparing percutaneous radiofrequency ablation (RFA) with partial hepatectomy for solitary, small (<5 cm) HCC tumors.[9,10] Although both studies demonstrate equivalence when comparing local ablative with resection therapies they are a highly selected group of patients representing fewer than 5% of patients presenting to their respective institutions with HCC. Both studies also suffer from relatively short mean follow-up time (under 3 years in both studies) and small patient numbers (38 and 90, respectively) that may have masked potential differences in treatment. Unless medical comorbidities or hepatic dysfunction are present, hepatic resection should be considered the treatment of choice. Further larger trials with longer follow-up are needed to fully address the use of favoring percutaneous ablative techniques over partial hepatectomy.

Despite the increased efficacy of surveillance programs using alpha fetoprotein and abdominal ultrasonography only 25% to 30% of HCC tumors are amenable to curative surgical therapies because of underlying hepatic dysfunction or tumor multifocality. Percutaneous ablative therapies provide an additional approach to unresectable HCC tumors. The ideal local ablative therapy has been addressed in multiple trials comparing RFA with PEI in patients with unresectable HCC. Shiina and colleagues[11] randomized 232 patients with HCC who had three or fewer lesions, each 3 cm or less in size with a Child-Pugh class of A or B, that either were deemed surgical unresectable or refused resection, to either ablation with RFA or PEI. The clinical characteristics of the two groups were similar with most patients having positive hepatitis C serology and tumors between 2 and 3 cm in size. Overall survival at 4 years in the RFA group (74%) was significantly higher than the PEI group (57%). Overall recurrence at 3 years was also significantly improved in the RFA (60%) group compared with the PEI (80%) group. Local tumor progression or recurrence was significantly increased (11% versus 2%) in the PEI group versus the RFA group. Both groups had similar rates of adverse events. This well done study by an experienced group demonstrates that RFA rather than PEI should be the choice for percutaneous local therapy in unresectable HCC.

ADJUVANT OR PALLIATIVE THERAPY

Attempts to reduce the 75% to 100% recurrence rate of HCC after partial hepatectomy with adjuvant, cytotoxic chemotherapy regimens have historically been unsuccessful. Two recent trials readdressed this question by giving adjuvant chemotherapy following OLT[12] or partial hepatectomy[13] for HCC demonstrating a lack of improvement in either overall or disease-free survival.

The use of adjuvant interferon therapy in patients with HCC secondary to chronic viral hepatitis hypothetically may improve disease-free survival and reduce recurrence rates caused by tumoricidal effects or suppression of viral hepatitis within the remnant liver. Five recent trials[14–20] have investigated this hypothesis with none showing conclusively that adjuvant interferon therapy following partial hepatectomy in viral hepatitis–linked HCC improves either disease-free or overall survival. All of the studies have demonstrated significant levels of adverse events associated with interferon use even in these highly selected noncirrhotic patient populations.

Two other trials[19,20] demonstrated that the administration of menatetrenone, a vitamin K_2 analog, reduced the rates of recurrence following partial hepatectomy or local ablative therapies for HCC. Unfortunately, none of these studies demonstrated a survival benefit, which may be explained by the low patient enrollment in both studies. Further, larger confirmatory studies are needed.

Sorafenib is a molecular targeted therapy that inhibits the serine-threonine kinases, Raf-1 and B-raf; the receptor tyrosine kinase activity of vascular endothelial growth factor receptors 1, 2, and 3; and platelet-derived growth factor β. Llovet and colleagues[21] randomized 599 patients with advanced-stage HCC, most secondary to chronic viral hepatitis, and Child-Pugh class A status to either oral sorafenib or placebo. Median overall survival was 10.7 months in the sorafenib group and 7.9 months in the placebo group ($P<.001$). Median time to radiologic progression was 5.5 months in the sorafenib group and 2.8 months in the placebo group ($P<.001$). The sorafenib group demonstrated a similar treatment response to the placebo group with only 2% and 1% partial response rates, respectively. Neither group demonstrated any complete responses by radiologic criteria. This is consistent with other studies examining molecular targeted therapy in solid tumors and demonstrates the need for developing other less traditional biomarkers than axial imaging to assess treatment response. The adverse event profile of sorafenib was similar to the placebo group with a similar rate of discontinuation of therapy. This and other studies have shown that sorafenib is poorly tolerated in patients with other than Child-Pugh class A cirrhosis.

Estrogen receptors are expressed in low concentration in HCC tumors and the administration of exogenous estrogens, in the form of birth control pills, promotes hepatocyte proliferation and is associated with an increased incidence of hepatic adenomas. Anecdotal case reports and small retrospective studies demonstrated the use of the antiestrogen receptor, tamoxifen, is associated with regression of HCC tumor burden. Two recent trials[22,23] failed to demonstrate an improvement in overall survival or response rate with tamoxifen in patients with advanced-stage, unresectable HCC.

Multiple trials addressed the use of octreotide alone[24,25] or in conjunction[26,27] with other chemotherapy regimens to induce tumor regression or provide symptomatic relief in HCC patients without any measurable success.

Because most patients with HCC present with advanced disease not amenable to curative therapies and the benefits of systemic chemotherapy regimens are unclear, alternative locoregional treatment approaches using transarterial embolization and chemoembolization techniques have been examined in RCTs. Llovet and colleagues[28] randomized 112 patients with unresectable HCC, most secondary to hepatitis C cirrhosis, preserved liver function, and no evidence of extrahepatic disease to either chemoembolization with Gelfoam and doxorubicin, embolization with Gelfoam, or best symptomatic therapy. Median overall survival was 28.7 months in the chemoembolization group and 17.9 months in the best symptomatic control group ($P = .009$). The trial was stopped because sequential inspection showed superiority in the chemoembolization group precluding a comparison between bland embolization and chemoembolization. In a similar trial, Lo and colleagues[29] randomized 79 patients with unresectable HCC, most with hepatitis B cirrhosis, preserved liver function, and no evidence of extrahepatic disease to either chemoembolization with cisplatin and Lipiodol or best symptomatic control. The 2-year overall survival was 31% in the chemoembolization group and 11% in the control group. The rate of objective tumor response in the measurable patients was significantly higher in the chemoembolization group than in the control group (39% versus 6%; $P = .014$). These two studies demonstrate in a carefully selected group of patients with preserved liver function and no evidence of extrahepatic spread, locoregional arterial embolization remains the preferred treatment method. Until RCTs currently underway are completed, however, the question of whether bland embolization or chemoembolization is the superior technique remains unanswered.

In one recent RCT, the combination of percutaneous ablative therapy with transarterial chemoembolization in patients with unresectable HCC demonstrated improved overall survival and response rates.[30] Performing transarterial chemoembolization before RFA increases the area of coagulation necrosis negating the heat sink effect mediated by the tissue perfusion of larger HCC tumors allowing the combination approach to provide a more effective treatment than RFA alone.

SURGERY

1. Abdominal drainage after hepatic resection is contraindicated in patients with chronic liver diseases. Liu CL, Fan ST, Lo CM, et al. Ann Surg 2004 Feb;239:194–201.[3]

Hypothesis: Routine abdominal drainage is beneficial after elective partial hepatectomy in patients with chronic underlying liver disease.

No. Patients Randomized	Study Groups	Stratification	Significance Demonstrated	% Change Identified in Trial
104	Drainage = 52 No drainage = 52	None	Yes; higher operative morbidity	RR 4.449 (95% CI, 1.700–11.64) drains associated with postoperative morbidity

Published abstract: Objective: The aim of this study was to determine whether abdominal drainage is beneficial after elective hepatic resection in patients with underlying chronic liver diseases. Summary background data: Traditionally, in patients with chronic liver diseases, an abdominal drainage catheter is routinely inserted after hepatic resection to drain ascitic fluid and to detect postoperative hemorrhage and bile leakage. The benefits of this surgical practice, however, have not been evaluated prospectively. Patients and methods: Between January 1999 and March 2002, 104 patients who had underlying chronic liver diseases were prospectively randomized to have either closed suction abdominal drainage (drainage group, N = 52) or no drainage (nondrainage group, N = 52) after elective hepatic resection. The operative outcomes of the two groups of patients were compared. Results: Fifty-seven (55%) patients had major hepatic resection with resection of three Coiunaud's segments or more. Sixty-nine (66%) patients had liver cirrhosis and 35 (34%) had chronic hepatitis. Demographic, surgical, and pathologic details were similar between both groups. The primary indication for hepatic resection was HCC (N = 100, 96%). There was no difference in hospital mortality between the two groups of patients (drainage group, 6% versus nondrainage group, 2%; $P = .618$). There was a significantly higher overall operative morbidity, however, in the drainage group (73% versus 38%; $P<.001$). This was related to a significantly higher incidence of wound complications in the drainage group compared with the nondrainage group (62% versus 21%; $P<.001$). In addition, a trend toward a higher incidence of septic complications in the drainage group was observed (33% versus 17%; $P = .07$). The mean ($\pm$ standard error of mean) postoperative hospital stay of the drainage group was 19 ± 2.2 days, which was significantly longer than that of the nondrainage group (12.5 ± 1.1 days; $P = .005$). With a median follow-up of 15 months, none of the 51 patients with HCC in the drainage group developed metastasis at the drain sites. On multivariate analysis, abdominal drainage, underlying liver cirrhosis, major hepatic resection, and intraoperative blood loss of greater than 1.5 L were independent and significant factors associated with postoperative morbidity. Conclusion: Routine abdominal drainage after hepatic resection is contraindicated in patients with chronic liver diseases. (Copyright 2004 Lippincott Williams & Wilkins. Reprinted with permission.)

Editor's summary and comments: This single institution RCT by an experienced HPB center is the first study to demonstrate that routine closed suction abdominal drainage following partial hepatectomy in patients with underlying liver dysfunction is associated with higher postoperative morbidity and length of hospital stay. The increased perioperative morbidity in the drainage group was caused by a higher incidence of wound complications. Most of these were caused by leakage of ascitic fluid for more than 3 days at either the incision or drain site (66%). The increase of perioperative morbidity in the drainage group corresponded to a significant increase in the length of hospital stay. Interestingly, although routine abdominal ultrasonography was performed at 7 days postoperatively, no difference in postoperative collections was seen between the two groups. Five patients in the drainage group required further radiologic-guided drainage procedures, however, compared with one patient in the nondrainage group. Whether the ultrasound was done too early in the postoperative period or ascending infection from the closed suction drainage was the etiology is unclear. It is the authors' policy to avoid closed suction drainage following partial hepatectomy; if either biliary-enteric anastomosis or thoracoabdominal incisions mandate their use it is preferred to use gravity drainage to avoid the pitfalls of negative pressure near the cut surface of the liver.

2. A randomized controlled trial of radiofrequency ablation with ethanol injection for small hepatocellular carcinoma. Shiina S, Teratani T, Obi S, et al. Gastroenterology 2005 Jul;129(1):122–30.[11]

Hypothesis: RFA is superior to PEI in terms of overall survival and recurrence rate for patients with small, unresectable HCC.

No. Patients Randomized	Study Groups	Stratification	Significance Demonstrated	% Change Identified in Trial
132	RFA = 114 PEI = 118	None	Yes; improved overall survival and decreased recurrence rate	4-year survival: RFA 74% (95% CI, 65%–84%) PEI 57% (95% CI, 45%–71%) $P = .01$

Published abstract: Background and aims: Percutaneous RFA is a recently introduced treatment for HCC, whereas PEI is now a standard therapy. Their long-term outcomes were compared. Methods: Two hundred thirty-two patients with HCC who had three or fewer lesions, each 3 cm or less in diameter, and liver function of Child-Pugh class A or B were entered onto a randomized controlled trial. The primary end point was survival, and the secondary end points were overall recurrence and local tumor progression. Results: One hundred eighteen patients were assigned to RFA and 114 to PEI. The number of treatment sessions was smaller (2.1 times versus 6.4 times, respectively; $P<.0001$) and the length of hospitalization was shorter (10.8 days versus 26.1 days, respectively; $P<.0001$) in RFA than in PEI. Four-year survival rate was 74% (95% CI, 65%–84%) in RFA and 57% (95% CI, 45%–71%) in PEI. RFA had a 46% smaller risk of death (adjusted relative risk, 0.54 [95% CI,

0.33–0.89]; $P = .02$), a 43% smaller risk of overall recurrence (adjusted relative risk 0.57 [95% CI, 0.41–0.80]; $P = .0009$), and an 88% smaller risk of local tumor progression (relative risk, 0.12 [95% CI, 0.03–0.55]; $P = .006$) than PEI. The incidence of adverse events was not different between the two therapies. Conclusions: Judging from higher survival but similar adverse events, RFA is superior to PEI for small HCC. (Copyright Elsevier 2005.)

Editor's summary and comments: This study by a group with extensive experience with both RFA and PEI demonstrates the superiority of RFA over PEI in a highly selected group of patients with small (<3 cm), predominantly hepatitis C cirrhosis–linked HCC with either Child-Pugh class A or B status. Patients in the PEI group received an average of 6.4 treatment sessions compared with 2.1 in the RFA group. Although axial imaging was done to ensure tumor necrosis after the percutaneous ablation, the PEI technique resulted in an 11.4% local progression rate compared with a 1.7% local progression rate in RFA-treated patients. The high rate of local progression questions the validity of radiologic follow-up as a marker of posttreatment tumor necrosis or the technique as an ablative therapy.

ADJUVANT OR PALLIATIVE THERAPY

3. Sorafenib in advanced hepatocellular carcinoma. Llovet JM, Ricci S, Mazzaferro V, et al. N Engl J Med 2008 Jul 24;359(4):378–90.[21]

Hypothesis: Single-agent sorafenib will have beneficial effect on overall survival in patients with advanced-stage HCC and Child-Pugh class A or B status.

No. Patients Randomized	Study Groups	Stratification	Significance Demonstrated	% Change Identified in Trial
599	Sorafenib = 297 Placebo = 302	Region, ECOG performance score and presence or absence of macroscopic vascular invasion or extrahepatic spread	Yes; improved overall survival	Median overall survival: Sorafenib: 10.7 mo Placebo: 7.9 mo $P<.001$

Published abstract: Background: No effective systemic therapy exists for patients with advanced HCC. A preliminary study suggested that sorafenib, an oral multikinase inhibitor of the vascular endothelial growth factor receptor, the platelet-derived growth factor receptor, and Raf may be effective in HCC. Methods: In this multicenter, phase 3, double-blind, placebo-controlled trial, 602 patients with advanced HCC who had not received previous systemic treatment were randomly assigned to receive either sorafenib (at a dose of 400 mg twice daily) or placebo. Primary outcomes were overall survival and the time to symptomatic progression. Secondary outcomes included the time to radiologic progression and safety. Results: At the second planned interim analysis, 321 deaths had occurred, and the study was stopped. Median overall survival was 10.7 months in the sorafenib group and 7.9 months in the placebo group (hazard ratio in the sorafenib group, 0.69; 95% CI, 0.55–0.87; $P<.001$). There was no significant difference between the two groups in the median time to symptomatic progression (4.1 months versus 4.9 months, respectively; $P = .77$). The median time to radiologic progression was 5.5 months in the sorafenib group and 2.8 months in the placebo group (P<.001). Seven patients in the sorafenib group (2%) and two patients in the placebo group (1%) had a partial response; no patients had a complete response. Diarrhea, weight loss, hand-foot skin reaction, and hypophosphatemia were more frequent in the sorafenib group. Conclusions: In patients with advanced HCC, median survival and the time to radiologic progression were nearly 3 months longer for patients treated with sorafenib than for those given placebo. (Copyright [2008] Massachusetts Medical Society. All rights reserved.)

Editor's summary and comments: This is the first large-scale RCT that has shown a significant survival benefit of medical therapy in advanced-stage HCC. In a highly selected group of patients with Child-Pugh class A status and a good performance status median survival was extended by 2.8 months with sorafenib treatment. This gain seems to be correlated to the 2.7-month delay in radiologic progression sorafenib group compared with the placebo group. Although 80% of patients in the sorafenib group, compared with 52% in the placebo group, experienced a treatment-related adverse event, the rate of discontinuation of treatment in the study group was similar to the control group (38% versus 37%). The excitement of the outcomes of this trial needs to be tempered by the fact that sorafenib, in the United States, costs on average $5400 per monthly treatment, and does not have widespread availability in areas of the world that are endemic for viral-linked hepatitis. Another area of concern is whether the results of this trial extrapolate to the cohort of patients commonly seen with advanced-stage HCC, patients with poor performance status with Child-Pugh class B or C status and viral-linked HCC. The etiology of HCC in this study was fairly well split between viral and non–viral-linked HCC and subgroup analysis was not done. Sorafenib is a dramatic first step in demonstrating molecular targeted therapy is efficacious in treating HCC. Many further trials investigating combination therapy with cytotoxic chemotherapy and other targeted therapies, more appropriate end point biomarkers, and treatment of patients with underlying liver dysfunction need to be completed and reported before it is considered standard therapy.

4. Arterial embolisation or chemoembolisation versus symptomatic treatment in patients with unresectable hepatocellular carcinoma: a randomized controlled trial. Llovet JM, Real MI, Montaña X, et al. Lancet 2002 May 18;359(9319):1734–9.[28]

Hypothesis: Transarterial chemoembolization in patients with unresectable HCC will provide a treatment-related survival benefit compared with best symptomatic therapy.

No. Patients Randomized	Study Groups	Stratification	Significance Demonstrated	% Change Identified in Trial
112	Embolization = 37 Chemoembolization = 40 Control treatment = 35	Center, tumor stage, Okuda stage	Yes; improved overall survival with chemoembolization	Mean overall survival: Chemoembolization: 28.7 mo Control treatment: 17.9 mo P = .009

Published abstract: Background: There is no standard treatment for unresectable HCC. Arterial embolization is widely used, but evidence of survival benefits is lacking. Methods: A randomized controlled trial was performed in patients with unresectable HCC not suitable for curative treatment, of Child-Pugh class A or B and Okuda stage I or II, to assess the survival benefits of regularly repeated arterial embolization (gelatin sponge) or chemoembolization (gelatin sponge plus doxorubicin) compared with conservative treatment. A total of 903 patients were assessed, and 112 (12%) patients were finally included in the study. The primary end point was survival. Analyses were by intention to treat. Findings: The trial was stopped when the ninth sequential inspection showed that chemoembolization had survival benefits compared with conservative treatment (hazard ratio of death 0.47 [95% CI, 0.25–0.91]; $P = .025$). A total of 25 of 37 patients assigned embolization, 21 of 40 assigned chemoembolization, and 25 of 35 assigned conservative treatments died. Survival probabilities at 1 year and 2 years were 75% and 50% for embolization; 82% and 63% for chemoembolization; and 63% and 27% for control (chemoembolization versus control; $P = .009$). Chemoembolization induced objective responses sustained for at least 6 months in 35%[14] of cases, and was associated with a significantly lower rate of portal-vein invasion than conservative treatment. Treatment allocation was the only variable independently related to survival (odds ratio 0.45 [95% CI, 0.25–0.81]; $P = .02$). Interpretation: Chemoembolization improved survival of stringently selected patients with unresectable HCC. (Copyright Elsevier 2002.)

Editor's summary and comments: This multicenter trial attempted to find a survival benefit using transarterial chemoembolization, which previous RCTs failed to demonstrate, by carefully selecting a group of patients with Child-Pugh class A status and good ECOG performance status not amenable to surgical therapy because of multifocality. Only 112 (12%) of 903 of patients registered with HCC met inclusion criteria. The patients were treated with an aggressive treatment approach with transarterial chemoembolization at baseline, at 2 months, at 6 months, and every 6 months thereafter until disease progression or patient request. Although chemoembolization had a significant survival benefit compared with best symptomatic control, a direct comparison with bland transarterial embolization could not be performed because of early stoppage of the trial. This is the first multicenter trial demonstrating a clear survival benefit with transarterial chemoembolization; however, the stringent inclusion criteria used to highlight the benefit might preclude its extrapolation to patients with a higher degree of liver dysfunction or more progressive disease.

5. Randomized controlled trial of transarterial lipiodol chemoembolization for unresectable hepatocellular carcinoma. Lo CM, Ngan H, Tso WK, et al. Hepatology. 2002 May;35(5):1164–71.[29]

Hypothesis: Transarterial chemoembolization with Lipiodol provided superior overall survival compared with symptomatic control in patients with unresectable HCC.

No. Patients Randomized	Study Groups	Stratification	Significance Demonstrated	% Change Identified in Trial
79	Chemoembolization = 40 Control treatment = 39	None	Yes; improved 1-year overall survival with chemoembolization	1-year overall survival: Chemoembolization: 57% Control treatment: 32% $P = .005$

Published abstract: This randomized, controlled trial assessed the efficacy of transarterial Lipiodol (Lipiodol Ultrafluide, Laboratoire Guerbet, Aulnay-Sous-Bois, France) chemoembolization in patients with unresectable HCC. From March 1996 to October 1997, 80 out of 279 Asian patients with newly diagnosed unresectable HCC fulfilled the entry criteria and randomly were assigned to treatment with chemoembolization using a variable dose of an emulsion of cisplatin in Lipiodol and gelatin-sponge particles injected through the hepatic artery (chemoembolization group, 40 patients) or symptomatic treatment (control group, 40 patients). One patient assigned to the control group secondarily was excluded because of unrecognized systemic metastasis. Chemoembolization was repeated every 2 to 3 months unless there was evidence of contraindications or progressive disease. Survival was the main end point. The chemoembolization group received a total of 192 courses of chemoembolization with a median of 4.5 (range, 1–15) courses per patient. Chemoembolization resulted in a marked tumor response, and the actuarial survival was significantly better in the chemoembolization group (1 year, 57%; 2 years, 31%; 3 years, 26%) than in the control group (1 year, 32%; 2 years, 11%; 3 years, 3%; P = .002). When adjustments for baseline variables that were prognostic on univariate analysis were made with a multivariate Cox model, the survival benefit of chemoembolization remained significant (relative risk of death, 0.49; 95% CI, 0.29–0.81; P = .006). Although death from liver failure was more frequent in patients who received chemoembolization, the liver functions of the survivors were not significantly different. In Asian patients with unresectable HCC, transarterial Lipiodol chemoembolization significantly improves survival and is an effective form of treatment. (Copyright 2002 John Wiley & Sons.)

Editor's summary and comments: This single-institution trial by an experienced center selected a group of patients with predominantly hepatitis B–linked HCC and well-preserved hepatic function to undergo cisplatin-Lipiodol transarterial chemoembolization. The treatment was performed at baseline and then every 2 or 3 months until disease progression or patient request. Contrary to other studies, the dose of cisplatin used was adjusted to tumor size. A significant benefit was demonstrated in the chemoembolization group with a minimal rate of adverse events seen in similar studies. Tumor size greater than 5 cm and unilobar portal vein occlusion were independent prognostic factors of worse overall survival in the chemoembolization group. As seen in similar studies because of strict inclusion criteria less than 25% of patients registered with HCC in their center were eligible.

DISCLOSURE

Authors have nothing to disclose.

REFERENCES

1. Parkin DM, Bray F, Ferlay J, et al. Global cancer statistics, 2002. CA Cancer J Clin 2005;55(22):74–108.
2. Fong Y, Brennan MF, Brown K, et al. Drainage is unnecessary after elective liver resection. Am J Surg 1996;171(1):158–62.
3. Liu CL, Fan ST, Lo CM, et al. Abdominal drainage after hepatic resection is contraindicated in patients with chronic liver diseases. Ann Surg 2004;239(2):194–201.
4. Melendez JA, Arslan V, Fischer ME, et al. Perioperative outcomes of major hepatic resections under low central venous pressure anesthesia: blood loss, blood transfusion, and the risk of postoperative renal dysfunction. J Am Coll Surg 1998;187(6):620–5.
5. Wang WD, Liang LJ, Huang XQ, et al. Low central venous pressure reduces blood loss in hepatectomy. World J Gastroenterol 2006;12(6):935–9.

6. Shi M, Guo RP, Lin XJ, et al. Partial hepatectomy with wide versus narrow resection margin for solitary hepatocellular carcinoma: a prospective randomized trial. Ann Surg 2007;245(1):36–43.
7. Liu CL, Fan ST, Cheung ST, et al. Anterior approach versus conventional approach right hepatic resection for large hepatocellular carcinoma: a prospective randomized controlled study. Ann Surg 2006;244(2):194–203.
8. Huang GT, Lee PH, Tsang YM, et al. Percutaneous ethanol injection versus surgical resection for the treatment of small hepatocellular carcinoma: a prospective study. Ann Surg 2005;242(1):36–42.
9. Chen MS, Li JQ, Zheng Y, et al. A prospective randomized trial comparing percutaneous local ablative therapy and partial hepatectomy for small hepatocellular carcinoma. Ann Surg 2006;243(3):321–8.
10. Koda M, Murawaki Y, Mitsuda A, et al. Combination therapy with transcatheter arterial chemoembolization and percutaneous ethanol injection compared with percutaneous ethanol injection alone for patients with small hepatocellular carcinoma: a randomized control study. Cancer 2001;92(6):1516–24.
11. Shiina S, Teratani T, Obi S, et al. A randomized controlled trial of radiofrequency ablation with ethanol injection for small hepatocellular carcinoma. Gastroenterology 2005;129(1):122–30.
12. Lu W, Li YH, Yu ZJ, et al. A comparative study of damage to liver function after TACE with use of low-dose versus conventional-dose of anticancer drugs in hepatocellular carcinoma. Hepatogastroenterology 2007;54(77):1499–502.
13. Gish RG, Porta C, Lazar L, et al. Phase III randomized controlled trial comparing the survival of patients with unresectable hepatocellular carcinoma treated with nolatrexed or doxorubicin. J Clin Oncol 2007;25(21):3069–75.
14. Lo CM, Liu CL, Chan SC, et al. A randomized, controlled trial of postoperative adjuvant interferon therapy after resection of hepatocellular carcinoma. Ann Surg 2007;245:831–42.
15. Mazzaferro V, Romito R, Schiavo M, et al. Prevention of hepatocellular carcinoma recurrence with alpha-interferon after liver resection in HCV cirrhosis. Hepatology 2006;44(6):1543–54.
16. Lin SM, Lin CJ, Hsu CW, et al. Prospective randomized controlled study of interferon-alpha in preventing hepatocellular carcinoma recurrence after medical ablation therapy for primary tumors. Cancer 2004;100(2):376–82.
17. Kubo S, Nishiguchi S, Hirohashi K, et al. Randomized clinical trial of long-term outcome after resection of hepatitis C virus-related hepatocellular carcinoma by postoperative interferon therapy. Br J Surg 2002;89(4):418–22.
18. Sun HC, Tang ZY, Wang L, et al. Postoperative interferon alpha treatment postponed recurrence and improved overall survival in patients after curative resection of HBV-related hepatocellular carcinoma: a randomized clinical trial. J Cancer Res Clin Oncol 2006;132(7):458–65.
19. Kakizaki S, Sohara N, Sato K, et al. Preventive effects of vitamin K on recurrent disease in patients with hepatocellular carcinoma arising from hepatitis C viral infection. J Gastroenterol Hepatol 2007;22(4):518–22.
20. Mizuta T, Ozaki I, Eguchi Y, et al. The effect of menatetrenone, a vitamin K2 analog, on disease recurrence and survival in patients with hepatocellular carcinoma after curative treatment: a pilot study. Cancer 2006;106(4):867–72.
21. Llovet JM, Ricci S, Mazzaferro V, et al. Sorafenib in advanced hepatocellular carcinoma. N Engl J Med 2008;359(4):378–90.
22. Barbare JC, Bouche O, Bonnetain F, et al. Randomized controlled trial of tamoxifen in advanced hepatocellular carcinoma. J Clin Oncol 2005;23(19):4338–46.

23. Chow PK, Tai BC, Tan CK, et al. High-dose tamoxifen in the treatment of inoperable hepatocellular carcinoma: a multicenter randomized controlled trial. Hepatology 2002;36(5):1221–6.

24. Becker G, Allgaier HP, Olschewski M, et al. Long-acting octreotide versus placebo for treatment of advanced HCC: a randomized controlled double-blind study. Hepatology 2007;45(1):9–15.

25. Dimitroulopoulos D, Xinopoulos D, Tsamakidis K, et al. Long acting octreotide in the treatment of advanced hepatocellular cancer and overexpression of somatostatin receptors: randomized placebo-controlled trial. World J Gastroenterol 2007;13(23):3164–70.

26. Treiber G, Rocken C, Wex T, et al. Octreotide alone or in combination with rofecoxib as palliative treatment for advanced hepatocellular cancer. Z Gastroenterol 2007;45(5):369–77.

27. Verset G, Verslype C, Reynaert H, et al. Efficacy of the combination of long-acting release octreotide and tamoxifen in patients with advanced hepatocellular carcinoma: a randomised multicentre phase III study. Br J Cancer 2007;97(5): 582–8.

28. Llovet JM, Real MI, Montana X, et al. Arterial embolisation or chemoembolisation versus symptomatic treatment in patients with unresectable hepatocellular carcinoma: a randomised controlled trial. Lancet 2002;359(9319):1734–9.

29. Lo CM, Ngan H, Tso WK, et al. Randomized controlled trial of transarterial lipiodol chemoembolization for unresectable hepatocellular carcinoma. Hepatology 2002;35(5):1164–71.

30. Li Q, Wang J, Sun Y, et al. Efficacy of postoperative transarterial chemoembolization and portal vein chemotherapy for patients with hepatocellular carcinoma complicated by portal vein tumor thrombosis: a randomized study. World J Surg 2006;30(11):2004–11.

An Update on Randomized Clinical Trials in Advanced and Metastatic Colorectal Carcinoma

Shishir K. Maithel, MD, Michael I. D'Angelica, MD*

KEYWORDS

- Metastatic colorectal cancer • Randomized controlled trials
- Chemotherapy • Liver metastases

It is estimated that approximately 150,000 new colorectal cancers are diagnosed each year in the United States and approximately 50% of patients eventually develop liver metastases.[1] During the past 8 years, there have been significant advances in the treatment and outcome of patients with metastatic colorectal cancer (MCRC). This is likely the result of improved imaging, staging, chemotherapy, and surgery. After conducting a standardized MEDLINE literature search, this article reviews the prospective randomized controlled trials in advanced colorectal cancer published between May 2001 and October 2008. There are a total of 96 studies and all are chemotherapy-related trials. They are divided into five categories based on each trial's focus: (1) types of chemotherapy (N = 55); (2) Administration of adjuvant or neoadjuvant chemotherapy for resectable liver metastases (N = 5); (3) regional chemotherapy with hepatic arterial infusion (HAI) (N = 11); (4) molecular markers of chemotherapy efficacy (N = 2); and (5) duration, dosing, and sequencing of chemotherapy (N = 23).

TRIALS USING DIFFERENT TYPES OF CHEMOTHERAPY

The time period of the previous report[2] primarily included trials that focused on 5-fluorouracil (5-FU) as the primary chemotherapeutic agent. Many of these trials investigated whether infusional 5-FU had any oncologic advantage over bolus administration and if comodulation with leucovorin (LV) was beneficial. The results of these previous trials resulted in infusional 5-FU administered with LV being the standard regimen offered to patients.[3,4]

Disclosure: See last page of article.
Hepatopancreatobiliary Service, Department of Surgery, Memorial Sloan-Kettering Cancer Center, 1275 York Avenue, New York, NY 10065, USA
* Corresponding author.
E-mail address: dangelim@mskcc.org (M.I. D'Angelica).

Surg Oncol Clin N Am 19 (2010) 163–181
doi:10.1016/j.soc.2009.09.013
1055-3207/09/$ – see front matter © 2010 Elsevier Inc. All rights reserved.

After multiple failed attempts to improve on the results of 5-FU–LV, the addition of irinotecan demonstrated superior response rates and survival for patients with MCRC and became the new standard first-line therapy.[5] It should be noted, however, that this regimen (irinotecan, bolus 5-FU, LV[IFL], Saltz regimen) used bolus 5-FU as opposed to infusional 5-FU, the latter of which had demonstrated superiority to the bolus preparation. As oxaliplatin emerged as an effective agent for MCRC, numerous trials examined the comparative affects of oxaliplatin versus irinotecan-based chemotherapeutic regimens. However, initial trials compared FOLFOX with the IFL regimen, which used the bolus preparation of 5-FU. Although some studies have reported FOLFOX to be superior to irinotecan-based regimens, these studies may have failed to accurately compare the efficacy of oxaliplatin with irinotecan because different administrations of 5-FU were used.[6,7] Level Ia trials that do compare FOLFOX with irinotecan, infusional 5-FU, LV (FOLFIRI), however, report equivalent tumor response and patient outcomes with an approximate median survival of 21 months.[8,9] Most oncologists today choose first-line treatment based on the toxicity profile of the regimen as it applies to each individual patient given equivalent oncologic efficacy.

For those patients not able to receive 5-FU chemotherapy because of toxicity, the combination of oxaliplatin with irinotecan has demonstrated manageable toxicity and oncologic efficacy as well with a median survival of 20.4 months when used as first-line therapy in advanced colorectal cancer.[10] Irinotecan administered alone also demonstrated similar response rates as 5-FU–LV,[5] but the use of oxaliplatin as a monotherapy seems to have minimal effect and should be discouraged as first-line therapy.[11] Most recently, new targeted antibody therapies, such as bevacizumab (Avastin) and cetuximab (Erbitux), have been added to the armamentarium of agents to combat advanced colorectal cancer. Although the data in support are not that convincing (discussed in detail later), bevacizumab is frequently added to either FOLFOX or FOLFIRI as first-line therapy. Cetuximab has mainly been used as third-line therapy for those patients who have progressed through standard cytotoxic chemotherapy (ie, FOLFOX and FOLFIRI).

Studies have also investigated the efficacy of an oral 5-FU analog (capecitabine, Xeloda), and they suggest that the oral preparation has similar oncologic benefit as the intravenous form and may actually be preferred by some patients.[12–15] This finding has led to the widespread use of capecitabine for the treatment of MCRC (discussed in more detail in the level Ia evidence section).

Lastly, multiple trials have investigated the use of coadministering immunotherapy and other agents, such as mitomycin C, celecoxib, methotrexate, and carbamazepine, with standard chemotherapeutic regimens to improve survival outcomes and reduce patient toxicity.[16] None of these trials have demonstrated improved outcomes and have not changed standard management. There is some suggestion that Marimastat, a metalloproteinase inhibitor, may offer a survival advantage in a select group of patients that demonstrate musculoskeletal side effects from the drug and warrants further study.[17]

TRIALS ON NEOADJUVANT AND ADJUVANT CHEMOTHERAPY FOR RESECTABLE LIVER METASTASES

There have been few randomized studies assessing the use of administering chemotherapy either before or after complete resection of liver metastases. Portier and colleagues[18] investigated the use of adjuvant 5-FU–LV after complete resection of liver metastases and reported an increased 5-year disease-free survival in patients receiving chemotherapy compared with those patients who did not (33.5% versus

26.7%; $P = .028$). There was no significant difference in overall survival (OS) between the two groups. This trial, however, was closed prematurely because of slow accrual. A pooled analysis of two trials addressing this issue of administering adjuvant 5-FU–LV after hepatic resection, one of which includes the Portier and colleagues[18] study, found that adjuvant 5-FU–LV was independently associated with both prolonged progression-free survival (PFS) and OS in multivariable analysis (median OS: chemotherapy group, 62.2 months; surgery alone, 47.3 months).[19] Kemeny and colleagues[20] investigated the use of adjuvant combined regional (FUDR) and systemic chemotherapy (infusional 5-FU) after complete resection of limited hepatic metastases (≤ 3 lesions) compared with surgery alone and found that patients receiving chemotherapy had a significantly improved 4-year recurrence-free survival (46% versus 25%; $P = .04$) and 4-year liver recurrence-free rate (67% versus 43%; $P = .03$). Finally, Kemeny and colleagues[21] have previously reported an improvement in PFS and OS at 2 years when HAI therapy is combined with systemic chemotherapy after resection compared with systemic therapy alone. It should be noted, however, that all of these studies were conducted before the era of modern chemotherapy and did not incorporate oxaliplatin- or irinotecan-based regimens. The EORTC Intergroup trial that addressed perioperative FOLFOX chemotherapy for resectable liver metastases[22] is discussed in detail in the level Ia evidence section.

TRIALS FOR HAI REGIONAL CHEMOTHERAPY

The rationale for delivering HAI chemotherapy for liver metastases is based on the fact that metastases derive their blood supply from the hepatic artery and chemotherapy can be delivered in higher doses.[2] Trials that have investigated the use of HAI have differed in the chemotherapeutic agent used for regional infusion ranging from FUDR (90% hepatic extraction rate) to 5-FU (variable hepatic extraction rate ranging from 19%–90%) so that the delivery of chemotherapy has not been standardized among trials. The second problem is that some studies have concurrently administered systemic therapy along with regional therapy, whereas others have compared regional therapy in isolation. Regional therapy to the liver with a high extraction rate has minimal impact on the progression of extrahepatic disease. Trials have been conflicting and difficult to compare because eight previous trials using HAI for unresectable hepatic metastases yielded mixed results.[2] There are two trials during the more recent time period included in this article that were ranked as Ia trials (discussed in detail later).

TRIALS ON MOLECULAR MARKERS OF CHEMOTHERAPY EFFICACY

In this generation of new chemotherapeutic agents and novel monoclonal antibodies directed at specific membrane receptors, it seems logical that the initiative has been to shift from a one-size-fits-all disease-based chemotherapy to individual tumor-directed therapy. The literature is populated with many retrospective studies that describe associations of chemotherapeutic response and patient survival outcomes with certain tumor genetic signatures, protein expression levels, or molecular markers. There is only a single study by Karapetis and colleagues[23] that has investigated such an association in a prospective randomized fashion, however, and it has defined the use of cetuximab and other epidermal growth factor receptor (EGFR) receptor inhibitors for patients with tumors that possess K-ras wild-type genotype. This study is discussed in detail in the level Ia evidence section.

TRIALS ON THE DURATION, DOSING, AND SEQUENCING OF CHEMOTHERAPY

Studies in this subject area have focused on using different dosages, durations, and schedules of delivering chemotherapy. There is not one single recipe for dosage, sequence, and duration that defines the standard administration of chemotherapy for all patients. Tournigand and colleagues[9] demonstrated similar results when FOL-FOX and FOLFIRI are interchanged as first-line and second-line therapy, suggesting that either order can be used. This trial also provided further support for the notion that FOLFOX and FOLFIRI have equivalent efficacy in advanced colorectal cancer. Two large trials recently published in 2007 (CAIRO study and MRC FOCUS study) reported that a sequential treatment strategy of 5-FU followed by either oxaliplatin- or irinotecan-based regimens after failure yielded similar patient survival outcomes as initiating treatment with a combination regimen as first-line therapy.[24,25] This strategy has not permeated into most oncologists' clinical practice today, however, because most patients are offered either FOLFOX or FOLFIRI as first-line therapy barring any toxicity contraindications.

LEVEL IA EVIDENCE RANDOMIZED CLINICAL TRIALS
Trials Using Different Types of Chemotherapy

1. Oral capecitabine versus intravenous 5-fluorouracil and leucovorin: integrated efficacy data and novel analyses from two large, randomized, phase III trials. Van Cutsem E, Hoff PM, Harper P, et al. Br J Cancer 2004 Mar 22;90(6):1190–7.[15]

Hypothesis: Oral capecitabine has similar efficacy as IV 5-FU for advanced colorectal cancer.

No. Patients Randomized	Study Groups	Stratification	Significance Demonstrated	% Change Identified in Trial
1207	Capecitabine N = 603 Bolus 5-FU–LV N = 604	None	No difference in OS	Median OS: 12.9 versus 12.8 mo

Published abstract: This study evaluates the efficacy of capecitabine using data from a large, well-characterized population of patients with MCRC treated in two identically designed phase III studies. A total of 1207 patients with previously untreated MCRC were randomized to either oral capecitabine (1250 mg m[-2] twice daily, days 1–14 every 21 days; N = 603) or IV bolus 5-FU–LV (Mayo Clinic regimen; N = 604). Capecitabine demonstrated a statistically significant superior response rate compared with 5-FU–LV (26% versus 17%; $P<.0002$). Subgroup analysis demonstrated that capecitabine consistently resulted in superior response rates ($P<.05$), even in patient subgroups with poor prognostic indicators. The median time to response and duration of response were similar and time to progression (TTP) was equivalent in the two arms (hazard ratio [HR] 0.997; 95% confidence interval [CI], 0.885–1.123; $P = .95$; median 4.6 versus 4.7 months with capecitabine and 5-FU–LV, respectively). Multivariate Cox regression analysis identified younger age, liver metastases, multiple metastases, and poor Karnofsky performance status as independent prognostic indicators for poor TTP. Overall survival was equivalent in the two arms (HR 0.95; 95% CI, 0.84–1.06; $P = .48$; median 12.9 versus 12.8 months, respectively). Capecitabine results in superior response rate, equivalent TTP and OS, an improved safety profile, and improved convenience compared with IV 5-FU–LV as first-line treatment for MCRC. For patients in whom fluoropyrimidine monotherapy is indicated, capecitabine should be strongly considered. Following encouraging results from phase I and II trials, randomized trials are evaluating capecitabine in combination with irinotecan, oxaliplatin, and radiotherapy. Capecitabine is a suitable replacement for IV 5-FU as the backbone of colorectal cancer therapy. (Copyright 2004 Nature Publishing Group; reprinted with permission.)

Editor's summary and comments: Although this is a pooled analysis of two identically designed studies, it secured a spot for oral capecitabine in the treatment of advanced colorectal cancer. It seems that the oral preparation has similar efficacy, less toxicity, and increased ease for patients. This trial must be interpreted in the context of the control group, however, consisting of bolus 5-FU as opposed to infusional 5-FU, of which the latter is the standard of care today.

2. Randomized phase III study of capecitabine plus oxaliplatin compared with fluorouracil/folinic acid plus oxaliplatin as first-line therapy for metastatic colorectal cancer. Cassidy J, Clarke S, Díaz-Rubio E, et al. J Clin Oncol 2008 Apr 20;26(12):2006–12.[12]

Hypothesis: Capecitabine plus oxaliplatin (XELOX) is not inferior to FOLFOX4 as first-line therapy in MCRC colorectal cancer.

No. Patients Randomized	Study Groups	Stratification	Significance Demonstrated	% Change Identified in Trial
2035	XELOX N = 1017 FOLFOX4 N = 1018	None	No difference in PFS or OS	Median PFS: 8 versus 8.5 mo Median OS: 19.8 versus 19.6 mo

Published abstract: The purpose is to evaluate whether XELOX is noninferior to FOLFOX4 as first-line therapy in MCRC. Patients and methods: The initial design of this trial was a randomized, two-arm, noninferiority, phase III comparison of XELOX with FOLFOX4. After patient accrual had begun, the trial design was amended in 2003 after bevacizumab phase III data became available. The resulting 2×2 factorial design randomly assigned patients to XELOX versus FOLFOX4, and then to also receive either bevacizumab or placebo. The results of the analysis of the XELOX versus FOLFOX4 arms are reported here. The analysis of bevacizumab versus placebo with oxaliplatin-based chemotherapy is reported separately. The prespecified primary end point for the noninferiority analysis was PFS. Results: The intent-to-treat population comprised 634 patients from the original two-arm portion of the study, plus an additional 1400 patients after the start of the amended 2×2 design, for a total of 2034 patients. The median PFS was 8 months in the pooled XELOX-containing arms versus 8.5 months in the FOLFOX4-containing arms (HR, 1.04; 97.5% CI, 0.93–1.16). The median OS was 19.8 months with XELOX versus 19.6 months with FOLFOX4 (HR, 0.99; 97.5% CI, 0.88–1.12). FOLFOX4 was associated with more grade 3 to 4 neutropenia-granulocytopenia and febrile neutropenia than XELOX, and XELOX with more grade 3 diarrhea and grade 3 hand-foot syndrome than FOLFOX4. Conclusion: XELOX is noninferior to FOLFOX4 as a first-line treatment for MCRC, and may be considered as a routine treatment option for appropriate patients. (Copyright 2008 American Society of Clinical Oncology; reprinted with permission.)

Editor's summary and comments: This multicenter trial compared the efficacy of oral capecitabine with infusional 5-FU in combination with oxaliplatin chemotherapy.

The trial was amended in 2003, however, to include the addition of bevacizumab as a 2 × 2 factorial design. The XELOX and FOLFOX groups each contain three subgroups of patients: those who received (1) the assigned chemotherapy, (2) chemotherapy plus placebo, and (3) chemotherapy plus bevacizumab. Although the authors state that treatment interaction was ruled out to assess for the effect of bevacizumab, the results of this trial are based on a pooled analysis of these groups. Nevertheless, assuming that the effect of bevacizumab was equal in both groups, capecitabine demonstrated oncologic noninferiority compared with standard infusional 5-FU.

3. A randomized controlled trial of fluorouracil plus leucovorin, irinotecan, and oxaliplatin combinations in patients with previously untreated metastatic colorectal cancer. Goldberg RM, Sargent DJ, Morton RF, et al. J Clin Oncol 2004 Jan 1;22(1):23–30.[6]

Hypothesis: Oxaliplatin-based chemotherapy is superior to the IFL regimen.

No. Patients Randomized	Study Groups	Stratification	Significance Demonstrated	% Change Identified in Trial
795	FOLFOX N = 267 IFL N = 264 IROX N = 264	Performance status, prior chemotherapy, prior immunotherapy, age, randomizing location	FOLFOX improved PFS, tumor response rate, and OS compared with IFL and IROX	Median PFS: 8.7 versus 6.9 versus 6.5 mo Tumor response rate: 45% versus 31% versus 35% Median OS: 19.5 versus 15 versus 17.4 mo

Published abstract: Three agents with differing mechanisms of action are available for treatment of advanced colorectal cancer: (1) FU, (2) irinotecan, and (3) oxaliplatin. This study compares the activity and toxicity of three different two-drug combinations in patients with MCRC who had not been treated previously for advanced disease. Patients and methods: Patients were concurrently randomly assigned to receive IFL (control combination); FOLFOX; or irinotecan and oxaliplatin (IROX). The primary end point was TTP, with secondary end points of response rate, survival time, and toxicity. Results: A total of 795 patients were randomly assigned between May 1999 and April 2001. A median TTP of 8.7 months, response rate of 45%, and median survival time of 19.5 months were observed for FOLFOX. These results were significantly superior to those observed for IFL for all end points (6.9 months, 31%, and 15 months, respectively) or for IROX (6.5 months, 35%, and 17.4 months, respectively) for TTP and response. The FOLFOX regimen had significantly lower rates of severe nausea, vomiting, diarrhea, febrile neutropenia, and dehydration. Sensory neuropathy and neutropenia were more common with the regimens containing oxaliplatin. Conclusion: The FOLFOX regimen was active and comparatively safe. It should be considered as a standard therapy for patients with advanced colorectal cancer. (Copyright 2004 American Society of Clinical Oncology; reprinted with permission.)

Editor's summary and comments: In the year 2000, the IFL regimen became the standard of care chemotherapeutic regimen in the United States for MCRC.[5] The multicenter trial reported previously (N9741) compared FOLFOX with IROX and IFL regimens in terms of PFS, tumor response, and OS. Although the median follow-up was only 20.4 months, the FOLFOX regimen performed better in all three end points.

To the authors' credit, a recent update after 5-year follow-up reported consistent findings.[26] The authors concluded that FOLFOX should replace irinotecan-based regimens as the standard therapy for advanced colorectal cancer. It must be stressed, however, that not all irinotecan regimens are the same; IFL, which uses bolus-FU, is distinct from FOLFIRI, which includes infusional 5-FU.

4. Phase III randomized trial of FOLFIRI versus FOLFOX4 in the treatment of advanced colorectal cancer: a multicenter study of the Gruppo Oncologico Dell'Italia Meridionale. Colucci G, Gebbia V, Paoletti G, et al. J Clin Oncol 2005 Aug 1;23(22):4866–75.[8]

Hypothesis: FOLFOX and FOLFIRI have equivalent tumor response rates.

No. Patients Randomized	Study Groups	Stratification	Significance Demonstrated	% Change Identified in Trial
360	FOLFIRI N = 178 FOLFOX4 N = 182	None	Similar overall response rate, TTP, and OS	Overall response rates: 31% versus 34% Median PFS: 7 versus 7 mo Median OS: 14 versus 15 mo

Published abstract: This phase III study was performed to compare the FOLFIRI with the FOLFOX4 in previously untreated patients with advanced colorectal cancer. Patients and methods: A total of 360 chemotherapy-naive patients were randomly assigned to receive, every 2 weeks, either arm A (FOLFIRI: irinotecan, 180 mg/m², on day 1 with LV, 100 mg/m², administered as a 2-hour infusion before FU, 400 mg/m², administered as an IV bolus injection, and FU, 600 mg/m², as a 22-hour infusion immediately after FU bolus injection on days 1 and 2 [LV5FU2]) or arm B (FOLFOX4: oxaliplatin, 85 mg/m², on day 1 with LV5FU2 regimen). Results: One hundred sixty-four and 172 patients were assessable in arm A and B, respectively. Overall response rates were 31% in arm A (95% CI, 24.6–38.3) and 34% in arm B (95% CI, 27.2–41.5; $P = .60$). In both arms A and B, median TTP (7 versus 7 months, respectively), duration of response (9 versus 10 months, respectively), and OS (14 versus 15 months, respectively) were similar, without any statistically significant difference. Toxicity was mild in both groups: alopecia and gastrointestinal disturbances were the most common toxicities in arm A; thrombocytopenia and neurosensorial were the most common toxicities in arm B. Grade 3 to 4 toxicities were uncommon in both arms, and no statistical significant difference was observed. Conclusion: There is no difference in overall response rates, TTP, and OS for patients treated with the FOLFIRI or FOLFOX4 regimen. Both therapies seemed effective as first-line treatment in these patients. The difference between these two combination therapies is mainly in the toxicity profile. (Copyright 2005 American Society of Clinical Oncology; reprinted with permission.)

Editor's summary and comments: This Italian study describes equivalent efficacy of oxaliplatin and irinotecan, namely that FOLFIRI and FOLFOX have similar tumor response rates, PFS, and OS. It is worth highlighting that this trial used irinotecan in combination with infusional 5-FU and reported its equivalent efficacy to FOLFOX as opposed to what has been previously reported for the IFL regimen (bolus 5-FU). Most oncologists today choose first-line treatment based on the toxicity profile of the regimen as it applies to each individual patient rather than a superior oncologic efficacy of one regimen over the other.

5. Bevacizumab plus irinotecan, fluorouracil, and leucovorin for metastatic colorectal cancer. Hurwitz H, Fehrenbacher L, Novotny W, et al. N Engl J Med 2004 Jun 3;350(23):2335–42.[27]

Hypothesis: Bevacizumab improves the efficacy of IFL.

No. Patients Randomized	Study Groups	Stratification	Significance Demonstrated	% Change Identified in Trial
813	IFL/Bev N = 402 IFL/placebo N = 411	None	Improved PFS and OS	Median PFS: 10.6 versus 6.2 mo Median OS: 20.3 versus 15.6 mo

Published abstract: Bevacizumab, a monoclonal antibody against vascular endothelial growth factor, has shown promising preclinical and clinical activity against MCRC, particularly in combination with chemotherapy. Methods: Of 813 patients with previously untreated MCRC, 402 were randomly assigned to receive IFL plus bevacizumab (5 mg per kilogram of body weight every 2 weeks) and 411 to receive IFL plus placebo. The primary end point was OS. Secondary end points were PFS, the response rate, the duration of the response, safety, and the quality of life. Results: The median duration of survival was 20.3 months in the group given IFL plus bevacizumab, compared with 15.6 months in the group given IFL plus placebo, corresponding to a HR for death of 0.66 (P<.001). The median duration of PFS was 10.6 months in the group given IFL plus bevacizumab, compared with 6.2 months in the group given IFL plus placebo (HR for disease progression, 0.54; P<.001); the corresponding rates of response were 44.8% and 34.8% (P = .004). The median duration of the response was 10.4 months in the group given IFL plus bevacizumab, compared with 7.1 months in the group given IFL plus placebo (HR for progression, 0.62; P = .001). Grade 3 hypertension was more common during treatment with IFL plus bevacizumab than with IFL plus placebo (11% versus 2.3%) but was easily managed. Conclusions: The addition of bevacizumab to FU-based combination chemotherapy results in statistically significant and clinically meaningful improvement in survival among patients with MCRC. (Copyright [2004] Massachusetts Medical Society. All rights reserved.)

Editor's summary and comments: This trial reported an increased survival of over 4 months with the addition of bevacizumab that led to a significant increase in the use of Avastin. These results must be interpreted with caution, however, because IFL chemotherapy was used as opposed to either FOLFOX or FOLFIRI, which have emerged as the standard first-line chemotherapeutic regimens. The reported survival of 20.3 months in this trial is now achieved with FOLFOX or FOLFIRI alone without the addition of bevacizumab. Also, the side effects and complications of Avastin, which include but are not limited to hypertension, bleeding, poor wound healing, and bowel perforation, must be considered before administering this to patients.

6. Bevacizumab in combination with oxaliplatin-based chemotherapy as first-line therapy in metastatic colorectal cancer: a randomized phase III study. Saltz LB, Clarke S, Díaz-Rubio E, et al. J Clin Oncol 2008 Apr 20;26(12):2013–9.[28]

Hypothesis: Bevacizumab improves the efficacy of capecitabine plus oxaliplatin (XELOX) and FOLFOX4.

No. Patients Randomized	Study Groups	Stratification	Significance Demonstrated	% Change Identified in Trial
1401	Chemo/Bev N = 700 Chemo/Placebo N = 701	None	Improved PFS but no difference in OS	Median PFS: 9.4 versus 8 mo Median OS: 21.3 versus 19.9 mo

Published abstract: The purpose is to evaluate the efficacy and safety of bevacizumab when added to first-line oxaliplatin-based chemotherapy (XELOX or FOL-FOX4) in patients with MCRC. Patients and methods: Patients with MCRC were randomly assigned, in a 2 × 2 factorial design, to XELOX versus FOLFOX4, and then to bevacizumab versus placebo. The primary end point was PFS. Results: A total of 1401 patients were randomly assigned in this 2 × 2 analysis. Median PFS was 9.4 months in the bevacizumab group and 8 months in the placebo group (HR, 0.83; 97.5% CI, 0.72–0.95; $P = .0023$). Median OS was 21.3 months in the bevacizumab group and 19.9 months in the placebo group (HR, 0.89; 97.5% CI, 0.76–1.03; $P = .077$). Response rates were similar in both arms. Analysis of treatment withdrawals showed that, despite protocol allowance of treatment continuation until disease progression, only 29% and 47% of bevacizumab and placebo recipients, respectively, were treated until progression. The toxicity profile of bevacizumab was consistent with that documented in previous trials. Conclusion: The addition of bevacizumab to oxaliplatin-based chemotherapy significantly improved PFS in this first-line trial in patients with MCRC. Overall survival differences did not reach statistical significance, and response rate was not improved by the addition of bevacizumab. Treatment continuation until disease progression may be necessary to optimize the contribution of bevacizumab to therapy. (Copyright 2008 American Society of Clinical Oncology; reprinted with permission.)

Editor's summary and comments: This multicenter trial investigated the efficacy of adding bevacizumab to XELOX or FOLFOX4 chemotherapy. This trial used a 2 × 2 factorial design; the bevacizumab and placebo groups included patients who received either XELOX or FOLFOX chemotherapy. The authors concurrently demonstrated noninferiority of XELOX compared with FOLFOX, so presumably the difference observed in PFS is related to bevacizumab administration. Although there was no difference observed in OS between the two groups, the authors suggest that the duration of therapy may be a factor. Nevertheless, the benefit of adding bevacizumab to cytotoxic chemotherapy is much less impressive in this trial than reported elsewhere by Hurwitz and colleagues,[27] which used the IFL regimen, and the TREE-2 study (abstract to follow).[29]

7. Safety and efficacy of oxaliplatin and fluoropyrimidine regimens with or without bevacizumab as first-line treatment of metastatic colorectal cancer: results of the TREE Study. Hochster HS, Hart LL, Ramanathan RK, et al. J Clin Oncol 2008 Jul 20;26(21):3523–9.[29]

Hypothesis: Bevacizumab improves the efficacy of oxaliplatin-based regimens.

No. Patients Randomized	Study Groups	Stratification	Significance Demonstrated	% Change Identified in Trial
373	Tree-1 (no bev) N = 150 Tree-2 (bev) N = 223	Three different oxaliplatin-based regimens: (1) FOLFOX6, (2) oxaliplatin with bolus 5-FU, (3) CapeOx	Improved overall response rate, PFS, and OS	FOLFOX6 ± Bev Overall response rates: 52% versus 41% Median PFS: 9.9 versus 8.7 mo Median OS: 26.1 versus 19.2 mo

Published abstract: The purpose is to evaluate the safety and efficacy of three oxaliplatin and fluoropyrimidine regimens, with or without bevacizumab, as first-line treatment for MCRC. Patients and methods: Patients with histologically documented metastatic or recurrent CRC and no prior treatment for advanced disease were randomly assigned to mFOLFOX6, bFOL (bolus FU and low-dose LV with oxaliplatin), or CapeOx (capecitabine with oxaliplatin), respectively (three regimens of eloxatin evaluation [TREE-1]). The study was later modified such that subsequent patients were randomized to the same regimens plus bevacizumab (TREE-2). Results: A total of 150 and 223 patients were randomly assigned in the TREE-1 and TREE-2 cohorts, respectively. Incidence of grade 3 to 4 treatment-related adverse events during the first 12 weeks of treatment were 59%, 36%, and 67% for mFOLFOX6, bFOL, and CapeOx, respectively (TREE-1); and 59%, 51%, and 56% for the corresponding treatments plus bevacizumab (TREE-2, primary end point). CapeOx toxicity in TREE-1 included grade 3 to 4 diarrhea (31%) and dehydration (27%); capecitabine dose reduction to 1700 $mg/m^2/d$ in TREE-2 resulted in improved tolerance. Overall response rates were 41%, 20%, and 27% (TREE-1) and 52%, 39%, and 46% (TREE-2); median OS was 19.2, 17.9, and 17.2 months (TREE-1) and 26.1, 20.4, and 24.6 months (TREE-2). For all treated patients, median OS was 18.2 months (95% CI, 14.5–21.6; TREE-1) and 23.7 months (95% CI, 21.3–26.8; TREE-2). Conclusion: The addition of bevacizumab to oxaliplatin and fluoropyrimidine regimens is well tolerated as first-line treatment of MCRC and does not markedly change overall toxicity. CapeOx tolerability and efficacy is improved with reduced-dose capecitabine. First-line oxaliplatin and fluoropyrimidine-based therapy plus bevacizumab resulted in a median OS of approximately 2 years. (Copyright 2008 American Society of Clinical Oncology; reprinted with permission.)

Editor's summary and comments: The two major studies that investigated the use of adding bevacizumab to standard first-line FOLFOX chemotherapy have yielded different results. Saltz and colleagues[28] reported a nonsignificant increase in OS of only 1.4 months, whereas the TREE-2 study reports a benefit of almost 7 months. The TREE study, however, is limited by a small number of patients and compares the results of patients treated with and without bevacizumab from sequential time periods as opposed to conducting a true randomization for patients to receive therapy with and without bevacizumab; the results should be interpreted with caution. Given the substantial cost and toxicity profile of Avastin, this discrepancy in findings between these two trials must be resolved before the addition of bevacizumab to FOLFOX-FOLFIRI becomes the recommended standard of care for patients with advanced colorectal cancer.

8. Cetuximab for the treatment of colorectal cancer. Jonker DJ, O'Callaghan CJ, Karapetis CS, et al. N Engl J Med 2007 Nov 15;357(20):2040–8.[30]

Hypothesis: Cetuximab improves survival in patients with EGFR expressing advanced colorectal cancer refractory to standard chemotherapeutic regimens.

No. Patients Randomized	Study Groups	Stratification	Significance Demonstrated	% Change Identified in Trial
572	Cetuximab N = 287 Best supportive care N = 285	ECOG performance status and center	Improved OS	Median OS: 6.1 versus 4.6 mo

Published abstract: Cetuximab, an IgG1 chimeric monoclonal antibody against EGFR, has activity against colorectal cancers that express EGFR. Methods: From December 2003 to August 2005, 572 patients who had colorectal cancer expressing immunohistochemically detectable EGFR and who had been previously treated with fluoropyrimidine, irinotecan, and oxaliplatin or had contraindications to treatment with these drugs underwent randomization to an initial dose of 400 mg of cetuximab per square meter of body-surface area followed by a weekly infusion of 250 mg/m^2 plus best supportive care (287 patients) or best supportive care alone (285 patients). The primary end point was OS. Results: Compared with best supportive care alone, cetuximab treatment was associated with a significant improvement in OS (HR for death, 0.77; 95% CI, 0.64–0.92; $P = .005$) and in PFS (HR for disease progression or death, 0.68; 95% CI, 0.57–0.80; $P<.001$). These benefits were robust after adjustment in a multivariable Cox proportional-hazards model. The median OS was 6.1 months in the cetuximab group and 4.6 months in the group assigned to supportive care alone. Partial responses occurred in 23 patients (8%) in the cetuximab group but in none in the group assigned to supportive care alone ($P<.001$); the disease was stable in an additional 31.4% of patients assigned to cetuximab and in 10.9% of patients assigned to supportive care alone ($P<.001$). Quality of life was better preserved in the cetuximab group, with less deterioration in physical function and global health status scores (both $P<.05$). Cetuximab treatment was associated with a characteristic rash; a rash of grade 2 or higher was strongly associated with improved survival (HR for death, 0.33; 95% CI, 0.22–0.50; $P<.001$). The incidence of any adverse event of grade 3 or higher was 78.5% in the cetuximab group and 59.1% in the group assigned to supportive care alone ($P<.001$). Conclusions: Cetuximab improves OS and PFS and preserves quality-of-life measures in patients with colorectal cancer in whom other treatments have failed. (Copyright [2007] Massachusetts Medical Society. All rights reserved.)

Editor's summary and comments: Although the prolongation in survival was modest compared with best supportive care, this trial secured a place for cetuximab as third-line therapy in the armamentarium of drugs to treat EGFR expressing advanced colorectal cancer. Interestingly, its oncologic efficacy is related to the grade of skin rash that is induced, because higher grades of rash (grade 2 > grade 1 > grade 0) are associated with an increased survival.

Trials for Neoadjuvant and Adjuvant Chemotherapy for Resectable Liver Metastases

9. Perioperative chemotherapy with FOLFOX4 and surgery versus surgery alone for resectable liver metastases from colorectal cancer (EORTC Intergroup trial 40,983): a randomized controlled trial. Nordlinger B, Sorbye H, Glimelius B, et al. Lancet 2008 Mar 22;371(9617):1007–16.[22]

Hypothesis: Perioperative chemotherapy improves survival compared with surgery alone.

No. Patients Randomized	Study Groups	Stratification	Significance Gemonstrated	% Change Identified in Trial
364	Perioperative chemo N = 182 Surgery alone N = 182	None	Increased 3-y PFS	All patients: 7.3% (P = .058) Resected patients: 9.2% (P = .025)

Published abstract: Surgical resection alone is regarded as the standard of care for patients with liver metastases from colorectal cancer, but relapse is common. The combination of perioperative chemotherapy and surgery compared with surgery alone for patients with initially resectable liver metastases from colorectal cancer was assessed. Methods: This parallel-group study reports the trial's final data for PFS for a protocol unspecified interim time-point, whereas OS is still being monitored. A total of 364 patients with histologically proved colorectal cancer and up to four liver metastases were randomly assigned to either six cycles of FOLFOX4 before and six cycles after surgery or to surgery alone (182 in perioperative chemotherapy group versus 182 in surgery group). Patients were centrally randomized by minimization, adjusting for center and risk score. The primary objective was to detect a HR of 0.71 or less for PFS. Primary analysis was by intention to treat. Analyses were repeated for all eligible (171 versus 171) and resected patients (151 versus 152). This trial is registered with ClinicalTrials.gov, number NCT00006479. Findings: In the perioperative chemotherapy group, 151 (83%) patients were resected after a median of six (range 1–6) preoperative cycles and 115 (63%) patients received a median six (range 1–8) postoperative cycles. A total of 152 (84%) patients were resected in the surgery group. The absolute increase in rate of PFS at 3 years was 7.3% (from 28.1% [95.66% CI, 21.3–35.5] to 35.4% [28.1–42.7]; HR 0.79 [0.62–1.02]; P = .058) in randomized patients; 8.1% (from 28.1% [21.2–36.6] to 36.2% [28.7–43.8]; HR 0.77 [0.60–1.00]; P = .041) in eligible patients; and 9.2% (from 33.2% [25.3–41.2] to 42.4% [34.0–50.5]; HR 0.73 [0.55–0.97]; P = .025) in patients undergoing resection. A total of 139 patients died (64 in perioperative chemotherapy group versus 75 in surgery group). Reversible postoperative complications occurred more often after chemotherapy than after surgery (40 [25%] of 159 versus 27 [16%] of 170; P = .04). After surgery two deaths were recorded in the surgery alone group and one was recorded in the perioperative chemotherapy group. Interpretation: Perioperative chemotherapy with FOLFOX4 is compatible with major liver surgery and reduces the risk of events of PFS in eligible and resected patients. (Copyright Elsevier 2008.)

Editor's summary and comments: This study addresses the question of administering chemotherapy as an adjunct to surgery using PFS as the primary end point. It must be stressed that this trial does not assess the timing of chemotherapy before or after a potentially curative resection because the control group was randomized to surgery alone and did not receive any chemotherapy. In an intention-to-treat analysis, there was a nonsignificant increase in the 3-year PFS rate of 7.3% in the chemotherapy group compared with the surgery only group (35.4% versus 28.1%; P = .058) along with a trend toward increased postoperative morbidity in those patients who received preoperative chemotherapy. Progression in either group that occurred within the first 20 weeks of randomization was recorded as a progression of disease at 10 weeks, which in effect combines all early recurrences to the same time point. The rate of nontherapeutic laparotomy caused by findings of unresectable disease at exploration, which was recorded as disease progression, in the chemotherapy group and surgery group was 5% and 11%, respectively. This 6% difference at the time of operation nearly completely accounts for the 7.3% difference in PFS. Furthermore, if one examines the survival curves in the manuscript, the curves separate at the first time point of 10 weeks and then remain nearly parallel for the duration of follow-up. Perhaps preoperative chemotherapy improved patient selection for resection accounting for the improved PFS. Regardless, this trial cannot be used to support the routine use of preoperative chemotherapy for resectable metastases. Rather, this trial supports combined modality therapy as evidenced by a subset secondary analysis that showed a 9.2% increase in 3-year PFS in those patients receiving both surgical resection and chemotherapy compared with surgery alone.

Trials for Regional Chemotherapy

10. Intrahepatic arterial versus intravenous fluorouracil and folinic acid for colorectal cancer liver metastases: a multicentre randomized trial. Kerr DJ, McArdle CS, Ledermann J, et al. Lancet 2003 Feb 1;361(9355):368–73.[31]

Hypothesis: Intrahepatic arterial (IHA) therapy is not superior to IV systemic chemotherapy.

No. Patients Randomized	Study Groups	Stratification	Significance Demonstrated	% Change Identified in Trial
290	IHA N = 145 Systemic chemo N = 145	None	No change in OS	None

Published abstract: The liver is the most frequent site for metastases of colorectal cancer, which is the second largest contributor to cancer deaths in Europe. A randomized trial was performed to compare an IHA fluorouracil and folinic acid regimen with the standard intravenous de Gramont FU and folinic acid regimen for patients with adenocarcinoma of the colon or rectum, with metastases confined to the liver. Methods: A total of 290 patients from 16 centers were randomly allocated to receive either IV chemotherapy (folinic acid, 200 mg/m^2, FU bolus, 400 mg^2, and 22-hour infusion, 600 mg/m^2, day 1 and 2, repeated every 14 days), or IHA chemotherapy designed to be equitoxic (folinic acid, 200 mg/m^2, FU, 400 mg/m^2 over 15 minutes and 22-hour infusion, 1600 mg/m^2, day 1 and 2, repeated every 14 days). The primary end point was OS, and analysis was by intention to treat. Findings: A total of 50 (37%) patients allocated to IHA did not start their treatment, and another 39 (29%) had to stop before receiving six cycles of treatment because of catheter failure. The IHA group received a median of two cycles (0–6), compared with 8.5 (6–12) for the intravenous group. A total of 45 (51%) IHA patients who did not start or did not receive six cycles switched to IV treatment. In both groups, grade 3 or 4 toxicity was uncommon. Median OS was 14.7 months for the IHA group and 14.8 months for the intravenous group (HR 1.04 [95% CI, 0.80–1.33]; log-rank test $P = .79$). Similarly, there was no significant difference in PFS. Interpretation: The results showed no evidence of an advantage in PFS or OS for the IHA group; continued use of this regimen cannot be recommended outside of a clinical trial. (Copyright Elsevier 2003.)

Editor's summary and comments: This trial failed to show any improvement in OS with the use of IHA chemotherapy beyond that achieved with the de Gramont regimen (systemic 5-FU–LV). The results of this study must be interpreted with caution, however, for the following three reasons: (1) the trial was stopped early because of slow accrual and did not reach its target recruitment of 312 patients; (2) the investigators used 5-FU as opposed to FUDR for intra-arterial therapy, of which the former has a significantly decreased hepatic extraction rate; and (3) the median number of cycles received in the IHA group was only two, whereas patients in the IV chemotherapy group received a median of 8.5 cycles. Fifty patients in the IHA group never received any intra-arterial chemotherapy during the study period. Although this may speak to the difficulty in administering intra-arterial therapy to patients, this has not been the experience at the authors' institution (Memorial Sloan-Kettering Cancer Center).

11. Hepatic arterial infusion versus systemic therapy for hepatic metastases from colorectal cancer: a randomized trial of efficacy, quality of life, and molecular markers (CALGB 9481). Kemeny NE, Niedzwiecki D, Hollis DR, et al. J Clin Oncol 2006 Mar 20;24(9):1395–403.[32]

Hypothesis: IHA therapy is superior to IV systemic chemotherapy.

No. Patients Randomized	Study Groups	Stratification	Significance Demonstrated	% Change Identified in Trial
135	HAI N = 68 Systemic chemo N = 67	None	Increased OS with HAI therapy	HAI: 24.4 mo Systemic: 20 mo

Published abstract: Hepatic metastases derive most of their blood supply from the hepatic artery; for patients with hepatic metastases from colorectal cancer, HAI of chemotherapy may improve outcome. Methods: In a multi-institutional trial, 135 patients were randomly assigned to receive HAI versus systemic bolus FU and LV. The primary end point was survival; secondary end points were response, recurrence, toxicity, quality of life, cost, and the influence of molecular markers. Results: Overall survival was significantly longer for HAI versus systemic treatment (median, 24.4 versus 20 months; $P = .0034$), as were response rates (47% and 24%; $P = .012$) and time to hepatic progression (9.8 versus 7.3 months; $P = .034$). Time to extrahepatic progression (7.7 versus 14.8 months; $P = .029$) was significantly shorter in the HAI group. Quality-of-life measurements showed improved physical functioning in the HAI group at the 3- and 6-month follow-up assessments. Toxicity included grade greater than or equal to 3 neutropenia (2% and 45%; $P<.01$), stomatitis (0% and 24%; $P<.01$), and bilirubin elevation (18.6% and 0%; $P<.01$) in the HAI and systemic treatment groups, respectively. A greater proportion of men versus women receiving HAI experienced biliary toxicity (37% and 15%, respectively; $P = .05$). For HAI patients with thymidylate synthase levels in tumor less than or equal to 4, the median survival was 24 and 14 months, respectively ($P = .17$). Conclusion: HAI therapy increased OS, response rate, and time to hepatic progression, and was associated with better physical functioning compared with systemic therapy. Additional studies need to address the overall benefit and cost of new chemotherapy agents versus HAI alone or the combination of HAI with new agents. (Copyright 2006 American Society of Clinical Oncology; reprinted with permission.)

Editor's summary and comments: In this multi-institutional trial, HAI therapy alone resulted in a greater tumor response rate and a 4.4-month improvement in survival compared with standard systemic chemotherapy. Only nine patients in each group did not receive their intended therapy. Although there was a shorter time to extrahepatic disease progression in the HAI group, the improved OS of patients receiving HAI therapy underscores the importance of liver-directed therapy and hepatic disease control. The inability of HAI therapy to control extrahepatic disease suggests, however, that it should be used in combination with systemic therapy and not in isolation.

Trials on Molecular Markers of Chemotherapy Efficacy

12. K-ras mutations and benefit from cetuximab in advanced colorectal cancer. Karapetis CS, Khambata-Ford S, Jonker DJ, et al. N Engl J Med 2008 Oct 23;359(17):1757–65.[23]

Hypothesis: Tumor K-ras gene mutational status is an independent prognostic factor for patients receiving supportive care for MCRC.

No. Patients Randomized	Study Groups	Stratification	Significance Demonstrated	% Change Identified in Trial
394	Cetuximab (C) N = 198 Supportive care (S) N = 196	K-ras mutational status	Cetuximab plus wild-type K-ras had increased OS, PFS, and tumor response rate	OS C/WT: 9.5 mo C/Mutated: 4.5 mo S/WT: 4.8 mo S/Mutated: 4.6 mo

Published abstract: Treatment with cetuximab, a monoclonal antibody directed against EGFR, improves OS and PFS and preserves the quality of life in patients with colorectal cancer that has not responded to chemotherapy. The mutation status of the K-ras gene in the tumor may affect the response to cetuximab and have treatment-independent prognostic value. Methods: Tumor samples were analyzed, obtained from 394 (68.9%) of 572 patients with colorectal cancer who were randomly assigned to receive cetuximab plus best supportive care or best supportive care alone, to look for activating mutations in exon 2 of the K-ras gene. Assessed was whether the mutation status of the K-ras gene was associated with survival in the cetuximab and supportive-care groups. Results: Of the tumors evaluated for K-ras mutations, 42.3% had at least one mutation in exon 2 of the gene. The effectiveness of cetuximab was significantly associated with K-ras mutation status ($P = .01$ and $P<.001$ for the interaction of K-ras mutation status with OS and PFS, respectively). In patients with wild-type K-ras tumors, treatment with cetuximab as compared with supportive care alone significantly improved OS (median, 9.5 versus 4.8 months; HR for death, 0.55; 95% CI, 0.41–0.74; $P<.001$) and PFS (median, 3.7 months versus 1.9 months; HR for progression or death, 0.40; 95% CI, 0.30–0.54; $P<.001$). Among patients with mutated K-ras tumors, there was no significant difference between those who were treated with cetuximab and those who received supportive care alone with respect to OS (HR, 0.98; $P = .89$) or PFS (HR, 0.99; $P = .96$). In the group of patients receiving best supportive care alone, the mutation status of the K-ras gene was not significantly associated with OS (HR for death, 1.01; $P = .97$). Conclusions: Patients with a colorectal tumor bearing mutated K-ras did not benefit from cetuximab, whereas patients with a tumor bearing wild-type K-ras did benefit from cetuximab. The mutation status of the K-ras gene had no influence on survival among patients treated with best supportive care alone. (Copyright [2008] Massachusetts Medical Society. All rights reserved.)

Editor's summary and comments: This landmark study has set the bar for other translational researchers and has demonstrated the need to shift from a one-size-fits-all chemotherapeutic approach to a specific tumor-directed strategy. This trial clearly shows how a downstream mutation in a receptor's signaling cascade, in this case K-ras, can render a therapeutic agent completely ineffective. The authors found that K-ras was mutated in approximately 40% of patients. One can extrapolate from this study that cetuximab and other EGFR inhibitors are not effective in nearly half of patients with MCRC, highlighting the importance of checking tumor K-ras mutational status before its administration. This also underscores the need for further biomarker discovery that help predict the efficacy of other commonly administered chemotherapeutic agents, such as oxaliplatin and irinotecan.

Trials on the Duration, Dosing, and Sequencing of Chemotherapy

13. FOLFIRI followed by FOLFOX6 or the reverse sequence in advanced colorectal cancer: a randomized GERCOR study. Tournigand C, André T, Achille E, et al. J Clin Oncol 2004 Jan 15;22(2):229–37.[9]

Hypothesis: FOLFOX and FOLFIRI are equivalent in terms of oncologic efficacy.

No. Patients Randomized	Study Groups	Stratification	Significance Demonstrated	% Change Identified in Trial
226	FOLFIRI N = 113 FOLFOX6 N = 113	None	Similar PFS and OS for either sequence	Median PFS: 8.5 versus 8 mo Median OS: 21.5 versus 20.6 mo

Published abstract: In MCRC, phase III studies have demonstrated the superiority of FU with LV in combination with irinotecan or oxaliplatin over FU and LV alone. This phase III study investigated two sequences: FOLFIRI followed by FOLFOX6 (arm A), and FOLFOX6 followed by FOLFIRI (arm B). Patients and methods: Previously untreated patients with assessable disease were randomly assigned to receive a 2-hour infusion of l-LV, 200 mg/m^2, or dl-LV, 400 mg/m^2, followed by a FU bolus, 400 mg/m^2, and 46-hour infusion, 2400 to 3000 mg/m^2, every 46 hours every 2 weeks, either with irinotecan, 180 mg/m^2, or with oxaliplatin, 100 mg/m^2, as a 2-hour infusion on day 1. At progression, irinotecan was replaced by oxaliplatin (arm A), or oxaliplatin by irinotecan (arm B). Result: Median survival was 21.5 months in 109 patients allocated to FOLFIRI then FOLFOX6 versus 20.6 months in 111 patients allocated to FOLFOX6 and then FOLFIRI ($P = .99$). Median second PFS was 14.2 months in arm A versus 10.9 in arm B ($P = .64$). In first-line therapy, FOLFIRI achieved 56% response rate and 8.5 months median PFS, versus FOLFOX6, which achieved 54% response rate and 8 months median PFS ($P = .26$). Second-line FOLFIRI achieved 4% response rate and 2.5 months median PFS, versus FOLFOX6, which achieved 15% response rate and 4.2 month PFS. In first-line therapy, National Cancer Institute Common Toxicity Criteria grade 3 to 4 mucositis, nausea, and vomiting, and grade 2 alopecia were more frequent with FOLFIRI, and grade 3 to 4 neutropenia and neurosensory toxicity were more frequent with FOLFOX6. Conclusion: Both sequences achieved a prolonged survival and similar efficacy. The toxicity profiles were different. (Copyright 2004 American Society of Clinical Oncology; reprinted with permission.)

Editor's summary and comments: This important multicenter trial demonstrated equivalent efficacy between FOLFIRI and FOLFOX6 as first-line therapy for advanced colorectal cancer. Both groups had similar times to first progression, similar tumor response rates, and similar OS. This trial also demonstrated that regardless of the sequence used, the tumor response and patient outcomes for second-line therapy are substantially reduced. The toxicity profiles for these two regimens are distinct and largely form the basis for choosing one regimen over the other.

DISCLOSURE

Authors have nothing to disclose.

REFERENCES

1. Abdalla EK, Vauthey JN, Ellis LM, et al. Recurrence and outcomes following hepatic resection, radiofrequency ablation, and combined resection/ablation for colorectal liver metastases. Ann Surg 2004;239(6):818–25 [discussion: 825–7].
2. Dangelica MI, Shoup MC, Nissan A. Randomized clinical trials in advanced and metastatic colorectal carcinoma. Surg Oncol Clin N Am 2002;11(1):173–91, ix.
3. Modulation of fluorouracil by leucovorin in patients with advanced colorectal cancer: evidence in terms of response rate. Advanced Colorectal Cancer Meta-Analysis Project. J Clin Oncol 1992;10(6):896–903.
4. de Gramont A, Bosset JF, Milan C, et al. Randomized trial comparing monthly low-dose leucovorin and fluorouracil bolus with bimonthly high-dose leucovorin and fluorouracil bolus plus continuous infusion for advanced colorectal cancer: a French Intergroup Study. J Clin Oncol 1997;15(2):808–15.
5. Saltz LB, Cox JV, Blanke C, et al. Irinotecan plus fluorouracil and leucovorin for metastatic colorectal cancer. Irinotecan Study Group. N Engl J Med 2000; 343(13):905–14.
6. Goldberg RM, Sargent DJ, Morton RF, et al. A randomized controlled trial of fluo-rouracil plus leucovorin, irinotecan, and oxaliplatin combinations in patients with previously untreated metastatic colorectal cancer. J Clin Oncol 2004;22(1):23–30.
7. Dy GK, Krook JE, Green EM, et al. Impact of complete response to chemotherapy on overall survival in advanced colorectal cancer: results from Intergroup N9741. J Clin Oncol 2007;25(23):3469–74.
8. Colucci G, Gebbia V, Paoletti G, et al. Phase III randomized trial of FOLFIRI versus FOLFOX4 in the treatment of advanced colorectal cancer: a multicenter study of the Gruppo Oncologico Dell'Italia Meridionale. J Clin Oncol 2005;23(22):4866–75.
9. Tournigand C, Andre T, Achille E, et al. FOLFIRI followed by FOLFOX6 or the reverse sequence in advanced colorectal cancer: a randomized GERCOR study. J Clin Oncol 2004;22(2):229–37.
10. Becouarn Y, Senesse P, Thezenas S, et al. A randomized phase II trial evaluating safety and efficacy of an experimental chemotherapy regimen (irinotecan + oxaliplatin, IRINOX) and two standard arms (LV5 FU2 + irinotecan or LV5 FU2 + oxaliplatin) in first-line metastatic colorectal cancer: a study of the Digestive Group of the Federation Nationale des Centres de Lutte Contre le Cancer. Ann Oncol 2007;18(12):2000–5.
11. Zori Comba A, Blajman C, Richardet E, et al. A randomised phase II study of oxaliplatin alone versus oxaliplatin combined with 5-fluorouracil and folinic acid (Mayo Clinic regimen) in previously untreated metastatic colorectal cancer patients. Eur J Cancer 2001;37(8):1006–13.

12. Cassidy J, Clarke S, Diaz-Rubio E, et al. Randomized phase III study of capecitabine plus oxaliplatin compared with fluorouracil/folinic acid plus oxaliplatin as first-line therapy for metastatic colorectal cancer. J Clin Oncol 2008;26(12):2006–12.

13. Nogue M, Salud A, Batiste-Alentorn E, et al. Randomised study of tegafur and oral leucovorin versus intravenous 5-fluorouracil and leucovorin in patients with advanced colorectal cancer. Eur J Cancer 2005;41(15):2241–9.

14. Twelves C, Gollins S, Grieve R, et al. A randomised cross-over trial comparing patient preference for oral capecitabine and 5-fluorouracil/leucovorin regimens in patients with advanced colorectal cancer. Ann Oncol 2006;17(2):239–45.

15. Van Cutsem E, Hoff PM, Harper P, et al. Oral capecitabine vs intravenous 5-fluorouracil and leucovorin: integrated efficacy data and novel analyses from two large, randomised, phase III trials. Br J Cancer 2004;90(6):1190–7.

16. Chong G, Bhatnagar A, Cunningham D, et al. Phase III trial of 5-fluorouracil and leucovorin plus either 3H1 anti-idiotype monoclonal antibody or placebo in patients with advanced colorectal cancer. Ann Oncol 2006;17(3):437–42.

17. King J, Zhao J, Clingan P, et al. Randomised double blind placebo control study of adjuvant treatment with the metalloproteinase inhibitor, Marimastat in patients with inoperable colorectal hepatic metastases: significant survival advantage in patients with musculoskeletal side-effects. Anticancer Res 2003;23(1B):639–45.

18. Portier G, Elias D, Bouche O, et al. Multicenter randomized trial of adjuvant fluorouracil and folinic acid compared with surgery alone after resection of colorectal liver metastases: FFCD ACHBTH AURC 9002 trial. J Clin Oncol 2006;24(31):4976–82.

19. Mitry E, Fields AL, Bleiberg H, et al. Adjuvant chemotherapy after potentially curative resection of metastases from colorectal cancer: a pooled analysis of two randomized trials. J Clin Oncol 2008;26(30):4906–11.

20. Kemeny MM, Adak S, Gray B, et al. Combined-modality treatment for resectable metastatic colorectal carcinoma to the liver: surgical resection of hepatic metastases in combination with continuous infusion of chemotherapy–an intergroup study. J Clin Oncol 2002;20(6):1499–505.

21. Kemeny N, Huang Y, Cohen AM, et al. Hepatic arterial infusion of chemotherapy after resection of hepatic metastases from colorectal cancer. N Engl J Med 1999;341(27):2039–48.

22. Nordlinger B, Sorbye H, Glimelius B, et al. Perioperative chemotherapy with FOLFOX4 and surgery versus surgery alone for resectable liver metastases from colorectal cancer (EORTC Intergroup trial 40983): a randomised controlled trial. Lancet 2008;371(9617):1007–16.

23. Karapetis CS, Khambata-Ford S, Jonker DJ, et al. K-ras mutations and benefit from cetuximab in advanced colorectal cancer. N Engl J Med 2008;359(17):1757–65.

24. Koopman M, Antonini NF, Douma J, et al. Sequential versus combination chemotherapy with capecitabine, irinotecan, and oxaliplatin in advanced colorectal cancer (CAIRO): a phase III randomised controlled trial. Lancet 2007;370(9582):135–42.

25. Seymour MT, Maughan TS, Ledermann JA, et al. Different strategies of sequential and combination chemotherapy for patients with poor prognosis advanced colorectal cancer (MRC FOCUS): a randomised controlled trial. Lancet 2007;370(9582):143–52.

26. Sanoff HK, Sargent DJ, Campbell ME, et al. Five-year data and prognostic factor analysis of oxaliplatin and irinotecan combinations for advanced colorectal cancer: N9741. J Clin Oncol 2008;26(35):5721–7.
27. Hurwitz H, Fehrenbacher L, Novotny W, et al. Bevacizumab plus irinotecan, fluorouracil, and leucovorin for metastatic colorectal cancer. N Engl J Med 2004; 350(23):2335–42.
28. Saltz LB, Clarke S, Diaz-Rubio E, et al. Bevacizumab in combination with oxaliplatin-based chemotherapy as first-line therapy in metastatic colorectal cancer: a randomized phase III study. J Clin Oncol 2008;26(12):2013–9.
29. Hochster HS, Hart LL, Ramanathan RK, et al. Safety and efficacy of oxaliplatin and fluoropyrimidine regimens with or without bevacizumab as first-line treatment of metastatic colorectal cancer: results of the TREE Study. J Clin Oncol 2008; 26(21):3523–9.
30. Jonker DJ, O'Callaghan CJ, Karapetis CS, et al. Cetuximab for the treatment of colorectal cancer. N Engl J Med 2007;357(20):2040–8.
31. Kerr DJ, McArdle CS, Ledermann J, et al. Intrahepatic arterial versus intravenous fluorouracil and folinic acid for colorectal cancer liver metastases: a multicentre randomised trial. Lancet 2003;361(9355):368–73.
32. Kemeny NE, Niedzwiecki D, Hollis DR, et al. Hepatic arterial infusion versus systemic therapy for hepatic metastases from colorectal cancer: a randomized trial of efficacy, quality of life, and molecular markers (CALGB 9481). J Clin Oncol 2006;24(9):1395–403.

Randomized Clinical Trials in Colon Cancer

Heather B. Neuman, MD, MS*, Jason Park, MD, MEd,
Martin R. Weiser, MD

KEYWORDS

- Colon cancer • Surgery • Adjuvant
- Randomized controlled trial

Significant advances have been made in the treatment of colon cancer in recent years. Surgery remains the mainstay of treatment and surgical resection alone results in 5-year survival in more than 60% of patients.[1] However, the use of fluorouracil (5-FU)-based adjuvant chemotherapy for patients at high risk of recurrence further prolongs disease-free survival (DFS) and has become the standard of care. New areas of research focus on decreasing the surgical trauma with minimally invasive approaches, improving the surgical staging of patients with colon cancer, and improving adjuvant treatment regimens. In this article, we review those randomized controlled trials (RCTs) that have most impacted the clinical management of patients with colon cancer in 2009 (**Table 1**).

SURGERY

Surgical resection is the mainstay of treatment for colon cancer. At the time of the last chapter[7], only four level Ia randomized controlled surgical trials had been published in the literature.[8–11] These trials provide some of the rationale supporting current surgical decision making in colon cancer. Early vascular ligation with a no-touch isolation technique has long been advocated as a means of improving outcomes. Although the only RCT to address this question failed to demonstrate a statistically significant difference with the technique when compared with standard practices, a trend toward improved DFS with the no-touch technique was observed.[8] The no-touch isolation technique was used in another RCT evaluating the extent of dissection necessary for patients presenting with descending colon cancer.[9] In this trial with a minimum of 5-year follow-up, survival after segmental colectomy and more radical left hemicolectomy with routine inferior mesenteric artery ligation was equivalent, indicating high ligation

Disclosure: See last page of article.
Department of Surgery, Memorial Sloan-Kettering Cancer Center, 1275 York Avenue, H1206, New York, NY 10065, USA
* Corresponding author.
E-mail address: neuman@surgery.wisc.edu (H.B. Neuman).

Surg Oncol Clin N Am 19 (2010) 183–204
doi:10.1016/j.soc.2009.09.010
1055-3207/09/$ – see front matter © 2010 Elsevier Inc. All rights reserved.

Table 1
Key randomized controlled trials establishing role of adjuvant therapy in stage III and high-risk stage II colon cancer

Author	Year of Study	Experimental Arms	Trial Outcome	Contribution to Patient Care
Windle et al[2]	1987	5-FU vs 5-FU + lev vs observation	Improved DSS (52% vs 32%) with 5-FU + lev	Suggested an additive effect of levamisole when used in combination with 5-FU
Moertel et al[3]	1995	5-FU + lev vs lev alone vs observation	33% reduction in death rate with 5-FU + lev	Established benefit of adjuvant therapy in stage III colon cancer
Wolmark et al[4] (NSABP C-03)	1993	5-FU + LV vs MOF	32% reduction in mortality and 30% improvement in DFS with 5-FU + LV	Contributed to establishment of 5-FU based adjuvant therapy as preferred regimen
O'Connell et al[1]	1997	5-FU + LV vs observation	Improved OS (74% vs 63%) with 5-FU + LV	Established that 6 months of adjuvant therapy improves outcomes and defined a standard of care
O'Connell et al[5]	1998	5-FU + lev vs 5-FU + LV + lev, 6 vs 12 months	Improved OS (70% vs 60%) with 6 months of 5-FU + LV + lev	Established the added benefit associated with LV; confirmed survival benefit seen with 6 months of therapy
Wolmark et al[6] (NSABP C-04)	1999	5-FU + LV vs 5-FU + lev vs 5-FU + LV + lev	Improved DFS (65% vs 60%) favoring regimens with 5-FU + LV, no added benefit with lev	Established 5-FU + LV as the preferred adjuvant regimen

Abbreviations: DFS, disease-free survival; DSS, disease-specific survival; 5-FU, 5-fluorouracil; lev, levamisole; LV, leucovorin; MOF, lomustine, vincristine, and 5-FU; OS, overall survival.

of the inferior mesenteric artery is not necessary. In the third trial highlighted in the last review,[7] the question of hand-sewn versus stapled anastomosis for colon cancer was addressed.[10] This RCT demonstrated that hand-sewn anastomosis was associated with an increased rate of radiologically detected leak. No conclusions could be drawn with regard to likelihood of local recurrence with either anastomotic technique. The final RCT evaluated the necessity of nasogastric tube usage after colon resection[11] and concluded that the routine use of nasogastric tube drainage was unnecessary.

Four RCTs were highlighted in the last review[7] that addressed the optimal postoperative surveillance schedule for patients with completely resected colon cancer.[12–15] These trials evaluated intensive versus less intensive surveillance strategies and attempted to identify a benefit with early detection and intervention for either local or distant recurrence. Although no survival difference was observed in any of the studies, all were underpowered and therefore no definitive conclusions could be made. No new data have been published and current postoperative surveillance schedules are based on expert opinion. A large, multicenter RCT is currently ongoing which, if accrual goals are met, will be adequately powered to answer this question.[16]

More than 24 RCTs addressing the surgical care of patients with colon cancer have been published; this includes five level Ia RCTs. Most of these address the role of laparoscopy in the treatment of colon cancer.[17–21] Although it quickly became clear within the surgical community that laparoscopic colon resections were technically feasible, the oncologic merits of laparoscopy were less certain. The adequacy of lymph node staging with a laparoscopic approach, the effect of abdominal insufflation on tumor dissemination, and risk of trochar site implants were unknown. To address these concerns, a number of RCTs have been conducted comparing laparoscopic and open colon resections. The first large, single-institution RCT to report results for laparoscopy-assisted colectomy in patients with colon cancer was initially reported in 2002.[17] In this trial, short-term outcomes such as return of bowel function and length of stay were improved in the laparoscopy cohort and cancer-related survival was also higher. This trial suggested that oncologic outcomes associated with laparoscopic surgery are at least equivalent, if not better, to those observed with open procedures.

Since this initial report, several other multi-institutional RCTs have reported both short- and long-term outcomes. On pathologic review, lymph node retrieval with laparoscopy was adequate, with 10 to 12 nodes per specimen harvested,[18–20] and adequate margins were also achievable.[18,20] Only the United Kingdom Medical Research Council Conventional versus Laparoscopic-Assisted Surgery in Colorectal Cancer (CLASICC) trial, which included patients with rectal cancer, noted a slightly increased rate of positive circumferential margins in the laparoscopic cohort, although this did not reach the level of statistical significance.[22] This did not correlate to an increase in tumor recurrence with longer follow-up, however, and may have minimal clinical significance.[19]

Long-term oncologic outcomes evaluated in trials of laparoscopic colectomy have varied, but include DFS, cancer-related survival, and time to recurrence. Most, because of power-size calculations, have been designed as noninferiority trials. No other trial[19,20,23] has reproduced the survival benefit with minimally invasive colectomy initially reported by Lacy and colleagues.[17] Additionally, the survival benefit observed by Lacy and colleagues[24] was not maintained with longer follow-up. All RCTs reported to date with long-term follow-up have found laparoscopic and open resections to be equivalent with regard to survival and recurrence.

Minimally invasive surgery is associated with short-term benefits. Blood loss is less after laparoscopic resection.[17–19,21,25] Additionally, patients tend to require fewer narcotics and return to bowel function is quicker; this correlates to a 1- to 2-day shorter length of stay.[17–19,21,25] Despite these observations, very little difference in quality of life (QOL) has been observed between the two procedures. Three trials have used validated questionnaires to assess QOL.[19,26,27] Short-term QOL after laparoscopy was slightly improved in two of the studies,[26,27] with one study demonstrating a slight difference in global QOL[26] and the other a benefit in social and role functioning 2 weeks following surgery.[27] These findings were not observed with longer follow-up (2- and 3-month). The third study evaluated both short-term and long-term (3-year) QOL with no differences seen.[19] It is noteworthy that in one of these RCTs,[27] patients with body mass index (BMI) higher than 30 were excluded. As obese patients may be those most likely to have short-term QOL benefits from laparoscopic resection, exclusion of these patients from the trial may have diluted any potential QOL benefit. Alternatively, the failure to demonstrate a QOL benefit with laparoscopy may relate to the inherent difficulty in measuring postoperative QOL and limited responsiveness of the utilized instruments to important postoperative factors. Some drawbacks to laparoscopic resection exist, as the procedure is associated with longer operative times.[17–19,21,25]

In summary, five large, multicenter trials have demonstrated the equivalency of laparoscopic and open colectomy in patients with colon cancer.[17–21] Laparoscopic colectomy in the setting of colon cancer should currently be considered an acceptable and equivalent alternative to an open resection in the hands of experienced surgeons. However, little is known about the learning curve surrounding laparoscopic colectomy or how this technique (and the outcomes observed in the setting of a RCT setting) will translate into community practice.

Sentinel lymph node (SLN) biopsy has dramatically changed nodal staging for melanoma and breast cancer by allowing the identification of the first lymph node to receive lymphatic drainage, and potential metastases, from a tumor. The SLN concept has been applied to colon cancer in an attempt to enhance pathologic identification of nodal metastases. One RCT has compared the likelihood of pathologic upstaging when standard versus enhanced pathologic evaluation through SLN mapping was performed.[28] In this trial, the false negative rate of SLN biopsy was 9.8% and enhanced pathologic evaluation upstaged 10.7% of patients; most of these patients had micrometastases. Although the clinical significance of micrometastases is currently unknown, this may represent a cohort of patients who would previously have been classified as stage II but may be at increased risk of recurrence. Unfortunately, the low false negative rate observed in this study has not been consistently reported in the literature; in four other prospective, nonrandomized multicenter trials, the false negative rate of SLN in colon cancer ranged from 7% to 54%.[29–32] Therefore, further study is required to confirm both the validity of the SLN concept in colon cancer as well as the clinical relevance of micrometastases identified through this technique.

ADJUVANT THERAPY

It is widely accepted that adjuvant chemotherapy is associated with improved survival in patients with stage III and possibly high-risk stage II colon cancer (see **Table 1**). The efficacy of adjuvant therapy, specifically 5-FU–based regimens, was first established in a multicenter, cooperative group trial evaluating 5-FU plus levamisole versus levamisole alone versus observation alone.[2] A series of RCTs followed, which have further defined the role of 5-FU modulators such as leucovorin (LV) or levamisole, as well as the optimal duration of therapy.[1,3–5] In NSABP C-04, the efficacy of 5-FU + LV versus 5-FU + levamisole versus 5-FU + LV + levamisole was evaluated.[6] The outcome of this trial established 6 months of 5-FU + LV as the preferred adjuvant regimen for patients with stage III or high-risk stage II disease.

Although the benefit of adjuvant therapy for patients with stage III disease is well accepted, the role of chemotherapy for patients with completely resected stage II disease is controversial. At the time of the last review, one RCT addressing the role of adjuvant therapy in patients with stage II colon cancer had been reported but was underpowered to detect small survival differences.[33] Three meta-analyses addressing the question were subsequently reported with conflicting findings. The first, a review of four National Surgical Adjuvant Breast and Bowl Project (NSABP) adjuvant studies, concluded that a survival advantage existed for stage II disease that was similar in scope to that for stage III disease.[34] In contrast, the International Multicentre Pooled Analysis of B2 Colon Cancer Trials (IMPACT B2) study failed to identify a benefit in survival or recurrence.[35] A final meta-analysis, which included only studies comparing 5-FU + LV or levamisole to observation alone, suggested a benefit in stage II disease, although smaller in magnitude than that seen in patients with stage III disease.[36]

Two RCTs have recently been reported that were specifically designed to address the question of adjuvant therapy for stage II colon cancer. One, unfortunately, was closed early because of difficulty in accrual and, like the prior RCT, was inadequately powered.[37] The second trial, however, is a multicenter trial that accrued more than 3000 patients who, in the opinion of each patient's clinician, did not have a clear indication for chemotherapy. These patients consisted primarily of patients with stage II disease.[38] The trial was powered to have an 80% chance of detecting a 5% improvement in survival. A small but statistically significant advantage to the use of adjuvant chemotherapy for stage II disease was observed. Unfortunately, central pathologic review was not a part of the study design and further exploratory analyses to identify characteristics of patients who may benefit most from adjuvant therapy are unable to be performed. Adjuvant treatment for patients with stage II colon cancer remains controversial.

Two new chemotherapeutic agents, both with efficacy in the metastatic setting, have been explored as adjuvant treatments in colon cancer. The first, irinotecan, was evaluated in a number of RCTs as an addition to 5-FU and LV. Disappointingly, in a multicenter trial coordinated through the Cancer and Leukemia Group B (CALGB), no survival benefit was associated with the addition of irinotecan to the adjuvant treatment of patients with stage III disease.[39] These findings have been preliminarily confirmed in two other large, multicenter trials that have been presented only in abstract form; we await the final results of these trials.[40,41]

The second agent considered as an addition to regimens of 5-FU and LV was oxaliplatin. Two large RCTs have been performed evaluating these regimens and long-term results reported.[42,43] In both trials, 3-year DFS with the addition of oxaliplatin is improved by an estimated 5%. This benefit was observed in both stage II and III colon cancer, but the magnitude of the benefit was most significant in patients with stage III disease. As a result of these trials, oxaliplatin has been established as the new standard of care in the adjuvant treatment of patients with surgically resected stage III colon cancer.

In addition to exploring agents to add in combination with intravenous fluorouracil regimens, several RCTs have explored oral fluorouracil analogues as a means of simplifying chemotherapy administration for patients and minimizing toxicity. Capecitabine is currently the only oral agent approved by the Food and Drug Administration (FDA) for the adjuvant treatment of colon cancer and has been demonstrated to be an effective alternative to intravenous regimens.[44] Similar findings were found with oral uracil and tegafur used in combination with LV[45]; this regimen, however, is not currently approved in the United States.

RCTs have been conducted evaluating the role of regional adjuvant systemic therapy as an addition to systemic therapy. Regional administrations have included both intraperitoneal and intraportal infusions.[46–48] Consistently, these trials have all failed to demonstrate a benefit in survival or local recurrence with the use of regional therapies, although most were underpowered to detect small survival differences.[46,47]

The prospective RCTs that are highlighted in the text that follows do not represent all of the trials that have contributed to our current knowledge of the optimal care of the patient with colon cancer. Rather, we have highlighted those trials that have served to define the standard of care in 2009. Only trials that have been published in a peer-reviewed format are considered.

SURGICAL TRIALS

(1) Laparoscopy-assisted colectomy versus open colectomy for treatment of non-metastatic colon cancer: a randomized trial. Lacy AM, Garcia-Valdecasa JC, Delgado S, et al. Lancet 2002;359:2224.[17]

Hypothesis: Cancer-related survival is equivalent between laparoscopy-assisted colectomy (LAC) and open colectomy.

No. Patients Randomized	Study Groups	Stratification	Significance Demonstrated	% Change Identified in Trial
219	Open colectomy = 108 LAC = 111	Site of primary	Yes Cancer-related survival	HR 0.38 (CI 0.16–0.91) favoring LAC; 84% vs 73%

Abbreviations: CI, confidence interval; HR, hazard ratio; LAC, laparoscopy-assisted colectomy.

Published Abstract: BACKGROUND: Although early reports on laparoscopy-assisted colectomy (LAC) in patients with colon cancer suggested that it reduces perioperative morbidity, its influence on long-term results is unknown. Our study aimed to compare efficacy of LAC and open colectomy (OC) for treatment of nonmetastatic colon cancer in terms of tumour recurrence and survival. METHODS: From November 1993 to July 1998 all patients with adenocarcinoma of the colon were assessed for entry in this randomized trial. Adjuvant therapy and postoperative follow-up were the same in both groups. The main end point was cancer-related survival. Data were analyzed according to the intention-to-treat principle. FINDINGS: A total 219 patients took part in the study (111 LAC group, 108 OC group). Patients in the LAC group recovered faster than those in the OC group, with shorter peristalsis-detection ($P = .001$) and oral-intake times ($P = .001$), and shorter hospital stays ($P = .005$). Morbidity was lower in the LAC group ($P = .001$), although LAC did not influence perioperative mortality. Probability of cancer-related survival was higher in the LAC group ($P = .02$). The Cox model showed that LAC was independently associated with reduced risk of tumor relapse (hazard ratio 0.39, 95% CI 0.19–0.82), death from any cause (0.48, 0.23–1.01), and death from a cancer-related cause (0.38, 0.16–0.91) compared with OC. This superiority of LAC was due to differences in patients with stage III tumors ($P = .04$, $P = .02$, and $P = .006$, respectively). INTERPRETATION: LAC is more effective than OC for treatment of colon cancer in terms of morbidity, hospital stay, tumor recurrence, and cancer-related survival. (Copyright Elsevier 2002. Reprinted with permission.)

Editor's Summary and Comments: This single-institution RCT was the first to report long-term outcomes of LAC versus open colectomy. LAC was associated with quicker return of bowel function, shorter hospital stay, and less morbidity. In the initial report, cancer-related survival was significantly higher in the laparoscopy-assisted group.[17] With longer follow-up (median 95 months), a trend toward improved overall survival (OS), cancer-related survival, and tumor recurrence was observed but was no longer statistically significant.[24] These findings have not been replicated in other, larger trials.

(2) A comparison of laparoscopically assisted and open colectomy for colon cancer. The Clinical Outcomes of Surgical Therapy Study Group. N Engl J Med 2004;350:2050.[18]

Hypothesis: Time to recurrence is equivalent between LAC and open colectomy (noninferiority trial).

No. Patients Randomized	Study Groups	Stratification	Significance Demonstrated	% Change Identified in Trial
872	Open colectomy = 437	Site of primary	No	HR 0.86(CI 0.63–
		ASA class	Time to	1.17)
	LAC = 435	Surgeon	recurrence	

Abbreviations: ASA, American Society of Anesthesiologists'; CI, confidence interval; HR, hazard ratio; LAC, laparoscopy-assisted colectomy.

Published Abstract: BACKGROUND: Minimally invasive, laparoscopically assisted surgery was first considered in 1990 for patients undergoing colectomy for cancer. Concern that this approach would compromise survival by failing to achieve a proper oncologic resection or adequate staging or by altering patterns of recurrence (based on frequent reports of tumor recurrences within surgical wounds) prompted a controlled trial evaluation. METHODS: We conducted a noninferiority trial at 48 institutions and randomly assigned 872 patients with adenocarcinoma of the colon to undergo open or laparoscopically assisted colectomy performed by credentialed surgeons. The median follow-up was 4.4 years. The primary end point was the time to tumor recurrence. RESULTS: At 3 years, the rates of recurrence were similar in the two groups—16% among patients in the group that underwent laparoscopically assisted surgery and 18% among patients in the open-colectomy group (two-sided $P = .32$; hazard ratio for recurrence, 0.86; 95% confidence interval, 0.63 to 1.17). Recurrence rates in surgical wounds were less than 1% in both groups ($P = .50$). The overall survival rate at 3 years was also very similar in the two groups (86% in the laparoscopic-surgery group and 85% in the open-colectomy group; $P = .51$; hazard ratio for death in the laparoscopic-surgery group, 0.91; 95% confidence interval, 0.68 to 1.21), with no significant difference between groups in the time to recurrence or overall survival for patients with any stage of cancer. Perioperative recovery was faster in the laparoscopic-surgery group than in the open-colectomy group, as reflected by a shorter median hospital stay (5 days versus 6 days, $P < .001$) and briefer use of parenteral narcotics (3 days versus 4 days, $P < .001$) and oral analgesics (1 day versus 2 days, $P = .02$). The rates of intraoperative complications, 30-day postoperative mortality, complications at discharge and 60 days, hospital readmission, and reoperation were very similar between groups. CONCLUSIONS: In this multi-institutional study, the rates of recurrent cancer were similar after laparoscopically assisted colectomy and open colectomy, suggesting that the laparoscopic approach is an acceptable alternative to open surgery for colon cancer. (Copyright [2004] Massachusetts Medical Society. All rights reserved. Reprinted with permission.)

Editor's Summary and Comments: The COST trial was the first reported multi-institution RCT of LAC versus open colectomy.[18] Surgeon participation required credentialing and surgical quality control was performed throughout the study period by an external monitoring committee. Time to tumor recurrence was the primary outcome, but survival, complications, and QOL end points were also considered. This was a well-conducted trial, with the major criticism being that they failed to reach accrual goals. However, statistical power was sufficient to report LAC as noninferior to open colectomy. These findings persist with the more recently reported 5-year data (OS 74.6% versus 76.4%).[23] Short-term and QOL benefits associated with laparoscopy were modest.[18,26] Although time to bowel function and length of stay were improved with laparoscopy, a difference in QOL between the two groups was not detectable using currently available standardized instruments. Those patients who required conversion from laparoscopic to open procedures (21%) reported the lowest QOL.

(3) Randomized trial of laparoscopic-assisted resection of colorectal carcinoma: 3-year results of the UK MRC CLASICC Trial Group. Jayne DG, Guillou PJ, Thorpe H, Quirek P, et al. J Clin Oncol 2007;25:3071.[19]

Hypothesis: A difference exists between the two procedures with regard to primary end points of 3-year OS, DFS, and local recurrence (LR).

No. Patients Randomized	Study Groups	Stratification	Significance Demonstrated	% Change Identified in Trial
794	Open colectomy = 268 LAC = 526	Site of primary Surgeon Liver metastases Preoperative XRT	No OS, DFS, local recurrence	Difference in: OS-1.8% DFS −1.4%, LR −0.8%.

Abbreviations: DFS, disease-free survival; LAC, laparoscopy-assisted colectomy; OS, overall survival; XRT, radiation.

Published Abstract: PURPOSE: The aim of the current study is to report the long-term outcomes after laparoscopic-assisted surgery compared with conventional open surgery within the context of the UK MRC CLASICC trial. Results from randomized trials have indicated that laparoscopic surgery for colon cancer is as effective as open surgery in the short term. Few data are available on rectal cancer, and long-term data on survival and recurrence are now required. METHODS: The United Kingdom Medical Research Council Conventional versus Laparoscopic-Assisted Surgery in Colorectal Cancer (UK MRC CLASICC; clinical trials number ISRCTN 74883561) trial study comparing conventional versus laparoscopic-assisted surgery in patients with cancer of the colon and rectum. The randomization ratio was 2:1 in favor of laparoscopic surgery. Long-term outcomes (3-year overall survival [OS], disease-free survival [DFS], local recurrence, and quality of life [QoL]) have now been determined on an intention-to-treat basis.

RESULTS: Seven hundred ninety-four patients were recruited (526 laparoscopic and 268 open). Overall, there were no differences in the long-term outcomes. The differences in survival rates were OS of 1.8% (95% CI, −5.2% to 8.8%; P = .55), DFS of −1.4% (95% CI, −9.5% to 6.7%; P = .70), local recurrence of −0.8% (95% CI, −5.7% to 4.2%; P = .76), and QoL (P > .01 for all scales). Higher positivity of the circumferential resection margin was reported after laparoscopic anterior resection (AR), but it did not translate into an increased incidence of local recurrence. CONCLUSION: Successful laparoscopic-assisted surgery for colon cancer is as effective as open surgery in terms of oncological outcomes and preservation of QoL. Long-term outcomes for patients with rectal cancer were similar in those undergoing abdominoperineal resection and AR, and support the continued use of laparoscopic surgery in these patients. (Copyright 2007 American Society of Clinical Oncology. Reprinted with permission.)

Editor's Summary and Comments: The CLASICC trial is the first, multicenter trial to include rectal cancer patients in the cohort.[19] The planned sample size of 1000 patients did not provide enough power to evaluate equivalency between the two procedures; therefore, the absolute difference for each short- and long-term trial end point was instead evaluated. Pathology was reviewed centrally and the trial required a minimum of 20 laparoscopic resections before surgeon participation. In short-term follow-up, no differences in any study end points were observed. However, there was a nonsignificant trend toward increased rate of positive circumferential margin for patients undergoing laparoscopic anterior resection[22]; this did not translate into an increased rate of LR when 3-year outcomes were reported. A trend toward poorer male sexual functioning after laparoscopic rectal surgery was also observed.[49] There were no differences in 3-year OS (67.8%) or DFS (66.8%).[19] Overall, this trial confirms the equivalency of laparoscopy and open procedures for colon cancer and is the first to evaluate the use of laparoscopic resection in patients with rectal cancer. It does suggest that further study on nononcologic outcomes such as sexual and bladder function after laparoscopic rectal surgery is warranted.

(4) Survival after laparoscopic surgery versus open surgery for colon cancer: long-term outcomes of a randomized clinical trial. The Colon Cancer Laparoscopic or Open Resection Study Group, Buunen M, Veldkamp R, Hop WC, et al. Lancet Oncol 2009;10:44.[20]

Hypothesis: Three-year DFS is equivalent between LAC and open colectomy (noninferiority trial).

No. Patients Randomized	Study Groups	Stratification	Significance Demonstrated	% Change Identified in Trial
1248	Open colectomy = 621 LAC = 627	Participating center Site of primary	No DFS	HR 0.92 (CI 0.74–1.15)

Abbreviations: CI, confidence interval; DFS, disease-free survival; HR, hazard ratio; LAC, laparoscopy-assisted colectomy.

Published Abstract: BACKGROUND: Laparoscopic surgery for colon cancer has been proven safe, but debate continues over whether the available long-term survival data justify implementation of laparoscopic techniques in surgery for colon cancer. The aim of the COlon cancer Laparoscopic or Open Resection (COLOR) trial was to compare 3-year disease-free survival and overall survival after laparoscopic and open resection of solitary colon cancer. METHODS: Between March 7, 1997, and March 6, 2003, patients recruited from 29 European hospitals with a solitary cancer of the right or left colon and a body mass index up to 30 kg/m² were randomly assigned to either laparoscopic or open surgery as curative treatment in this noninferiority randomized trial. Disease-free survival at 3 years after surgery was the primary outcome, with a pre-specified noninferiority boundary at 7% difference between groups. Secondary outcomes were short-term morbidity and mortality, number of positive resection margins, local recurrence, port-site or wound-site recurrence, and blood loss during surgery. Neither patients nor health care providers were blinded to patient groupings. Analysis was by intention to treat. This trial is registered with ClinicalTrials.gov, number NCT00387842. FINDINGS: During the recruitment period, 1248 patients were randomly assigned to either open surgery (n = 621) or laparoscopic surgery (n = 627); 172 were excluded after randomisation, mainly because of the presence of distant metastases or benign disease, leaving 1076 patients eligible for analysis (542 assigned open surgery and 534 assigned laparoscopic surgery). Median follow-up was 53 months (range 0.03–60.00). Positive resection margins, number of lymph nodes removed, and morbidity and mortality were similar in both groups. The combined 3-year disease-free survival for all stages was 74.2% (95% CI 70.4 – 78.0) in the laparoscopic group and 76.2% (72.6–79.8) in the open-surgery group (P = .70 by log-rank test); the difference in disease-free survival after 3 years was 2.0% (95% CI−3.2 to 7.2). The hazard ratio (HR) for disease-free survival (open versus laparoscopic surgery) was 0.92 (95% CI 0.74–1.15). The combined 3-year overall survival for all stages was 81.8% (78.4 – 85.1) in the laparoscopic group and 84.2% (81.1 – 87.3) in the open-surgery group (P = .45 by log-rank test); the difference in overall survival after 3 years was 2.4% (95% CI −2.1 to 7.0; HR 0.95 [0.74–1.22]). INTERPRETATION: Our trial could not rule out a difference in disease-free survival at 3 years in favor of open colectomy because the upper limit of the 95% CI for the difference just exceeded the predetermined noninferiority boundary of 7%. However, the difference in disease-free survival between groups was small and, we believe, clinically acceptable, justifying the implementation of laparoscopic surgery into daily practice. Further studies should address whether laparoscopic surgery is superior to open surgery in this setting. (Copyright Elsevier 2009. Reprinted with permission.)

Editor's Summary and Comments: This trial failed to meet its primary end point of demonstrating noninferiority between LAC and open colectomy, as the P value for the noninferiority test exceeded the predetermined significance level of .025 (P = .030). However, the 3-year DFS after LAC or open colectomy was comparable (74.2% versus 76.2%) and the authors therefore concluded that the actual survival difference between the groups was small enough as to not be clinically significant. The reported conversion rate in this study was 17% and was higher in patients with T4 cancers. Of note, this study excluded patients with a body mass index greater than 30 kg/m².

(5) Prospective randomized study comparing sentinel lymph node evaluation with standard pathologic evaluation for the staging of colon carcinoma: results from the United States Military Cancer Institute Clinical Trials Group Study GI-01. Stojadinovic A, Nissan A, Protic M, et al. Ann Surg 2007;245:846.[28]

Hypothesis: A 25% difference in the rate of nodal metastasis will exist between conventional histopathologic staging and SLN ultrastaging.

No. Patients Randomized	Study Groups	Stratification	Significance Demonstrated	% Change -dentified in Trial
175	Conventional histopathology = 82 SLN/ ultrastaging = 93	Stage (I/II vs III) Extent of resection	Yes Rate of positive node	Control 38.7% vs SLN 57.3%

Abbreviation: SLN, sentinel lymph node.

Published Abstract: BACKGROUND: The principal role of sentinel lymph node (SLN) sampling and ultrastaging in colon cancer is enhanced staging accuracy. The utility of this technique for patients with colon cancer remains controversial. PURPOSE: This multicenter randomized trial was conducted to determine if focused assessment of the SLN with step sectioning and immunohistochemistry (IHC) enhances the ability to stage the regional nodal basin over conventional histopathology in patients with resectable colon cancer. PATIENTS AND METHODS: Between August 2002 and April 2006 we randomly assigned 161 patients with stage I-III colon cancer to standard histopathologic evaluation or SLN mapping (ex vivo, subserosal, peritumoral, 1% isosulfan blue dye) and ultrastaging with pan-cytokeratin IHC in conjunction with standard histopathology. SLN-positive disease was defined as individual tumor cells or cell aggregates identified by hematoxylin and eosin (H&E) and/or IHC. Primary end point was the rate of nodal upstaging. RESULTS: Significant nodal upstaging was identified with SLN ultrastaging (control versus SLN: 38.7% versus 57.3%, $P = .019$). When SLNs with cell aggregates of 0.2 mm or less in size were excluded, no statistically significant difference in node-positive rate was apparent between the control and SLN arms (38.7% versus 39.0%, $P = .97$). However, a 10.7% (6/56) nodal upstaging was identified by evaluation of H&E-stained step sections of SLNs among study arm patients who would have otherwise been staged node-negative (N0) by conventional pathologic assessment alone. CONCLUSION: SLN mapping, step sectioning, and IHC identifies small volume nodal disease and improves staging in patients with resectable colon cancer. A prospective trial is ongoing to determine the clinical significance of colon cancer micrometastasis in SLNs. (Copyright 2007 Lippincott Williams & Wilkins. Reprinted with permission.)

Editor's Summary and Comments: This RCT evaluates the added benefit of SLN mapping when compared with standard pathologic evaluation of the colonic mesenteric nodes. This is a well-designed study with quality control for SLN mapping and harvest and central pathologic review. The false negative rate was 9.8%. The addition of an SLN upstaged six patients (10.7%) from node negative to positive, primarily through the identification of micrometastases (≤ 0.2 mm). All adjuvant treatment decisions in this trial were determined based only on standard pathologic evaluation, as the clinical significance of micrometastases in colon cancer is unknown.

It is noteworthy that the success of SLN mapping in other, prospective multicenter trials has been variable.[29-32] In one study, coordinated by the CALGB, 72 patients with stage I-III colon cancer underwent SLN mapping.[32] SLN localization was successful in 92%, yielding an average of 2.1 sentinel nodes per patient. However, in only two patients (3%) was the SLN the only positive node identified using standard pathologic techniques. Additionally, the false negative rate was 54% (13/24). The results of this study and others, where false negative rates have varied from as low as 7% to as high as 54%,[29-32] suggests that the application of the SLN technique to colon cancer requires more study.

(6) Oxaliplatin, fluorouracil, and leucovorin as adjuvant treatment for colon cancer. Andre T, Boni C, Mounedji-Boudiaf L, et al. N Engl J Med 2004; 350:2343.[42]

Hypothesis: The addition of oxaliplatin to fluorouracil and leucovorin will improve DFS.

No. Patients Randomized	Study Groups	Stratification	Significance Demonstrated	% Change Identified in Trial
2246	5-FU/LV/ OX = 1123 FU + LV = 1123	TNM stage Obstruction/ perforation Medical center	Yes DFS	78.2% vs 72.9% DFS at 3-years

Abbreviations: DFS, disease-free survival; 5-FU, 5-fluorouracil; LV, leucovorin; OX, oxaliplatin.

Published Abstract: BACKGROUND: The standard adjuvant treatment of colon cancer is fluorouracil plus leucovorin (FL). Oxaliplatin improves the efficacy of this combination in patients with metastatic colorectal cancer. We evaluated the efficacy of treatment with FL plus oxaliplatin in the postoperative adjuvant setting. METHODS: We randomly assigned 2246 patients who had undergone curative resection for stage II or III colon cancer to receive FL alone or with oxaliplatin for 6 months. The primary end point was disease-free survival. RESULTS: A total of 1123 patients were randomly assigned to each group. After a median follow-up of 37.9 months, 237 patients in the group given FL plus oxaliplatin had had a cancer-related event, as compared with 293 patients in the FL group (21.1% versus 26.1%; hazard ratio for recurrence, 0.77; $P = .002$). The rate of disease-free survival at 3 years was 78.2% (95% confidence interval, 75.6 to 80.7) in the group given FL plus oxaliplatin and 72.9% (95% confidence interval, 70.2 to 75.7) in the FL group ($P = .002$ by the stratified log-rank test). In the group given FL plus oxaliplatin, the incidence of febrile neutropenia was 1.8%, the incidence of gastrointestinal adverse effects was low, and the incidence of grade 3 sensory neuropathy was 12.4% during treatment, decreasing to 1.1% at 1 year of follow-up. Six patients in each group died during treatment (death rate, 0.5%). CONCLUSIONS: Adding oxaliplatin to a regimen of fluorouracil and leucovorin improves the adjuvant treatment of colon cancer. (Copyright [2004] Massachusetts Medical Society. All rights reserved. Reprinted with permission.)

Editor's Summary and Comments: This well-conducted trial has solidified the place of oxaliplatin in combination with 5-FU and LV as the preferred adjuvant regimen for patients with stage III colorectal cancer. Both stage II and stage III patients experienced improved DFS at 3 years (78.2% versus 72.9%). However, the benefit was greater for patients with stage III (hazard ratio 0.76 [0.62–0.92], 72.2% versus 65.3%) versus stage II (hazard ratio 0.80 [0.56–1.15], 87% versus 84.3%) disease. No difference in OS was observed (87.7% versus 86.6%). In an update of this trial (abstract only),[50] the benefit in DFS was maintained. Additionally, at a median 6 years of follow-up, an improved OS was seen in patients with stage III disease who received oxaliplatin.

(7) Capecitabine as adjuvant treatment for stage III colon cancer. Twelves C, Wong A, Nowacki MP, et al. N Engl J Med 2005;352:2696.[44]

Hypothesis: DFS is equivalent between oral capecitabine and bolus 5-FU and LV (noninferiority trial).

No. Patients Randomized	Study Groups	Stratification	Significance Demonstrated	% Change Identified in Trial
1987	Bolus 5-FU/LV = 983 Oral capecitabine = 1004		No No difference in DFS	HR 0.87 (CI 0.75–1.0); 64.2% vs 60.6% DFS at 3-years

Abbreviations: CI, confidence interval; DFS, disease-free survival; 5-FU, 5-fluorouracil; HR, hazard ratio; LV, leucovorin; OX, oxaliplatin.

Published Abstract: BACKGROUND: Intravenous bolus fluorouracil plus leucovorin is the standard adjuvant treatment for colon cancer. The oral fluoropyrimidine capecitabine is an established alternative to bolus fluorouracil plus leucovorin as first-line treatment for metastatic colorectal cancer. We evaluated capecitabine in the adjuvant setting. METHODS: We randomly assigned a total of 1987 patients with resected stage III colon cancer to receive either oral capecitabine (1004 patients) or bolus fluorouracil plus leucovorin (Mayo Clinic regimen; 983 patients) over a period of 24 weeks. The primary efficacy end point was at least equivalence in disease-free survival; the primary safety end point was the incidence of grade 3 or 4 toxic effects due to fluoropyrimidines. RESULTS: Disease-free survival in the capecitabine group was at least equivalent to that in the fluorouracil-plus-leucovorin group (in the intention-to-treat analysis, $P < .001$ for the comparison of the upper limit of the hazard ratio with the noninferiority margin of 1.20). Capecitabine improved relapse-free survival (hazard ratio, 0.86; 95% confidence interval, 0.74 to 0.99; $P = .04$) and was associated with significantly fewer adverse events than fluorouracil plus leucovorin ($P < .001$). CONCLUSIONS: Oral capecitabine is an effective alternative to intravenous fluorouracil plus leucovorin in the adjuvant treatment of colon cancer. (Copyright [2005] Massachusetts Medical Society. All rights reserved.)

Editor's Summary and Comments: In this RCT, oral capecitabine was found to be noninferior to an intravenous bolus regimen of 5-FU and LV in patients with surgically resected stage III colon cancer. Importantly, grade 3 and 4 toxicities were significantly reduced with capecitabine. This supports the use of capecitabine as an alternative, and possibly preferable, adjuvant regimen. An RCT is currently ongoing to determine whether capecitabine can be used in place of intravenous 5-FU in combination with oxaliplatin.[51]

(8) Adjuvant regional chemotherapy and systemic chemotherapy versus systemic chemotherapy alone in patients with stage II-III colorectal cancer: a multicentre randomized controlled phase III trial. Nordlinger B, Rougier P, Arnaud JP, et al. Lancet Oncol 2005;6:459–68.[48]

Hypothesis: The addition of adjuvant regional chemotherapy to a systemic regimen is more effective in terms of OS than systemic therapy alone.

No. Patients Randomized	Study Groups	Stratification	Significance Demonstrated	% Change Identified in Trial
1857	5-FU–based systemic therapy = 753 5-FU–based systemic therapy + IP = 748		No OS	HR 0.97 (CI 0.81–1.15) 72.3% vs 72% OS at 5 years

Abbreviations: CI, confidence interval; 5-FU, 5-fluorouracil; HR, hazard ratio; IP, intraperitoneal or intraportal; OS, overall survival.

Published Abstract: BACKGROUND: Systemic adjuvant chemotherapy can improve overall survival and reduce the incidence of distant metastases for patients with advanced colon cancer. This study aimed to investigate whether regional chemotherapy (given by intraperitoneal or intraportal methods) combined with systemic chemotherapy was more effective than was systemic chemotherapy alone in terms of survival and recurrence for patients with stage II-III colorectal cancer. The study also compared systemic chemotherapy with fluorouracil and folinic acid with that of fluorouracil and levamisole. METHODS: During surgery, 753 patients with stage II-III colorectal cancer were randomly assigned to systemic chemotherapy alone (379 with fluorouracil and folinic acid, and 374 with fluorouracil and levamisole), and 748 to postoperative regional chemotherapy with fluorouracil followed by systemic chemotherapy with fluorouracil and folinic acid (n = 368) or with fluorouracil and levamisole (n = 380). Regional chemotherapy was given intraperitoneally (n = 415) or intraportally (n = 235) according to institution. The primary end point was 5-year overall survival. Secondary end points were 5-year disease-free survival and toxic effects. Analyses were by intention to treat. FINDINGS: Median follow-up was 6.8 years (range 0.0–10.1). Five-year overall survival was 72.3% (95% CI 69.0–75.6) for patients assigned regional and systemic chemotherapy, compared with 72.0% (68.7–75.3) for those assigned systemic chemotherapy alone (hazard ratio [HR] 0.97 [0.81–1.15], $P = .69$). Five-year overall survival for all patients assigned fluorouracil and levamisole was 72.0% (68.7–75.2) compared with 72.3% (69.0–75.6) for all those assigned fluorouracil and folinic acid (HR 0.98 [0.82–1.17], $P = .81$). The hazard ratios for 5-year disease-free survival were 0.94 (0.80 – 1.10) for regional versus nonregional treatment, and 0.92 (0.79–1.08) for all fluorouracil and levamisole versus fluorouracil and folinic acid. Grade 3 – 4 toxic effects were low in all groups. INTERPRETATION: Fluorouracil-based regional chemotherapy adds no further benefit to that obtained with systemic chemotherapy alone in patients with advanced colorectal cancer. (Copyright Elsevier 2005. Reprinted with permission.)

Editor's Summary and Comments: This is the only study of adjuvant regional therapy adequately powered to detect a survival benefit. Although regional chemotherapy was well tolerated, no survival or recurrence benefit was seen. There is currently no role for regional chemotherapy in the adjuvant treatment of patients with completely resected colon cancer.

(9) Oral uracil and tegafur plus leucovorin compared with intravenous fluorouracil and leucovorin in stage II and III carcinoma of the colon: results from National Surgical Adjuvant Breast and Bowel Project Protocol C-06. Lembersky BC, Wieand HS, Petrelli NJ, et al. J Clin Oncol 2006;24:2059–64.[45]

Hypothesis: Five-year OS with oral uracil/tegafur plus LV is equal to intravenous 5-FU and LV.

No. Patients Randomized	Study Groups	Stratification	Significance Demonstrated	% Change Identified in Trial
1608	Oral UFT + LV = 805 5-FU + LV = 803	# of positive nodes	No OS	HR 1.01(CI 0.83–1.25) 78.7 *vs.* 78.5% OS at 5-years

Abbreviations: CI, confidence interval; 5-FU, 5-fluorouracil; HR, hazard ratio; OS, overall survival; UFT, uracil and tegafur.

Published Abstract: PURPOSE: The primary aim of this study was to compare the relative efficacy of oral uracil and tegafur (UFT) plus leucovorin (LV) with the efficacy of weekly intravenous fluorouracil (FU) plus LV in prolonging disease-free survival (DFS) and overall survival (OS) after primary surgery for colon carcinoma. PATIENTS AND METHODS: Between February 1997 and March 1999, 1608 patients with stage II and III carcinoma of the colon were randomly assigned to receive either oral UFT + LV or intravenous FU + LV. RESULTS: Of the total patients, 47% had stage II colon cancer, and 53% had stage III colon cancer. Median follow-up time was 62.3 months. The estimated hazard ratio (HR) for OS of patients who received UFT + LV versus that of patients who received FU + LV was 1.014 (95% CI, 0.825 to 1.246). The estimated HR for DFS was 1.004 (95% CI, 0.847 to 1.190). Cox proportional hazards model analyses with regard to age (< 60 versus ≥ 60 years), stage, or number of involved nodes (none versus one to three versus $\geq$ four nodes) revealed no interaction with OS or DFS. Toxicity was similar in the two groups. In the UFT + LV arm, 38.2% of patients experienced any grade 3 or 4 toxic event compared with 37.8% of patients in the FU + LV arm. Primary quality-of-life end points did not differ between the two regimens, although convenience of care analysis favored UFT + LV. CONCLUSION: UFT + LV achieved similar DFS and OS when compared with an intravenous, weekly, bolus FU + LV regimen. The two regimens were equitoxic and generally well tolerated (Copyright 2006 American Society of Clinical Oncology. Reprinted with permission.)

Editor's Summary and Comments: Tegafur is an oral prodrug of fluorouracil that is administered in combination with high-dose uracil to minimize first-pass metabolism by the liver. In this trial, OS and DFS after an adjuvant regimen of oral UFT + LV was shown to be equivalent to an IV, weekly bolus regimen of 5-FU and LV. Additionally, although no differences in QOL between the two regimens were observed, more patients receiving UFT found the regimen to be "very convenient."[52] Although UFT is widely used across the world as an adjuvant regimen, it is not currently FDA approved for use in the United States.

(10) Adjuvant chemotherapy versus observation in patients with colorectal cancer: a randomized study. QUASAR Collaborative Group. Lancet 2007;370:2020–29.[38]

Hypothesis: Adjuvant chemotherapy will improve all-cause mortality in patients with colorectal cancer who do not have clear indications for chemotherapy.

No. Patients Randomized	Study Groups	Stratification	Significance Demonstrated	% Change Identified in Trial
3239	Observation = 1617 Chemotherapy = 1622	Age Tumor site Stage Portal vein infusion Pre-op XRT Chemo schedule	Yes All-cause mortality	HR 0.82 (CI 0.7– 0.95) favoring chemotherapy

Abbreviations: CI, confidence interval; HR, hazard ratio; XRT, radiation.

Published Abstract: BACKGROUND: The aim of the QUASAR trial was to determine the size and duration of any survival benefit from adjuvant chemotherapy for patients with colorectal cancer at low risk of recurrence, for whom the indication for such treatment is unclear. METHODS: After apparently curative resections of colon or rectal cancer, 3239 patients (2963 [91%] with stage II [node-negative] disease, 2291 [71%] with colon cancer, median age 63 [IQR 56–68] years) enrolled between May 1994 and December 2003, from 150 centers in 19 countries were randomly assigned to receive chemotherapy with fluorouracil and folinic acid (n = 1622) or to observation (with chemotherapy considered on recurrence; n = 1617). Chemotherapy was delivered as six 5-day courses every 4 weeks or as 30 once-weekly courses of intravenous fluorouracil (370 mg/m^2) with high-dose (175 mg) L-folinic acid or low-dose (25 mg) L-folinic acid. Until 1997, levamisole (12 courses of 450 mg over 3 days repeated every 2 weeks) or placebo was added. After 1997, patients who were assigned to receive chemotherapy were given fluorouracil and low-dose folinic acid only. The primary outcome was all-cause mortality. Analyses were done by intention to treat. This trial is registered with the International Clinical Trial Registry, number ISRCTN82375386. FINDINGS: At the time of analysis, 61 (3.8%) patients in the chemotherapy group and 50 (3.1%) in the observation group had missing follow-up. After a median follow-up of 5.5 (range 0–10.6) years, there were 311 deaths in the chemotherapy group and 370 in the observation group; the relative risk of death from any cause with chemotherapy versus observation alone was 0.82 (95% CI 0.70–0.95; P = .008). There were 293 recurrences in the chemotherapy group and 359 in the observation group; the relative risk of recurrence with chemotherapy versus observation alone was 0.78 (0.67–0.91; P = .001). Treatment efficacy did not differ significantly by tumor site, stage, sex, age, or chemotherapy schedule. Eight (0.5%) patients in the chemotherapy group and four (0.25%) in the observation group died from non–colorectal cancer causes within 30 weeks of randomization; only one of these deaths was deemed to be possibly chemotherapy related. INTERPRETATION: Chemotherapy with fluorouracil and folinic acid could improve survival of patients with stage II colorectal cancer, although the absolute improvements are small: assuming 5-year mortality without chemotherapy is 20%, the relative risk of death seen here translates into an absolute improvement in survival of 3.6% (95% CI 1.0–6.0). (Copyright Elsevier 2007. Reprinted with permission.)

Editor's Summary and Comments: This large RCT was designed to evaluate the benefit of chemotherapy in patients with completely resected colon or rectal cancer who had an uncertain indication for adjuvant chemotherapy; in 91% of patients, this equated to node-negative disease. Colon primaries comprised 70% of the cohort. In this study, chemotherapy was associated with a small reduction in relative risk of death (0.82 [CI 0.70–0.95]) as well as recurrence (0.78 [CI 0.67–0.91]) when compared with observation alone; this translated into an absolute survival benefit of 3.6%. The treatment efficacy was seen for both colon and rectal primaries. One limitation of this study was the lack of central pathology review; as a result, those patients with high-risk features who may most benefit cannot be delineated. Overall, the absolute survival benefit observed with adjuvant chemotherapy in the study cohort was small.

(11) Irinotecan fluorouracil plus leucovorin is not superior to fluorouracil plus leucovorin alone as adjuvant treatment for stage III colon cancer: results of CALGB 89803. Saltz LB, Niedzwiecki D, Hollis D, et al. J Clin Oncol 2007;25:3456.[39]

Hypothesis: The addition of irinotecan to 5-FU and LV will increase median survival.

No. Patients Randomized	Study Groups	Stratification	Significance Demonstrated	% Change Identified in Trial
1264	5-FU/LV = 629 CPT-11 + FU + LV = 635	No. of positive nodes (1–3 vs 4 or more) Histology CEA level	No	OS 81% vs 80%

Abbreviations: CEA, carcinoembryonic antigen; CPT-11, irinotecan; 5-FU, 5-fluorouracil; LV, leucovorin; OS, overall survival.

Published Abstract: PURPOSE: Randomized studies have shown that irinotecan (CPT-11) extends survival in metastatic colorectal cancer patients when administered in second-line and when added to fluorouracil (FU) plus leucovorin (LV) in first-line therapy of metastatic colorectal cancer. When this study was initiated, FU plus LV was standard adjuvant treatment for stage III colon cancer. We evaluated the efficacy and safety of weekly bolus CPT-11 plus FU plus LV in the treatment of patients with completely resected stage III colon cancer. METHODS: A total of 1264 patients were randomly assigned to receive either standard weekly bolus FU plus LV regimen or weekly bolus CPT-11 plus FU plus LV. The primary end points of the study were overall survival (OS) and disease-free survival (DFS). RESULTS: Treatment arms were well-balanced for patient characteristics and prognostic variables. There were no differences in either DFS or OS between the two treatment arms. Toxicity, including lethal toxicity, was significantly higher on the CPT-11 plus FU plus LV arm. CONCLUSION: The addition of CPT-11 to weekly bolus FU plus LV did not result in improvement in DFS or OS in stage III disease, but did increase both lethal and nonlethal toxicity. This trial demonstrates that advances in the treatment of metastatic disease do not necessarily translate into advances in adjuvant treatment, and it reinforces the need for randomized controlled adjuvant studies. (Copyright 2007 American Society of Clinical Oncology. Reprinted with permission.)

Editor's Summary and Comments: This trial was initiated based on the survival advantage observed with the use of irinotecan in metastatic colorectal cancer. Unfortunately, the success in the metastatic setting did not translate to a benefit in the adjuvant setting. No difference in 5-year OS (81% versus 80%), DFS (69% versus 66%), or recurrence-free (71% versus 68%) survival was observed with the addition of irinotecan. This was a well-designed and conducted study; the two experimental arms were well balanced with regard to clinicopathologic variables and the outcomes for the control arm were comparable to those seen in other multicenter studies. The results of this study, as well as two other studies currently ongoing,[40,41] do not support the use of irinotecan in the setting of adjuvant treatment for stage III colon cancer.

(12) Oxaliplatin combined with weekly bolus fluorouracil and leucovorin as surgical adjuvant chemotherapy for stage II and III colon cancer: results from NSABP C-07. Kuebler JP, Wieand HS, O'Connell MJ, et al. J Clin Oncol 2007;25:2198.[43]

Hypothesis: The addition of oxaliplatin to fluorouracil and leucovorin will improve DFS.

No. Patients Randomized	Study Groups	Stratification	Significance Demonstrated	% Change Identified in Trial
2492	5-FU/LV/ OX = 1247 FU + LV = 1245	Medical center No. of positive nodes (0, 1–3, >4)	Yes DFS	76.1% vs 71.8% DFS at 3 years

Abbreviations: DFS, disease-free survival; 5-FU, 5-fluorouracil; LV, leucovorin; OX, oxaliplatin.

Published Abstract: PURPOSE: This phase III clinical trial evaluated the impact on disease-free survival (DFS) of adding oxaliplatin to bolus weekly fluorouracil (FU) combined with leucovorin as surgical adjuvant therapy for stage II and III colon cancer. PATIENTS AND METHODS: Patients who had undergone a potentially curative resection were randomly assigned to either FU 500 mg/m^2 intravenous (IV) bolus weekly for 6 weeks plus leucovorin 500 mg/m^2 IV weekly for 6 weeks during each 8-week cycle for three cycles (FULV), or the same FULV regimen with oxaliplatin 85 mg/m^2 IV administered on weeks 1, 3, and 5 of each 8-week cycle for three cycles (FLOX). RESULTS: A total of 2407 patients (96.6%) of the 2492 patients randomly assigned were eligible. Median follow-up for patients still alive is 42.5 months. The hazard ratio (FLOX v FULV) is 0.80 (95% CI, 0.69 to 0.93), a 20% risk reduction in favor of FLOX ($P < .004$). The 3- and 4-year disease-free survival (DFS) rates were 71.8% and 67.0% for FULV and 76.1% and 73.2% for FLOX, respectively. Grade 3 neurosensory toxicity was noted in 8.2% of patients receiving FLOX and in 0.7% of those receiving FULV ($P < .001$). Hospitalization for diarrhea associated with bowel wall thickening occurred in 5.5% of the patients receiving FLOX and in 3.0% of the patients receiving FULV ($P < .01$). A total of 1.2% of patients died as a result of any cause within 60 days of receiving chemotherapy, with no significant difference between regimens. CONCLUSION: The addition of oxaliplatin to weekly FULV significantly improved DFS in patients with stage II and III colon cancer. FLOX can be recommended as an effective option in clinical practice. (Copyright 2007 American Society of Clinical Oncology. Reprinted with permission.)

Editor's Summary and Comments: This trial, using a bolus regimen of 5-FU and LV with oxaliplatin, confirmed the findings of the MOSAIC trial where the addition of oxaliplatin in patients with stage II or III resected colon cancer resulted in improved DFS. In a recently presented update of this study with minimum of 5-year follow-up (abstract form only),[53] a trend toward improved OS with the inclusion of oxaliplatin was observed, but did not reach statistical significance ($P = .61$). The toxicity of the two regimens used in MOSAIC (FOLFOX) versus NSABP C-07 (FLOX) differed slightly, with FOLFOX being associated with more grade 3 neurotoxicity (12% versus 8.2%) and the FLOX regimen having more grade 3/4 diarrhea (38% versus 10.8%). However, either regimen is recommended for use in clinical practice.

DISCLOSURE

Authors have nothing to disclose.

REFERENCES

1. O'Connell MJ, Mailliard JA, Kahn MJ, et al. Controlled trial of fluorouracil and low-dose leucovorin given for 6 months as postoperative adjuvant therapy for colon cancer. J Clin Oncol 1997;15(1):246–50.

2. Windle R, Bell PR, Shaw D. Five year results of a randomized trial of adjuvant 5-fluorouracil and levamisole in colorectal cancer. Br J Surg 1987;74(7):569–72.
3. Moertel CG, Fleming TR, Macdonald JS, et al. Fluorouracil plus levamisole as effective adjuvant therapy after resection of stage III colon carcinoma: a final report. Ann Intern Med 1995;122(5):321–6.
4. Wolmark N, Rockette H, Fisher B, et al. The benefit of leucovorin-modulated fluorouracil as postoperative adjuvant therapy for primary colon cancer: results from National Surgical Adjuvant Breast and Bowel Project protocol C-03. J Clin Oncol 1993;11(10):1879–87.
5. O'Connell MJ, Laurie JA, Kahn M, et al. Prospectively randomized trial of postoperative adjuvant chemotherapy in patients with high-risk colon cancer. J Clin Oncol 1998;16(1):295–300.
6. Wolmark N, Rockette H, Mamounas E, et al. Clinical trial to assess the relative efficacy of fluorouracil and leucovorin, fluorouracil and levamisole, and fluorouracil, leucovorin, and levamisole in patients with Dukes' B and C carcinoma of the colon: results from National Surgical Adjuvant Breast and Bowel Project C-04. J Clin Oncol 1999;17(11):3553–9.
7. Shoup MC, Nissan A, Dangelica MI, Tschmelitsch J. Randomized clinical trials in colon cancer. Surg Oncol Clin N Am 2002;11(1):133–48.
8. Wiggers T, Jeekel J, Arends JW, et al. No-touch isolation technique in colon cancer: a controlled prospective trial. Br J Surg 1988;75(5):409–15.
9. Rouffet F, Hay JM, Vacher B, et al. Curative resection for left colonic carcinoma: hemicolectomy vs. segmental colectomy. A prospective, controlled, multicenter trial. French Association for Surgical Research. Dis Colon Rectum 1994;37(7):651–9.
10. Docherty JG, McGregor JR, Akyol AM, et al. Comparison of manually constructed and stapled anastomoses in colorectal surgery. West of Scotland and Highland Anastomosis Study Group. Ann Surg 1995;221(2):176–84.
11. Wolff BG, Pembeton JH, van Heerden JA, et al. Elective colon and rectal surgery without nasogastric decompression. A prospective, randomized trial. Ann Surg 1989;209(6):670–3 [discussion: 673–5].
12. Kjeldsen BJ, Kronborg O, Fenger C, et al. A prospective randomized study of follow-up after radical surgery for colorectal cancer. Br J Surg 1997;84(5):666–9.
13. Makela JT, Laitinen SO, Kairaluoma MI. Five-year follow-up after radical surgery for colorectal cancer. Results of a prospective randomized trial. Arch Surg 1995;130(10):1062–7.
14. Ohlsson B, Breland U, Ekberg H, et al. Follow-up after curative surgery for colorectal carcinoma. Randomized comparison with no follow-up. Dis Colon Rectum 1995;38(6):619–26.
15. Schoemaker D, Black R, Giles L, et al. Yearly colonoscopy, liver CT, and chest radiography do not influence 5-year survival of colorectal cancer patients. Gastroenterology 1998;114(1):7–14.
16. Grossmann EM, Johnson FE, Virgo KS, et al. Follow-up of colorectal cancer patients after resection with curative intent-the GILDA trial. Surg Oncol 2004;13(2–3):119–24.
17. Lacy AM, Garcia-Valdecasas JC, Delgado S, et al. Laparoscopy-assisted colectomy versus open colectomy for treatment of non-metastatic colon cancer: a randomised trial. Lancet 2002;359(9325):2224–9.
18. Clinical Outcomes of Surgical Therapy Study Group. A comparison of laparoscopically assisted and open colectomy for colon cancer. N Engl J Med 2004;350(20):2050–9.

19. Jayne DG, Guillou PJ, Thorpe H, et al. Randomized trial of laparoscopic-assisted resection of colorectal carcinoma: 3-year results of the UK MRC CLASICC Trial Group. J Clin Oncol 2007;25(21):3061–8.
20. Buunen M, Veldkamp R, Hop WC, et al. Survival after laparoscopic surgery versus open surgery for colon cancer: long-term outcome of a randomised clinical trial. Lancet Oncol 2009;10(1):44–52.
21. Hewett PJ, Allardyce RA, Bagshaw PF, et al. Short-term outcomes of the Australasian randomized clinical study comparing laparoscopic and conventional open surgical treatments for colon cancer: the ALCCaS trial. Ann Surg 2008;248(5): 728–38.
22. Guillou PJ, Quirke P, Thorpe H, et al. Short-term endpoints of conventional versus laparoscopic-assisted surgery in patients with colorectal cancer (MRC CLASICC trial): multicentre, randomised controlled trial. Lancet 2005;365(9472):1718–26.
23. Fleshman J, Sargent DJ, Green E, et al. Laparoscopic colectomy for cancer is not inferior to open surgery based on 5-year data from the COST Study Group trial. Ann Surg 2007;246(4):655–62 [discussion: 662–4].
24. Lacy AM, Delgado S, Castells A, et al. The long-term results of a randomized clinical trial of laparoscopy-assisted versus open surgery for colon cancer. Ann Surg 2008;248(1):1–7.
25. Veldkamp R, Kuhry E, Hop WC, et al. Laparoscopic surgery versus open surgery for colon cancer: short-term outcomes of a randomised trial. Lancet Oncol 2005; 6(7):477–84.
26. Weeks JC, Nelson H, Gelber S, et al. Short-term quality-of-life outcomes following laparoscopic-assisted colectomy vs open colectomy for colon cancer: a randomized trial. JAMA 2002;287(3):321–8.
27. Janson M, Lindholm E, Anderberg B, et al. Randomized trial of health-related quality of life after open and laparoscopic surgery for colon cancer. Surg Endosc 2007;21(5):747–53.
28. Stojadinovic A, Nissan A, Protic M, et al. Prospective randomized study comparing sentinel lymph node evaluation with standard pathologic evaluation for the staging of colon carcinoma: results from the United States Military Cancer Institute Clinical Trials Group Study GI-01. Ann Surg 2007;245(6): 846–57.
29. Bembenek AE, Rosenberg R, Wagler E, et al. Sentinel lymph node biopsy in colon cancer: a prospective multicenter trial. Ann Surg 2007;245(6):858–63.
30. Kelder W, Braat AE, Karrenbeld A, et al. The sentinel node procedure in colon carcinoma: a multi-centre study in The Netherlands. Int J Colorectal Dis 2007; 22(12):1509–14.
31. Bilchik AJ, DiNome M, Saha S, et al. Prospective multicenter trial of staging adequacy in colon cancer: preliminary results. Arch Surg 2006;141(6):527–33 [discussion: 533–4].
32. Bertagnolli M, Miedema B, Redston M, et al. Sentinel node staging of resectable colon cancer: results of a multicenter study. Ann Surg 2004;240(4):624–8 [discussion: 628–30].
33. Moertel CG, Fleming TR, Macdonald JS, et al. Intergroup study of fluorouracil plus levamisole as adjuvant therapy for stage II/Dukes' B2 colon cancer. J Clin Oncol 1995;13(12):2936–43.
34. Mamounas E, Wieand S, Wolmark N, et al. Comparative efficacy of adjuvant chemotherapy in patients with Dukes' B versus Dukes' C colon cancer: results from four National Surgical Adjuvant Breast and Bowel Project adjuvant studies (C-01, C-02, C-03, and C-04). J Clin Oncol 1999;17(5):1349–55.

35. Efficacy of adjuvant fluorouracil and folinic acid in B2 colon cancer. International Multicentre Pooled Analysis of B2 Colon Cancer Trials (IMPACT B2) Investigators. J Clin Oncol 1999;17(5):1356–63.
36. Gill S, Loprinzi CL, Sargent DJ, et al. Pooled analysis of fluorouracil-based adjuvant therapy for stage II and III colon cancer: who benefits and by how much? J Clin Oncol 2004;22(10):1797–806.
37. Schippinger W, Samonigg H, Schaberl-Moser R, et al. A prospective randomised phase III trial of adjuvant chemotherapy with 5-fluorouracil and leucovorin in patients with stage II colon cancer. Br J Cancer 2007;97(8):1021–7.
38. Quasar Collaborative Group, Gray R, Barnwell J, et al. Adjuvant chemotherapy versus observation in patients with colorectal cancer: a randomised study. Lancet 2007;370(9604):2020–9.
39. Saltz LB, Niedzwiecki D, Hollis D, et al. Irinotecan fluorouracil plus leucovorin is not superior to fluorouracil plus leucovorin alone as adjuvant treatment for stage III colon cancer: results of CALGB 89803. J Clin Oncol 2007;25(23):3456–61.
40. Yehou M, Raoul J, Douillard J. A phase III randomized trial of LV5FU2+CPT-11 vs. LV5FU2 alone in adjuvant high risk colon cancer (FNCLCC Accord02/FFCD9802). Proc Am Soc Clin Oncol 2005;23:3502 [abstract].
41. Cutsem EV, Labianca R, Hossfeld D. Randomized phase III trial comparing infused irinotecan/5-fluorouracil (5-FU)/folinic acid versus 5-FU/folinic acid in stage III colon cancer patients [abstract]. Proc Am Soc Clin Oncol 2005;23. LBA8.
42. Andre T, Boni C, Mounedji-Boudiaf L, et al. Oxaliplatin, fluorouracil, and leucovorin as adjuvant treatment for colon cancer. N Engl J Med 2004;350(23):2343–51.
43. Kuebler JP, Wieand HS, O'Connell MJ, et al. Oxaliplatin combined with weekly bolus fluorouracil and leucovorin as surgical adjuvant chemotherapy for stage II and III colon cancer: results from NSABP C-07. J Clin Oncol 2007;25(16):2198–204.
44. Twelves C, Wong A, Nowacki MP, et al. Capecitabine as adjuvant treatment for stage III colon cancer. N Engl J Med 2005;352(26):2696–704.
45. Lembersky BC, Wieand HS, Petrelli NJ, et al. Oral uracil and tegafur plus leuco-vorin compared with intravenous fluorouracil and leucovorin in stage II and III carcinoma of the colon: results from National Surgical Adjuvant Breast and Bowel Project Protocol C-06. J Clin Oncol 2006;24(13):2059–64.
46. Wolmark N, Rockette H, Wickerham DL, et al. Adjuvant therapy of Dukes' A, B, and C adenocarcinoma of the colon with portal-vein fluorouracil hepatic infusion: preliminary results of National Surgical Adjuvant Breast and Bowel Project Protocol C-02. J Clin Oncol 1990;8(9):1466–75.
47. Labianca R, Fossati R, Zaniboni A, et al. Randomized trial of intraportal and/or systemic adjuvant chemotherapy in patients with colon carcinoma. J Natl Cancer Inst 2004;96(10):750–8.
48. Nordlinger B, Rougier P, Arnaud JP, et al. Adjuvant regional chemotherapy and systemic chemotherapy versus systemic chemotherapy alone in patients with stage II-III colorectal cancer: a multicentre randomised controlled phase III trial. Lancet Oncol 2005;6(7):459–68.
49. Jayne DG, Brown JM, Thorpe H, et al. Bladder and sexual function following resection for rectal cancer in a randomized clinical trial of laparoscopic versus open technique. Br J Surg 2005;92(9):1124–32.
50. de Gramont A, Boni C, Navarro M, et al. Oxaliplatin/5FU/LV in adjuvant colon cancer: updated efficacy results of the MOSAIC trial, including survival, with a median follow-up of six years. Proc Am Soc Clin Oncol 2007;25(18):S4007.

51. Schmoll HJ, Cartwright T, Tabernero J, et al. Phase III trial of capecitabine plus oxaliplatin as adjuvant therapy for stage III colon cancer: a planned safety analysis in 1,864 patients. J Clin Oncol 2007;25(1):102–9.
52. Kopec JA, Yothers G, Ganz PA, et al. Quality of life in operable colon cancer patients receiving oral compared with intravenous chemotherapy: results from National Surgical Adjuvant Breast and Bowel Project Trial C-06. J Clin Oncol 2007;25(4):424–30.
53. Wolmark N, Wieand S, Kuebler PJ, et al. A phase III trial comparing FULV to FULV + oxaliplatin in stage II or III carcinoma of the colon: Survival results of NSABP Protocol C-07. J Clin Oncol 2008;26 [abstract LBA4005].

Randomized Clinical Trials in Rectal and Anal Cancers

Jason Park, MD, MEd, Heather B. Neuman, MD, MS,
Martin R. Weiser, MD, W. Douglas Wong, MD*

KEYWORDS

- Rectal cancer • Anal cancer • Surgery • Radiation
- Chemotherapy • Randomized trials

The modern management of rectal cancer involves multimodality therapy, and advances in each of the modalities have contributed to improved outcomes for patients with this disease. Surgery remains the cornerstone of curative treatment for rectal cancer. Surgical resection with total mesorectal excision (TME, defined as complete excision of the visceral mesorectum with pelvic nerve preservation) has gained widespread acceptance. This technique is associated with high rates of local control and increased disease-free survival (DFS).

Even with high-quality surgery, local and distant recurrences remain problematic, and adjuvant therapeutic approaches with radiation therapy (RT) and chemotherapy have been developed and applied to improve local control and potentially impact survival. Recent studies have attempted to further improve multimodality therapy by better defining the effects of RT and chemotherapy when optimal TME surgery is performed.

This article reviews randomized clinical trials (RCTs) published between April 2001 and November 2008 on the management of patients with rectal cancer. In total, the authors reviewed 78 RCTs on therapy for rectal cancer. Of these, five met the authors' criteria for level 1a evidence. Details of RCT selection for review and subsequent categorization for level of evidence are presented in the introductory article of this issue. The following summary discusses the major RCTs and relevant findings that have impacted clinical management most and includes most but not all RCTs on therapy for rectal cancer published during this period.

SURGERY

The previous review of prospective RCTs in rectal cancer identified 37 trials that focused on surgery.[1] Of these, the larger RCTs were directed at two main aspects

Disclosure: See last page of article.
Department of Surgery, Memorial Sloan-Kettering Cancer Center, 1275 York Avenue, New York, NY 10065, USA
* Corresponding author.
E-mail address: wongd@mskcc.org (W. Douglas Wong).

of rectal cancer surgery: sphincter preservation and colorectal reconstruction techniques. One major trial that compared low anterior resection (LAR) with abdominoperineal resection (APR) found comparable rates of recurrence and survival between the two operations.[2] Furthermore, multiple retrospective reviews suggested that LAR did not compromise oncologic outcomes, all of which supported sphincter preserving rectal cancer surgery when possible.[3,4] The previous review also presented multiple RCTs on reconstructive techniques after anterior resection, and these showed a benefit in functional outcomes for colonic J-pouches over straight anastomoses.[5,6] Interestingly, the TME technique for rectal cancer resection, which represents a significant advance in surgical technique, has never been assessed in any large, prospective RCTs. The locoregional failure rates in retrospective series (ranging from 3% to 7%), however, have been consistently lower with the TME technique compared with historic and contemporary controls.[7–9] Thus, surgical resection with TME has been established as the standard of care in the surgical management of rectal cancer.

The authors have identified 36 prospective RCTs comprising 42 articles evaluating different aspects of surgery for rectal cancer that have been published since the last review. The major topics examined in this period included: minimally invasive surgical approaches (10 RCTs), reconstruction techniques (17 RCTs) and defunctioning stomas after anterior resection (four RCTs), and local excision for rectal cancer (one RCT).

Minimally Invasive versus Open Resection

The application of minimally invasive approaches to rectal surgery represents a significant technical advance in the management of rectal cancer. The authors identified 10 studies that assessed minimally invasive approaches to surgery for rectal cancer. Of these, the only trial that fulfilled the authors' criteria for level 1a evidence was the Conventional versus Laparoscopic-Assisted Surgery in Colorectal Cancer (CLASICC) trial from the UK Medical Research Council. In this multicenter trial, 794 patients with colorectal cancer, of whom 381 (48%) had rectal primaries, were randomized to laparoscopic-assisted or open resection.[10,11] A TME technique was used in most patients in both groups. The short-term results demonstrated that the laparoscopic-assisted group had shorter hospital stays (by 2 days). In the subgroup of rectal cancer patients who underwent LAR, there was a trend toward a higher rate of positive circumferential margins in the laparoscopic-assisted compared with the open surgery group (12% versus 6%).[10] On long-term follow-up, however, this trend did not translate into any significant differences between groups with regard to local recurrence, 3-year DFS, or overall survival (OS).[11] Other findings from the CLASICC trial suggested a trend toward worse sexual function for men in the laparoscopic-assisted group.[12]

Other smaller RCTs have shown results similar to the CLASICC trial with regard to shorter postoperative hospitalizations,[13–16] but longer operating room times and higher costs for the laparoscopic groups.[14,15,17] In addition, these smaller studies have not demonstrated any differences in DFS and OS between laparoscopic and open approaches, although they are underpowered for these types of analyses.[14,17] Although the results of the CLASICC trial and these smaller studies are promising, the authors take the viewpoint that further data on the long-term oncologic outcomes of laparoscopic approaches are needed before minimally invasive surgery can be considered standard for mid- to low rectal cancers. Currently, the National Cancer Institutes-sponsored American College of Surgeons Oncology Group (ACOSOG) Z6051 multicenter RCT of laparoscopic-assisted rectal cancer resection is accruing patients to add further data to these issues.

Resection versus Local Excision

The authors identified one RCT comparing local excision with transanal endoscopic microsurgery (TEM) to laparoscopic resection (LAR or APR).[18,19] This trial randomized 70 patients with clinically staged T2N0, well- to moderately differentiated rectal tumors to TEM or laparoscopic resection after neoadjuvant chemoradiation. With a minimum follow-up of 5 years, no differences in local recurrence (two in the TEM and one in the resection group) or DFS were seen between the TEM and laparoscopic resection groups. These results are consistent with an earlier RCT, described in the previous review, which compared TEM with anterior resection in 50 patients with clinically staged T1N0 rectal cancers.[20] Even combined, however, these trials are severely underpowered. Furthermore, the length of follow-up needs to be taken into consideration, as data from Memorial Sloan-Kettering Cancer Center and the University of Minnesota suggest that greater than 5 years of follow-up are necessary to fully appreciate recurrence after local excision.[21–24] The results from these small RCTs therefore must be considered in conjunction with multiple large, retrospective studies that demonstrate high rates of recurrence after local excision of rectal cancers on long-term follow-up.[21–24]

Reconstructive Techniques after Anterior Resection

Reconstruction options to restore intestinal continuity following anterior resection were assessed in 17 RCTs. Seven RCTs comprising 506 patients compared functional outcomes of colonic J-pouches (CJPs) versus straight anastomoses (SA) after anterior resection. Of these seven trials, six reported better short-term functional outcomes with CJPs.[25–31] Three of the seven trials also included quality-of-life assessments, and, of these, one showed a difference in quality of life favoring the CPJ group.[28]

Two RCTs compared CJPs to side-to-end anastomoses and found similar functional outcomes between techniques.[32–34] Five RCTs compared CJPs with transverse coloplasty pouches (TCPs); in two of these trials, better functional outcomes were seen with CJPs,[25,31] while the other three RCTs showed comparable outcomes.[35–37] Additionally, Fazio and colleagues[25] compared TCPs with SA and found no differences in functional outcomes, although the analysis for this portion of the trial was underpowered. Considered together with previous RCTs,[6] these data on reconstructive techniques support a functional benefit to reconstruction with CJPs over SA. In the event that CJP reconstruction is not technically feasible, however, the benefit of TCPs over SA is uncertain.[25]

Defunctioning Stomas after Resection

Two large RCTs assessed whether defunctioning stomas reduced the rate of anastomotic leaks after rectal cancer surgery. In both of these studies, a lower incidence of anastomotic leaks was found when defunctioning loop stomas were performed after LAR.[38,39] Matthiessen and colleagues[39] showed a symptomatic leak rate of 10.3% in patients who underwent defunctioning stomas (compared with 28% for patients with no stomas). An interesting finding from this study was the low likelihood of stoma reversal in patients who developed anastomic leaks. Twenty-five patients in the nondefunctioned group developed a symptomatic leak, and of these patients, only eight were stoma-free after long-term follow-up. In comparison, 12 patients in the defunctioned group developed a leak, and seven of these patients were stoma-free on follow-up.

RADIATION

For the purposes of this article, the RT section includes trials that compared RT and surgery with surgery alone and different fractions and schedules of RT and chemoradiation. The authors have included trials comparing RT with RT and chemotherapy, in which the only independent variable was the addition of chemotherapy, in the chemotherapy section of this article.

The previous review presented randomized data supporting pre- or postoperative RT for rectal cancer. RT administered either preoperatively (short-course or long-course) or postoperatively was shown to reduce the rate of local recurrences over surgery alone in multiple (although not all) studies.[40–47] A minority of randomized trials also showed an improvement in OS with preoperative RT,[43,44] but multiple other studies have not replicated these findings. One additional RCT that compared preoperative short-course RT with postoperative long-course RT found a decrease in local recurrences with preoperative RT but no improvement in survival.[48] Taken together, these previous data strongly supported a role for RT, particularly in the preoperative setting, to improve local control in locally advanced, resectable rectal cancer.

The authors have identified 15 RCTs comprising 28 papers looking at different aspects of RT for rectal cancer that have been published since the last review. The major topics examined included: preoperative RT versus surgery (three RCTs), preoperative versus postoperative chemoradiation (four RCTs), and preoperative short course RT versus long course chemoradiation (1 RCT).

Preoperative Radiation versus Surgery Alone

Three large, randomized studies examined preoperative RT versus surgery alone. Of these, only the RCT from the Dutch Colorectal Cancer Group presented new data, while the other two provided long-term follow-up data.[49,50] The Dutch trial was a multicenter RCT that examined the added benefit of preoperative short-course RT to TME for rectal cancer. The authors included this trial as level 1a evidence because of its design and impact on practice. The distinguishing features of this trial were the rigorous efforts to standardize surgery with TME and the multiple measures instituted to ensure surgical and pathologic quality control. This level of standardization and quality control allowed the authors to address the key question of whether preoperative RT was beneficial when optimal surgical therapy with TME was performed. Patients (N = 1861) with resectable disease were randomized to short-course RT (5 × 5 Gy) followed by TME surgery or TME surgery alone. On short-term follow-up, the 2-year local recurrence rate was lower in the RT plus TME group compared with the TME alone group (2.4% versus 8.2%).[49] On longer follow-up, the 5-year local recurrence risk remained lower in the RT plus TME group (5.6% versus 10.9%), but no difference in 5-year OS was observed between groups (64.2% versus 63.5%).[50] Thus, these results showed that there was a benefit to preoperative RT even when optimal surgery was performed using a TME technique.

Two other RCTs reported long-term data on preoperative short-course RT for rectal cancer. The Stockholm II trial found that patients receiving preoperative RT had a lower incidence of pelvic recurrences compared with those who underwent surgery alone (12% versus 25%), but OS was not different between groups.[51,52] However, the Swedish Rectal Cancer Trial, which randomized 1168 patients with resectable disease to preoperative RT or surgery alone, found improved disease-specific survival (DSS) (72% versus 62%) and OS favoring the preoperative RT group.[44] These survival results differ from both the Dutch and the Stockholm II trials, which did not find a survival benefit with preoperative RT. Although subject to debate, some authors have pointed to the lack of standardization of TME surgery and high local recurrence rate in the Swedish trial as possible reasons for these contrasting results.

Multiple papers derived from the previously mentioned trials also have presented data related to the effects of preoperative RT on nononcologic outcomes. In terms of complications, these papers suggest a higher incidence of perioperative complications and wound problems,[53] and more long-term complications and small bowel obstructions (SBO) for patients receiving preoperative RT.[54,55] In terms of function and quality of life, patients who received preoperative RT report higher rates of sexual dysfunction and fecal incontinence, although these studies show few differences in overall health-related quality of life.[56,57]

Preoperative versus Postoperative Chemoradiation

Three large RCTs comparing preoperative versus postoperative chemoradiation for clinically resectable rectal cancer were initiated, but two of these (NSABP R-03 and INT 0147) were closed early because of low accrual. Fortunately, the third trial, from the German Rectal Cancer Group (CAO/ARO/AIO 94), was completed, and the authors have included this trial as 1a level of evidence. The German trial randomized 823 patients with locally advanced rectal cancer to preoperative or postoperative chemoradiation, consisting of long-course RT (50.4 Gy in 25 fractions) and infusional fluorouracil (FU).[58,59] The preoperative chemoradiation group was found to have fewer toxicities and an improved 5-year local recurrence rate compared with the postoperative chemoradiation group (6% versus 13%). There was no difference between groups with regard to 5-year OS, however.

Preoperative Short-Course Radiation versus Combined-Modality Therapy

A trial from the Polish Colorectal Group compared preoperative short-course RT with long course chemoradiation.[60] In this trial, 312 patients with clinical T3 or T4 rectal cancers were randomized to either preoperative RT (25 Gy in five fractions) and TME surgery within 7 days or long course chemoradiation (RT 50.4 Gy in 28 fractions and infusional 5-FU and leucovorin [LV]) followed by TME surgery 4 to 6 weeks later. The results showed a higher rate of grade 3 or 4 toxicities for the chemoradiation group (18% versus 3%) but no differences in rates of sphincter preservation or postoperative complications.[61,62] On long-term follow-up, there were no differences in the crude incidence of recurrence or 4-year DSS or OS between treatment groups.[60] Unfortunately, the study was powered to detect differences of 15% or greater, and therefore was unlikely by design to detect smaller differences between groups.

CHEMOTHERAPY

The previous review of RCTs in rectal cancer presented data supporting a survival benefit with postoperative adjuvant chemotherapy over observation and an improvement in local control with combined chemoradiation over RT alone.

Previous RCTs from the United States and Japan suggested that the addition of chemotherapy with intravenous or oral FU-based regimens in the postoperative period improved OS after surgery for locally advanced rectal cancer.[41,63] Furthermore, studies on postoperative combined chemoradiation suggested improved local control and DFS compared with observation or postoperative RT alone.[64,65] These studies subsequently formed the basis for the National Institutes of Health consensus recommendations for postoperative RT and chemotherapy to patients with stage 2 or 3 rectal cancers.[66]

Since the last review, the authors have identified 27 RCTs comprising 29 papers on chemotherapy for rectal cancer. The main topics assessed by these RCTs included: the addition of chemotherapy to RT, chemotherapy versus observation in the postoperative setting, and comparisons of various neoadjuvant or adjuvant chemotherapeutic agents.

Combined Chemoradiation versus Radiation

The European Organization for Research and Treatment of Cancer (EORTC) developed protocol 22921 to assess the effect of adding chemotherapy to preoperative RT and the value of postoperative chemotherapy in patients with rectal cancers.[67–69] In this trial, patients (N=1011) with clinical T3 or T4 rectal cancer were randomized to one of four arms:

1. Preoperative RT (45 Gy in 25 fractions)
2. Preoperative combined chemoradiation (RT plus 5-FU and LV)
3. Preoperative RT followed by postoperative chemotherapy
4. Preoperative combined chemoradiation followed by postoperative chemotherapy

The 5-year local recurrence rate was found to be significantly lower in all three arms that received any chemotherapy (preoperative and/or postoperative) compared with the preoperative RT-alone group (8% to 10% versus 17%), which suggests a benefit for chemotherapy regardless of when it is administered. The addition of chemotherapy to RT (preoperatively or postoperatively), however, did not impact survival.

The authors identified one additional large RCT comparing preoperative combined chemoradiation to RT. Federation Francophone de la Cancerologie Digestive (FFCD) protocol 9203 randomized 733 patients with T3-4 Nx rectal cancer to preoperative long-course RT with or without concurrent 5-FU and LV.[70] Consistent with EORTC 22921, this study showed a decrease in the 5-year local recurrence rate with combined chemoradiation over RT alone (8% versus 17%) but no difference in OS.[70] Thus, these most recent data from two large RCTs both demonstrate that the addition of 5-FU to RT improves local control but not survival. These results challenge previous findings of a survival benefit to postoperative RT with concurrent chemotherapy from the older and much smaller North Central Cancer Treatment Group (NCCTG) trial.[65]

One additional trial compared the effects of preoperative combined chemoradiation (RT plus 5-FU and LV) to RT alone in 207 patients with unresectable primary or recurrent rectal cancers. The authors defined unresectable tumors as those that were fixed on digital rectal examination or had computed tomography (CT) or magnetic resonance imaging evidence of sacral, pelvic sidewall/floor, base of bladder, or prostate invasion. The chemoradiation arm in this study had higher rates of R0 resection, local control, and DSS, although there was more toxicity in chemoradiation (CRT) group as well.[71,72]

Adjuvant Chemotherapy versus Surgery

The Quick and Simple and Reliable (QUASAR) trial was a multicenter trial that randomized 3239 patients with colorectal cancer (including 948 with rectal cancer), most of whom had stage 2 disease, to chemotherapy with intravenous FU or observation following curative surgical resection.[73] Approximately half of the rectal cancer patients in this trial received RT (either pre- or postoperatively). This study found that adjuvant chemotherapy was associated with a small reduction in the relative risk of recurrence and death when compared with observation alone, irrespective of site (colon versus rectal) or chemotherapy schedule.

However, a survival benefit with adjuvant chemotherapy in patients with locally advanced rectal cancer has not been a consistent finding in modern randomized trials when pre- or postoperative RT is given. EORTC 22921, described previously, found that the 5-year OS rate was not different for rectal cancer patients who received post-operative chemotherapy compared with those who did not receive postoperative chemotherapy (hazard ratio [HR] for death in the adjuvant chemotherapy group 0.85, 95% confidence interval [CI] 0.68 to 1.04). Another RCT of 1029 stage 2 or 3 colorectal patients (including 299 rectal cancer patients, of whom more than 50% received RT) failed to demonstrate a survival benefit with FU-based chemotherapy following surgery in the subset of rectal cancer patients.[74] Despite these data, postoperative intravenous chemotherapy still is considered standard treatment for patients who receive preoperative chemoradiation, while further trials and meta-analyses on adjuvant chemotherapy are being conducted.[75]

Several RCTs from Japan have investigated oral chemotherapy in the adjuvant setting. Consistent with previous results,[63] these RCTs have demonstrated higher DFS in patients with resected rectal cancers receiving oral uracil–tegafur over no chemotherapy, although the data on OS were more inconsistent.[76,77]

In addition to the previously mentioned RCTs on systemic (intravenous or oral) chemotherapy, the authors identified one large RCT that examined the role of regional chemotherapy (given by intraperitoneal or intraportal methods) combined with systemic chemotherapy for patients with stage 2 or 3 colorectal cancers.[78] In this study, FU-based regional chemotherapy did not add any benefit with regards to recurrence or survival over systemic chemotherapy alone.

Comparisons of Chemotherapeutic Regimens

One large RCT (N = 1917) compared infusional to bolus regimens of intravenous FU in patients with resected T3 to T4 or N1 rectal cancers who also were receiving concurrent RT. The regimens were found to be comparable in terms of local recurrence, DSS, and OS.[79] There were differences in the toxicity profiles, however, with patients receiving infusional FU experiencing fewer hematologic toxicities.

Another RCT assessed the addition of LV or levamisole, or both LV and levamisole with intravenous 5-FU alone in patients with stage 2 or 3 colorectal cancer. This trial failed to demonstrate a benefit in DFS or OS with the addition of any of these agents alone or in combination over 5-FU alone.[80,81]

Finally, in a comparison of oral versus intravenous FU, an RCT of patients with clinically staged T3 to T4 and/or N-positive rectal cancers found that those treated with preoperative oral uracil, tegafur, and LV concomitant with RT experienced fewer toxicities than those treated with intravenous 5-FU and LV plus RT, with no differences in local control or suvival.[82]

SUMMARY

The multimodality management of rectal cancer continues to evolve, with significant changes in all aspects of therapy related to surgery, radiation, and chemotherapy. Surgery remains the cornerstone of curative therapy, and resection with TME is the standard of care in the surgical management of rectal cancer. The standard approach to pelvic dissection for mid- to low rectal cancers remains open surgery. Recent studies, however, suggest that minimally invasive approaches that use a TME technique are feasible, although more data are awaited on oncologic outcomes with these approaches.

Neoadjuvant and adjuvant treatments have important roles in improving local control and potentially impacting survival. Recent, well-designed trials have demonstrated that:

RT reduces local recurrences even when optimal surgery with TME is performed.
Chemotherapy when given concurrently with RT has an additive benefit.
Preoperative RT with chemotherapy improves local control and is tolerated better than postoperative RT with chemotherapy.
Postoperative chemotherapy may have a survival benefit.

Together, these data support neoadjuvant combined long-course RT with chemotherapy followed by surgical resection with TME and then postoperative chemotherapy as the standard of care for patients with stage 2 or 3 rectal cancer.

RANDOMIZED CLINICAL TRIALS IN THE TREATMENT OF EPIDERMOID CANCERS OF THE ANAL CANAL

The initial observation that anal canal cancers were highly sensitive to chemoradiation drastically changed the treatment paradigm for this disease. Nigro and colleagues[83] reported on 28 patients treated with RT combined with chemotherapy, only a minority of whom went on to have an APR. This study found that 24 (86%) patients overall had a clinically complete response to RT with chemotherapy, and 22 (79%) had prolonged DFS, suggesting that chemoradiation could be effective as primary therapy for cancer of the anal canal.

The previous review identified three large RCTs on therapy for anal canal cancer. Of these, two RCTs established that concurrent chemoradiation had better local control and decreased colostomy rates compared with RT alone.[84,85] The third large RCT showed that the addition of mitomycin C (MMC) to 5-FU given concurrently with RT led to improved DFS and colostomy-free survival compared with 5-FU alone with RT.[86] These results established chemoradiation with 5-FU and MMC and concurrent RT as the standard of care for most patients with anal squamous cell cancer, with surgery reserved for circumstances when salvage is required.

The authors have identified three RCTs on squamous cell cancer of the anus that have been published since the previous review.[87–89] The largest of these was by the Radiation Therapy Oncology Group (RTOG, protocol 98-11), which randomized 644 patients to induction therapy with cisplatin and FU, followed by cisplatin and FU concurrent with RT, or standard therapy with MMC and FU and concurrent RT.[87] The cisplatin-based therapy failed to improve DFS and was associated a higher colostomy rate compared with standard MMC-based therapy, which argues against the use of the cisplatin regimen given in the RTOG study. Two other large RCTs using cisplatin and FU-based chemotherapy with concurrent RT are being conducted (Intergroup/ ACCORD 3 and Cancer Research United Kingdom Anal Cancer Trial [ACT II]), but the final results of these RCTs have yet to be published.

LEVEL 1A EVIDENCE: PROSPECTIVE RANDOMIZED CLINICAL TRIALS IN RECTAL CANCER

1. Randomized trial of laparoscopic-assisted resection of colorectal carcinoma: 3-year results of the UK MRC CLASICC Trial Group. Jayne DG, Guillou PJ, Thorpe H, et al. J Clin Onc 2007;25:3071.[11]

Hypothesis: Laparoscopic-assisted is as effective as open resection of colorectal carcinomas in terms of recurrence and survival. Please refer to the colon article of this issue for the abstract and editor's summary and review of this trial.

2. Preoperative radiotherapy combined with total mesorectal excision for resectable rectal cancer. Kapiteijn E, Marijnen CA, Nagtegaal ID, et al. N Engl J Med 2001;345(9):638–46.[49]

Hypothesis: The addition of preoperative RT improves local control in patients who undergo a standardized TME for rectal cancer.

# Patients Randomized	Study Groups	Stratification	Significance Demonstrated	% Change Identified in Trial
1861	TME N=937 Preoperative RT + TME N=924	Center Type of resection	Yes—local control	Local recurrence 2.4% versus 8.2% favoring RT + TME group

Published abstract: BACKGROUND: Short-term preoperative RT and total mesorectal excision have been shown to improve local control of disease in patients with resectable rectal cancer. The authors conducted a multicenter, randomized trial to determine whether the addition of preoperative RT increases the benefit of total mesorectal excision. METHODS: The authors randomly assigned 1861 patients with resectable rectal cancer either to preoperative RT (5 Gy on each of 5 days) followed by total mesorectal excision (924 patients) or to total mesorectal excision alone (937 patients). The trial was conducted with the use of standardization and quality-control measures to ensure the consistency of the RT, surgery, and pathologic techniques. RESULTS:Of the 1861 patients randomly assigned to one of the two treatment groups, 1805 were eligible to participate. The overall rate of survival at 2 years among the eligible patients was 82.0% in the group assigned to both RT and surgery and 81.8% in the group assigned to surgery alone ($P = .84$). Among the 1748 patients who underwent a macroscopically complete local resection, the rate of local recurrence at 2 years was 5.3%. The rate of local recurrence at 2 years was 2.4% in the RT plus surgery group and 8.2% in the surgery-only group ($P<.001$). CONCLUSIONS:The authors concluded that short-term preoperative RT reduces the risk of local recurrence in patients with rectal cancer who undergo a standardized total mesorectal excision. (Copyright 2001, Massachusetts Medical Society. All rights reserved. Reprinted with permission.)

Editor's summary and comments: This multicenter study from the Dutch Colorectal Cancer Group assessed whether there was a benefit to adding preoperative short-course RT to TME for rectal cancer. This study standardized surgery with a TME technique and instituted multiple measures to ensure that quality control was maintained with respect to surgery and pathologic assessment. This level of standardization and quality control allowed the authors to addresses the key question of whether preoperative RT was beneficial when optimal surgical therapy was performed. The 2-year local recurrence rate was found to be lower in the TME plus RT group compared with the TME group, but there were no differences between groups in OS. Long-term follow-up results, which were reported in 2007, were consistent with the previous data. The 5-year local recurrence risk was lower in the RT plus TME group compared with the TME alone group (5.6% versus 10.9%), and the 5-year OS was not different between groups (64.2% versus 63.5%). Overall, preoperative short-course RT offers a benefit in terms of local recurrence even when high-quality TME surgery is performed, although OS appears to be unaffected.

3. Preoperative versus postoperative chemoradiotherapy for rectal cancer. Sauer R, Becker H, Hohenberger W, et al. N Engl J Med 2004;351(17):1731–40.[58]

Hypothesis: Preoperative RT with chemotherapy improves overall survival compared with postoperative RT with chemotherapy.

# Patients Randomized	Study Groups	Stratification	Significance Demonstrated	% Change Identified in Trial
823	Preoperative chemoradiation N=421 Postoperative chemoradiation N=402	Surgeon	No—5-year OS Yes—5-year local recurrence rate	OS—76% preoperative versus 74% postoperative chemoradiation group Local recurrence—6% versus 13% favoring preoperative chemoradiation group

Published abstract: BACKGROUND: Postoperative chemoradiotherapy is the recommended standard therapy for patients with locally advanced rectal cancer. In recent years, encouraging results with preoperative RT have been reported. The authors compared preoperative chemoradiotherapy with postoperative chemoradiotherapy for locally advanced rectal cancer. METHODS: The authors randomly assigned patients with clinical stage T3 or T4 or node-positive disease to receive either preoperative or postoperative chemoradiotherapy. The preoperative treatment consisted of 5040 cGy delivered in fractions of 180 cGy/d, 5 d/wk, and fluorouracil, given in a 120-hour continuous intravenous infusion at a dose of 1000 mg per square meter of body surface area per day during the first and fifth weeks of RT. Surgery was performed 6 weeks after the completion of chemoradiotherapy. One month after surgery, four 5-day cycles of fluorouracil (500 mg per square meter per day) were given. Chemoradiotherapy was identical in the postoperative treatment group, except for the delivery of a boost of 540 cGy. The primary end point was overall survival. RESULTS: Four hundred twenty-one patients randomly were assigned to receive preoperative chemoradiotherapy, and 402 patients were assigned randomly to receive postoperative chemoradiotherapy. The overall 5-year survival rates were 76% and 74%, respectively ($P = .80$). The 5-year cumulative incidence of local relapse was 6% for patients assigned to preoperative chemoradiotherapy and 13% in the postoperative treatment group ($P = .006$). Grade 3 or 4 acute toxic effects occurred in 27% of the patients in the preoperative treatment group, as compared with 40% of the patients in the postoperative treatment group ($P = .001$). The corresponding rates of long-term toxic effects were 14% and 24%, respectively ($P = .01$). CONCLUSIONS: The authors concluded that preoperative chemoradiotherapy, as compared with postoperative chemoradiotherapy, improved local control and was associated with reduced toxicity but did not improve overall survival. (Copyright 2004, Massachusetts Medical Society. All rights reserved. Reprinted with permission.)

Editor's summary and comments: This large, prospective RCT compared the effects of preoperative with postoperative combined chemoradiation in patients with stage 2 and 3 rectal cancers. This was a very well-designed study that attempted to standardize preoperative staging (all patients underwent CT and endorectal ultrasound) and surgery with TME technique. Of note, 18% of patients assigned to the postoperative chemoradiation group were found to have stage 1 disease on pathology review after resection, which suggests tumor overstaging and overtreatment in a substantial number of patients in the preoperative treatment group, assuming random distribution. There was a significant decrease in local recurrence favoring the preoperative treatment group, but no difference in OS. Furthermore, the results also showed a benefit for preoperative chemoradiation in terms of increased compliance with treatment and reduced early and long-term toxicities. Thus, the risk of overtreatment with preoperative chemoradiation must be considered in light of these clinical benefits experienced by patients who undergo preoperative over postoperative treatment. The development of more accurate clinical staging modalities to improve patient selection for preoperative therapy is a key area of future work.

4. Chemotherapy with preoperative radiotherapy in rectal cancer. Bosset JF, Collette L, Calais G, et al. N Engl J Med 2006;355:1114–1123.[67]

Hypothesis: The addition of chemotherapy to preoperative RT improves overall survival.

# Patients Randomized	Study Groups	Stratification	Significance Demonstrated	% Change Identified in Trial
1011	Preoperative RT N=252 Preoperative chemoradiation N=253 Preoperative RT and postoperative chemotherapy N=253 Preoperative chemoradiation and postoperative chemotherapy N=253	Institution Sex T-stage Tumor distance from anal verge	No—DFS and OS between preoperative RT versus preoperative chemoradiation groups	HR for death in preoperative chemoradiation group 1.02 (0.83–1.26) Local recurrence–7.6 to 9.6% in groups that received chemotherapy versus 17.1% in preoperative RT alone group

Published abstract: BACKGROUND: Preoperative RT is recommended for selected patients with rectal cancer. The authors evaluated the addition of chemotherapy to preoperative RT and the use of postoperative chemotherapy in the treatment of rectal cancer. METHODS: The authors randomly assigned patients with clinical stage T3 or T4 resectable rectal cancer to receive preoperative RT, preoperative chemoradiotherapy, preoperative RT and postoperative chemotherapy, or preoperative chemoradiotherapy and postoperative chemotherapy. Radiotherapy consisted of 45 Gy delivered over a period of 5 weeks. One course of chemotherapy consisted of 350 mg of fluorouracil per square meter of body surface area per day and 20 mg of leucovorin per square meter per day, both given for 5 days. Two courses were combined with preoperative RT in the group receiving preoperative chemoradiotherapy and the group receiving preoperative chemoradiotherapy and postoperative chemotherapy. Four courses were planned postoperatively in the group receiving preoperative RT and postoperative chemotherapy and the group receiving preoperative chemoradiotherapy and postoperative chemotherapy. The primary end point was overall survival. RESULTS: The authors enrolled 1011 patients in the trial. There was no significant difference in overall survival between the groups that received chemotherapy preoperatively ($P = .84$) and those that received it postoperatively ($P = .12$). The combined 5-year overall survival rate for all four groups was 65.2%. The 5-year cumulative incidence rates for local recurrences were 8.7%, 9.6%, and 7.6% in the groups that received chemotherapy preoperatively, postoperatively, or both, respectively, and 17.1% in the group that did not receive chemotherapy ($P = .002$). The rate of adherence to preoperative chemotherapy was 82.0%, and for postoperative chemotherapy, the rate was 42.9%. CONCLUSIONS: The authors concluded that in patients with rectal cancer who receive preoperative RT, adding fluorouracil-based chemotherapy preoperatively or postoperatively has no significant effect on survival. Chemotherapy, regardless of whether it is administered before or after surgery, confers a significant benefit with respect to local control. (Copyright 2006, Massachusetts Medical Society. All rights reserved. Reprinted with permission.)

Editor's summary and comments: This study used a 2 × 2 factorial design to assess the effects of the addition of chemotherapy to preoperative RT versus RT alone and the use of postoperative chemotherapy in the treatment of rectal cancer. The primary outcome that the study was powered to detect was a difference in OS between the two preoperative and two postoperative treatments. The authors found that the addition of chemotherapy to RT did not have a significant effect on survival. Chemotherapy, however, was found to decrease local failures regardless of when it was given. The authors also found that the rate of adherence to preoperative chemotherapy was significantly higher compared with postoperative chemotherapy. Thus, although preoperative RT with chemotherapy may not confer a survival benefit over RT alone, receiving chemotherapy does appear to have a benefit with regard to local recurrence, and it appears to be better tolerated in the preoperative setting.

5. Adjuvant chemotherapy versus observation in patients with colorectal cancer: a randomized study. QUASAR Collaborative Group. Lancet 2007;370: 2020–29.[47]

Hypothesis: Adjuvant chemotherapy improves all-cause mortality in patients with colorectal cancer (mostly those with stage 2 or 3 disease). Please refer to the colon article of this issue for the abstract and editor's summary and review of this trial.

LEVEL 1A EVIDENCE: PROSPECTIVE RANDOMIZED CLINICAL TRIALS IN ANAL CANCER

6. Fluorouracil, mitomycin, and radiotherapy versus fluorouracil, cisplatin, and radiotherapy for carcinoma of the anal canal: a randomized controlled trial. Ajani JA, Winter KA, Gunderson LL, et al. JAMA 2008;299 (16):1914–21.[87]

Hypothesis: Cisplatin-based therapy improved DFS over mitomycin-based therapy in the treatment of anal canal carcinoma.

# Patients Randomized	Study Groups	Stratification	Significance Demonstrated	% Change Identified in Trial
644	Induction chemotherapy then chemoradiation with cisplatin N=341 Chemoradiation with MMC N=341	Sex Tumor size N-stage	No—DFS and OS	60% 5-year DFS in MMC group versus. 54% in cisplatin group

Published abstract: CONTEXT: Chemoradiation as definitive therapy is the preferred primary therapy for patients with anal canal carcinoma; however, the 5-year DFS rate from concurrent fluorouracil/mitomycin and radiation is only approximately 65%. OBJECTIVE: The objective was to compare the efficacy of cisplatin-based (experimental) therapy versus mitomycin-based (standard) therapy in treatment of anal canal carcinoma. DESIGN, SETTING, AND PARTICIPANTS: US Gastrointestinal Intergroup trial RTOG 98-11 was a multicenter, phase 3, randomized controlled trial comparing treatment with fluorouracil plus mitomycin and RT versus treatment with fluorouracil plus cisplatin and radiotherapy in 682 patients with anal canal carcinoma enrolled between Oct. 31, 1998, and June 27, 2005. Stratifications included sex, clinical nodal status, and tumor diameter. INTERVENTION: Participants were assigned randomly to one of two intervention groups: (1) The mitomycin-based group (n = 341), where patients received fluorouracil (1000 mg/m^2 on days 1 to 4 and 29 to 32) plus mitomycin (10 mg/m^2 on days 1 and 29) and radiotherapy (45 to 59 Gy) or (2) The cisplatin-based group (n = 341), where patients received fluorouracil (1000 mg/m^2 on days 1 to 4, 29 to 32, 57 to 60, and 85 to 88) plus cisplatin (75 mg/m^2 on days 1, 29, 57, and 85) and RT (45 to 59 Gy; start day = day 57). MAIN OUTCOME MEASURES: The primary end point was 5-year DFS; secondary end points were overall survival and time to relapse. RESULTS: Six hundred forty-four patients were assessable. The median follow-up for all patients was 2.51 years. Median age was 55 years; 69% were women; Twenty-seven percent had a tumor diameter greater than 5 cm, and 26% had clinically positive nodes. The 5-year DFS rate was 60% (95% CI, 53% to 67%) in the mitomycin-based group and 54% (95% CI, 46%to 60%) in the cisplatin-based group (P = .17). The 5-year overall survival rate was 75% (95% CI, 67% to 81%) in the mitomycin-based group and 70% (95% CI, 63% to 76%) in the cisplatin-based group (P = .10). The 5-year local–regional recurrence and distant metastasis rates were 25% (95% CI, 20% to 30%) and 15% (95% CI, 10% to 20%), respectively, for mitomycin-based treatment and 33% (95% CI, 27% to 40%) and 19% (95% CI, 14% to 24%), respectively, for cisplatin-based treatment. The cumulative rate of colostomy was significantly better for mitomycin-based than cisplatin-based treatment (10% versus 19%; P = .02). Severe hematologic toxicity was worse with mitomycin-based treatment (P<.001). CONCLUSIONS: The authors concluded that in this population of patients with anal canal carcinoma, cisplatin-based therapy failed to improve DFS compared with mitomycin-based therapy, but cisplatin-based therapy resulted in a significantly worse colostomy rate. These findings do not support the use of cisplatin in place of mitomycin in combination with fluorouracil and RT for treating anal canal carcinoma. (Copyright 2008, American Medical Association. All Rights Reserved. Reprinted with permission.)

Editor's summary and comments: This RCT found comparable DFS and OS in patients with anal cancer who underwent induction chemotherapy with cisplatin and FU, followed by cisplatin and FU and concurrent RT compared with standard therapy with MMC and FU and concurrent RT. The trial design, however, was not direct comparison of cisplatin to MMC-based chemotherapy, because the cisplatin group also underwent induction chemotherapy, which delayed RT in this group. Even though cisplatin-based chemotherapy is used in other squamous malignancies, these results do not support a survival benefit with cisplatin for anal cancer in the regimen described. Other large RCTs assessing the addition of cisplatin are ongoing, however.

DISCLOSURE

Authors have nothing to disclose.

REFERENCES

1. Nissan A, Dangelica MI, Shoup MC, et al. Randomized clinical trials in rectal and anal cancer. Surg Oncol Clin N Am 2002;11:149–72.
2. Ferulano GP, Dilillo S, La Manna S, et al. Influence of the surgical treatment on local recurrence of rectal cancer: a prospective study (1980–1992). J Surg Oncol 2000;74:153–7.
3. Moore HG, Riedel E, Minsky BD, et al. Adequacy of 1 cm distal margin after restorative rectal cancer resection with sharp mesorectal excision and preoperative combined-modality therapy. Ann Surg Oncol 2003;10:80–5.
4. Paty PB, Enker WE, Cohen AM, et al. Treatment of rectal cancer by low anterior resection with coloanal anastomosis. Ann Surg 1994;219:365–73.
5. Lazorthes F, Chiotasso P, Gamagami RA, et al. Late clinical outcome in a randomized prospective comparison of colonic J pouch and straight coloanal anastomosis. Br J Surg 1997;84:1449–51.
6. Hallbook O, Pahlman L, Krog M, et al. Randomized comparison of straight and colonic J pouch anastomosis after low anterior resection. Ann Surg 1996;224:58–65.
7. Enker WE, Thaler HT, Cranor ML, et al. Total mesorectal excision in the operative treatment of carcinoma of the rectum. J Am Coll Surg 1995;181:335–46.
8. MacFarlane JK, Ryall RD, Heald RJ. Mesorectal excision for rectal cancer. Lancet 1993;341:457–60.
9. Heald RJ, Ryall RD. Recurrence and survival after total mesorectal excision for rectal cancer. Lancet 1986;1:1479–82.
10. Guillou PJ, Quirke P, Thorpe H, et al. Short-term end points of conventional versus laparoscopic-assisted surgery in patients with colorectal cancer (MRC CLASICC trial): multicentre, randomised controlled trial. Lancet 2005;365:1718–26.
11. Jayne DG, Guillou PJ, Thorpe H, et al. Randomized trial of laparoscopic-assisted resection of colorectal carcinoma: 3-year results of the UK MRC CLASICC Trial Group. J Clin Oncol 2007;25:3061–8.
12. Jayne DG, Brown JM, Thorpe H, et al. Bladder and sexual function following resection for rectal cancer in a randomized clinical trial of laparoscopic versus open technique. Br J Surg 2005;92:1124–32.
13. Zhou ZG, Hu M, Li Y, et al. Laparoscopic versus open total mesorectal excision with anal sphincter preservation for low rectal cancer. Surg Endosc 2004;18:1211–5.
14. Braga M, Frasson M, Vignali A, et al. Laparoscopic resection in rectal cancer patients: outcome and cost–benefit analysis. Dis Colon Rectum 2007;50:464–71.

15. Braga M, Vignali A, Zuliani W, et al. Laparoscopic versus open colorectal surgery: cost-benefit analysis in a single-center randomized trial. Ann Surg 2005;242: 890–5.
16. Arteaga González I, Díaz Luis H, Martín Malagón A, et al. A comparative clinical study of short-term results of laparoscopic surgery for rectal cancer during the learning curve. Int J Colorectal Dis 2006;21:590–5.
17. Ng SS, Leung KL, Lee JF, et al. Laparoscopic-assisted versus open abdomino-perineal resection for low rectal cancer: a prospective randomized trial. Ann Surg Oncol 2008;15:2418–25.
18. Lezoche E, Guerrieri M, Paganini AM, et al. Transanal endoscopic versus total mesorectal laparoscopic resections of T2-N0 low rectal cancers after neoadjuvant treatment: a prospective randomized trial with a 3-years minimum follow-up period. Surg Endosc 2005;19:751–6.
19. Lezoche G, Baldarelli M, Guerrieri M, et al. A prospective randomized study with a 5-year minimum follow-up evaluation of transanal endoscopic microsurgery versus laparoscopic total mesorectal excision after neoadjuvant therapy. Surg Endosc 2008;22:352–8.
20. Winde G, Nottberg H, Keller R, et al. Surgical cure for early rectal carcinomas (T1). Transanal endoscopic microsurgery vs. anterior resection. Dis Colon Rectum 1996;39:969–76.
21. Paty PB, Nash GM, Baron P, et al. Long-term results of local excision for rectal cancer. Ann Surg 2002;236:522–9.
22. Bentrem DJ, Okabe S, Wong WD, et al. T1 adenocarcinoma of the rectum: transanal excision or radical surgery? Ann Surg 2005;242:472–7.
23. Nash GM, Weiser MR, Guillem JG, et al. Long-term survival after transanal excision of T1 rectal cancer. Dis Colon Rectum 2009;52:577–82.
24. Garcia-Aguilar J, Mellgren A, Sirivongs P, et al. Local excision of rectal cancer without adjuvant therapy: a word of caution. Ann Surg 2000;231:345–51.
25. Fazio VW, Zutshi M, Remzi FH, et al. A randomized multicenter trial to compare long-term functional outcome, quality of life, and complications of surgical procedures for low rectal cancers. Ann Surg 2007;246:481–8.
26. Liang JT, Lai HS, Lee PH, et al. Comparison of functional and surgical outcomes of laparoscopic-assisted colonic J-pouch versus straight reconstruction after total mesorectal excision for lower rectal cancer. Ann Surg Oncol 2007;14:1972–9.
27. Park JG, Lee MR, Lim SB, et al. Colonic J-pouch anal anastomosis after ultralow anterior resection with upper sphincter excision for low-lying rectal cancer. World J Gastroenterol 2005;11:2570–3.
28. Sailer M, Fuchs KH, Fein M, et al. Randomized clinical trial comparing quality of life after straight and pouch coloanal reconstruction. Br J Surg 2002;89: 1108–17.
29. Furst A, Burghofer K, Hutzel L, et al. Neorectal reservoir is not the functional principle of the colonic J-pouch: the volume of a short colonic J-pouch does not differ from a straight coloanal anastomosis. Dis Colon Rectum 2002;45:660–7.
30. Oya M, Komatsu J, Takase Y, et al. Comparison of defecatory function after colonic J-pouch anastomosis and straight anastomosis for stapled low anterior resection: results of a prospective randomized trial. Surg Today 2002;32:104–10.
31. Ho YH, Seow-Choen F, Tan M. Colonic J-pouch function at six months versus straight coloanal anastomosis at two years: randomized controlled trial. World J Surg 2001;25:876–81.
32. Jiang JK, Yang SH, Lin JK. Transabdominal anastomosis after low anterior resection: a prospective, randomized, controlled trial comparing long-term results

between side-to-end anastomosis and colonic J-pouch. Dis Colon Rectum 2005; 48:2100–8.

33. Machado M, Nygren J, Goldman S, et al. Functional and physiologic assessment of the colonic reservoir or side-to-end anastomosis after low anterior resection for rectal cancer: a two-year follow-up. Dis Colon Rectum 2005;48:29–36.

34. Machado M, Nygren J, Goldman S, et al. Similar outcome after colonic pouch and side-to-end anastomosis in low anterior resection for rectal cancer: a prospective randomized trial. Ann Surg 2003;238:214–20.

35. Furst A, Suttner S, Agha A, et al. Colonic J-pouch vs. coloplasty following resection of distal rectal cancer: early results of a prospective, randomized, pilot study. Dis Colon Rectum 2003;46:1161–6.

36. Ulrich AB, Seiler CM, Z'graggen K, et al. Early results from a randomized clinical trial of colon J-pouch versus transverse coloplasty pouch after low anterior resection for rectal cancer. Br J Surg 2008;95:1257–63.

37. Pimentel JM, Duarte A, Gregorio C, et al. Transverse coloplasty pouch and colonic J-pouch for rectal cancer—a comparative study. Colorectal Dis 2003;5: 465–70.

38. Chude GG, Rayate NV, Patris V, et al. Defunctioning loop ileostomy with low anterior resection for distal rectal cancer: should we make an ileostomy as a routine procedure? A prospective randomized study. Hepatogastroenterology 2008;55: 1562–7.

39. Matthiessen P, Hallbook O, Rutegard J, et al. Defunctioning stoma reduces symptomatic anastomotic leakage after low anterior resection of the rectum for cancer: a randomized multicenter trial. Ann Surg 2007;246:207–14.

40. Randomised trial of surgery alone versus radiotherapy followed by surgery for potentially operable locally advanced rectal cancer. Medical Research Council Rectal Cancer Working Party. Lancet 1996;348:1605–10.

41. Fisher B, Wolmark N, Rockette H, et al. Postoperative adjuvant chemotherapy or radiation therapy for rectal cancer: results from NSABP protocol R-01. J Natl Cancer Inst 1988;80:21–9.

42. Roswit B, Higgins GA, Keehn RJ. Preoperative irradiation for carcinoma of the rectum and rectosigmoid colon: report of a national Veterans Administration randomized study. Cancer 1975;35:1597–602.

43. Reis Neto JA, Quilici FA, Reis JA Jr. A comparison of nonoperative vs. preoperative radiotherapy in rectal carcinoma. A 10-year randomized trial. Dis Colon Rectum 1989;32:702–10.

44. Folkesson J, Birgisson H, Pahlman L, et al. Swedish Rectal Cancer Trial: long-lasting benefits from radiotherapy on survival and local recurrence rate. J Clin Oncol 2005;23:5644–50.

45. Cedermark B, Johansson H, Rutqvist LE, et al. The Stockholm I trial of preoperative short term radiotherapy in operable rectal carcinoma. A prospective randomized trial. Stockholm Colorectal Cancer Study Group. Cancer 1995;75: 2269–75.

46. Gerard A, Buyse M, Nordlinger B, et al. Preoperative radiotherapy as adjuvant treatment in rectal cancer. Final results of a randomized study of the European Organization for Research and Treatment of Cancer (EORTC). Ann Surg 1988; 208:606–14.

47. Colorectal Cancer Collaborative Group. Adjuvant radiotherapy for rectal cancer: a systematic overview of 8507 patients from 22 randomised trials. Lancet 2001; 358:1291–304.

48. Pahlman L, Glimelius B. Pre- or postoperative radiotherapy in rectal and rectosigmoid carcinoma. Report from a randomized multicenter trial. Ann Surg 1990;211: 187–95.
49. Kapiteijn E, Marijnen CA, Nagtegaal ID, et al. Preoperative radiotherapy combined with total mesorectal excision for resectable rectal cancer. N Engl J Med 2001;345:638–46.
50. Peeters KC, Marijnen CA, Nagtegaal ID, et al. The TME trial after a median follow-up of 6 years: increased local control but no survival benefit in irradiated patients with resectable rectal carcinoma. Ann Surg 2007;246:693–701.
51. Martling A, Holm T, Johansson H, et al. The Stockholm II trial on preoperative radiotherapy in rectal carcinoma: long-term follow-up of a population-based study. Cancer 2001;92:896–902.
52. Holm T, Johansson H, Rutqvist LE, et al. Tumour location and the effects of preoperative radiotherapy in the treatment of rectal cancer. Br J Surg 2001; 88:839–43.
53. Marijnen CA, Kapiteijn E, van de Velde CJ, et al. Acute side effects and complications after short-term preoperative radiotherapy combined with total mesorectal excision in primary rectal cancer: report of a multicenter randomized trial. J Clin Oncol 2002;20:817–25.
54. Birgisson H, Pahlman L, Gunnarsson U, et al. Late gastrointestinal disorders after rectal cancer surgery with and without preoperative radiation therapy. Br J Surg 2008;95:206–13.
55. Birgisson H, Pahlman L, Gunnarsson U, et al. Adverse effects of preoperative radiation therapy for rectal cancer: long-term follow-up of the Swedish Rectal Cancer Trial. J Clin Oncol 2005;23:8697–705.
56. Lange MM, den Dulk M, Bossema ER, et al. Risk factors for faecal incontinence after rectal cancer treatment. Br J Surg 2007;94:1278–84.
57. Marijnen CA, van de Velde CJ, Putter H, et al. Impact of short-term preoperative radiotherapy on health-related quality of life and sexual functioning in primary rectal cancer: report of a multicenter randomized trial. J Clin Oncol 2005;23: 1847–58.
58. Sauer R, Becker H, Hohenberger W, et al. Preoperative versus postoperative chemoradiotherapy for rectal cancer. N Engl J Med 2004;351:1731–40.
59. Sauer R, Fietkau R, Wittekind C, et al. Adjuvant vs. neoadjuvant radiochemotherapy for locally advanced rectal cancer: the German trial CAO/ARO/AIO-94. Colorectal Dis 2003;5:406–15.
60. Bujko K, Nowacki MP, Nasierowska-Guttmejer A, et al. Long-term results of a randomized trial comparing preoperative short-course radiotherapy with preoperative conventionally fractionated chemoradiation for rectal cancer. Br J Surg 2006;93:1215–23.
61. Bujko K, Nowacki MP, Kepka L, et al. Postoperative complications in patients irradiated pre-operatively for rectal cancer: report of a randomised trial comparing short-term radiotherapy vs chemoradiation. Colorectal Dis 2005;7:410–6.
62. Bujko K, Nowacki MP, Nasierowska-Guttmejer A, et al. Sphincter preservation following preoperative radiotherapy for rectal cancer: report of a randomised trial comparing short-term radiotherapy vs. conventionally fractionated radiochemotherapy. Radiother Oncol 2004;72:15–24.
63. Five-year results of a randomized controlled trial of adjuvant chemotherapy for curatively resected colorectal carcinoma. The Colorectal Cancer Chemotherapy Study Group of Japan. Jpn J Clin Oncol 1995;25:91–103.

64. Prolongation of the disease-free interval in surgically treated rectal carcinoma. Gastrointestinal Tumor Study Group. N Engl J Med 1985;312:1465–72.
65. Krook JE, Moertel CG, Gunderson LL, et al. Effective surgical adjuvant therapy for high-risk rectal carcinoma. N Engl J Med 1991;324:709–15.
66. NIH consensus conference. Adjuvant therapy for patients with colon and rectal cancer. JAMA 1990;264:1444–50.
67. Bosset JF, Collette L, Calais G, et al. Chemotherapy with preoperative radiotherapy in rectal cancer. N Engl J Med 2006;355:1114–23.
68. Bosset JF, Calais G, Mineur L, et al. Enhanced tumorocidal effect of chemotherapy with preoperative radiotherapy for rectal cancer: preliminary results–EORTC 22921. J Clin Oncol 2005;23:5620–7.
69. Bosset JF, Calais G, Daban A, et al. Preoperative chemoradiotherapy versus preoperative radiotherapy in rectal cancer patients: assessment of acute toxicity and treatment compliance. Report of the 22921 randomised trial conducted by the EORTC Radiotherapy Group. Eur J Cancer 2004;40:219–24.
70. Gerard JP, Conroy T, Bonnetain F, et al. Preoperative radiotherapy with or without concurrent fluorouracil and leucovorin in T3-4 rectal cancers: results of FFCD 9203. J Clin Oncol 2006;24:4620–5.
71. Frykholm GJ, Pahlman L, Glimelius B. Combined chemo- and radiotherapy vs. radiotherapy alone in the treatment of primary, nonresectable adenocarcinoma of the rectum. Int J Radiat Oncol Biol Phys 2001;50:427–34.
72. Braendengen M, Tveit KM, Berglund A, et al. Randomized phase III study comparing preoperative radiotherapy with chemoradiotherapy in nonresectable rectal cancer. J Clin Oncol 2008;26:3687–94.
73. Gray R, Barnwell J, McConkey C, et al. Quasar Collaborative Group. Adjuvant chemotherapy versus observation in patients with colorectal cancer: a randomised study. Lancet 2007;370:2020–9.
74. Taal BG, Van Tinteren H, Zoetmulder FA. Adjuvant 5FU plus levamisole in colonic or rectal cancer: improved survival in stage II and III. Br J Cancer 2001;85:1437–43.
75. Minsky BD, Guillem JG. Multidisciplinary management of resectable rectal cancer. New developments and controversies. Oncology (Williston Park) 2008;22:1430–7.
76. Akasu T, Moriya Y, Ohashi Y, et al. Adjuvant chemotherapy with uracil-tegafur for pathological stage III rectal cancer after mesorectal excision with selective lateral pelvic lymphadenectomy: a multicenter randomized controlled trial. Jpn J Clin Oncol 2006;36:237–44.
77. Kato T, Ohashi Y, Nakazato H, et al. Efficacy of oral UFT as adjuvant chemotherapy to curative resection of colorectal cancer: multicenter prospective randomized trial. Langenbecks Arch Surg 2002;386:575–81.
78. Nordlinger B, Rougier P, Arnaud JP, et al. Adjuvant regional chemotherapy and systemic chemotherapy versus systemic chemotherapy alone in patients with stage II-III colorectal cancer: a multicentre randomised controlled phase III trial. Lancet Oncol 2005;6:459–68.
79. Smalley SR, Benedetti JK, Williamson SK, et al. Phase III trial of fluorouracil-based chemotherapy regimens plus radiotherapy in postoperative adjuvant rectal cancer: GI INT 0144. J Clin Oncol 2006;24:3542–7.
80. Tsavaris N, Gennatas K, Kosmas C, et al. Leucovorin and fluorouracil vs levamisole and fluorouracil as adjuvant chemotherapy in rectal cancer. Oncol Rep 2004;12:927–32.

81. De Placido S, Lopez M, Carlomagno C, et al. Modulation of 5-fluorouracil as adjuvant systemic chemotherapy in colorectal cancer: the IGCS-COL multicentre, randomised, phase III study. Br J Cancer 2005;93:896–904.
82. de la Torre A, Garcia-Berrocal MI, Arias F, et al. Preoperative chemoradiotherapy for rectal cancer: randomized trial comparing oral uracil and tegafur and oral leucovorin vs. intravenous 5-fluorouracil and leucovorin. Int J Radiat Oncol Biol Phys 2008;70:102–10.
83. Nigro ND, Seydel HG, Considine B, et al. Combined preoperative radiation and chemotherapy for squamous cell carcinoma of the anal canal. Cancer 1983;51: 1826–9.
84. Epidermoid anal cancer: results from the UKCCCR randomised trial of radiotherapy alone versus radiotherapy, 5-fluorouracil, and mitomycin. UKCCCR Anal Cancer Trial Working Party. UK Coordinating Committee on Cancer Research. Lancet 1996;348:1049–54.
85. Bartelink H, Roelofsen F, Eschwege F, et al. Concomitant radiotherapy and chemotherapy is superior to radiotherapy alone in the treatment of locally advanced anal cancer: results of a phase III randomized trial of the European Organization for Research and Treatment of Cancer Radiotherapy and Gastrointestinal Cooperative Groups. J Clin Oncol 1997;15:2040–9.
86. Flam M, John M, Pajak TF, et al. Role of mitomycin in combination with fluorouracil and radiotherapy, and of salvage chemoradiation in the definitive nonsurgical treatment of epidermoid carcinoma of the anal canal: results of a phase III randomized intergroup study. J Clin Oncol 1996;14:2527–39.
87. Ajani JA, Winter KA, Gunderson LL, et al. Fluorouracil, mitomycin, and radiotherapy vs fluorouracil, cisplatin, and radiotherapy for carcinoma of the anal canal: a randomized controlled trial. JAMA 2008;299:1914–21.
88. Tournier-Rangeard L, Mercier M, Peiffert D, et al. Radiochemotherapy of locally advanced anal canal carcinoma: prospective assessment of early impact on the quality of life (randomized trial ACCORD 03). Radiother Oncol 2008;87:391–7.
89. Kouloulias V, Plataniotis G, Kouvaris J, et al. Chemoradiotherapy combined with intracavitary hyperthermia for anal cancer: feasibility and long-term results from a phase II randomized trial. Am J Clin Oncol 2005;28:91–9.

Index

Note: Page numbers of article titles are in **boldface** type.

A

Abdominal drainage, after hepatic resection, 159–160
Ablation, radiofrequency, for hepatocellular carcinoma, 160–161
Adenocarcinoma, pancreatic. *See* Pancreatic adenocarcinoma.
Adjuvant therapy, for colon cancer, 190–192, 198–204
    for esophageal carcinoma, 62–63, 66–67
    for gastric cancer, 85–86
    for hepatocellular carcinoma, 157–159, 161–164
    for high-risk melanoma, 15–16, 23–26
    for pancreatic adenocarcinoma, 119–128, 138–144
    for rectal cancer, 217–220
    for resectable liver metastases from colorectal carcinoma, 168–169, 178–179
Allogeneic tumor vaccine, for resected node-negative melanoma, 22–23
    melanoma lysate, with interferon alfa-2b for resected stage III cutaneous melanoma, 26–27
Anal cancer, randomized clinical trials in rectal and, **205–223**
    level IA evidence, 220–222
Anastrozole, with tamoxifen, for early-stage breast cancer, 53–55
Antibiotic prophylaxis, surgical site, in gastric cancer patients, 83
Arterial chemoembolization, in advanced hepatocellular carcinoma, 162–164
Axilla, in breast cancer, Level 1A evidence on evaluation and management of, 39–40
Axillary lymph node dissection, *vs.* sentinel node biopsy as staging procedure in breast cancer, 39–40

B

Bevcizumab, for metastatic colorectal cancer, 174–176
Biochemotherapy, for melanoma, 27–29
Breast cancer, randomized clinical trials in, **33–58**
    Level IA evidence, 33–55
        adjuvant radiation, 40–44
        endocrine therapy, 49–55
        evaluation and management of the axilla, 39–40
        polychemotherapy in operable cases, 44–49
        surgical trials, 33–39

C

Cancer, randomized clinical trials for, 1–227
    breast cancer, **33–58**
    colon cancer, **183–204**
    colorectal carcinoma, advanced and metastatic, **163–181**

Moving?

Make sure your subscription moves with you!

To notify us of your new address, find your **Clinics Account Number** (located on your mailing label above your name), and contact customer service at:

Email: journalscustomerservice-usa@elsevier.com

800-654-2452 (subscribers in the U.S. & Canada)
314-447-8871 (subscribers outside of the U.S. & Canada)

Fax number: 314-447-8029

Elsevier Health Sciences Division
Subscription Customer Service
3251 Riverport Lane
Maryland Heights, MO 63043

*To ensure uninterrupted delivery of your subscription, please notify us at least 4 weeks in advance of move.

Printed and bound by CPI Group (UK) Ltd, Croydon, CR0 4YY

03/10/2024

01040449-0003